Startle Modification

The startle response (response to a loud noise, for instance) is a reflex that is wired into the brain at a very basic level. Although everyone has such a reflex, the strength and quickness of the startle response is modified by a subject's underlying psychoneurological state. The nature of this modification, therefore, is now seen as an accurate, objective measure of very deep neurological processes.

This book is the first comprehensive volume devoted to startle modification and offers a unique overview of the methods, measurement, physiology, and psychology of the phenomenon, particularly modification of the human startle eyeblink. Chapters are written by many of the world's leading investigators in the field and include coverage of elicitation and recording of the startle blink; issues in measurement and quantification; the neurophysiological basis of the basic startle response and its modification by attentional and affective processes; psychological processes underlying short and long lead interval modification (including prepulse inhibition); applications of startle modification to the study of psychopathology, including schizophrenia, affective disorders, and psychopathy; developmental processes; and relationships with event-related potentials and behavioral measures of information processing.

This book will be an invaluable reference for graduate students and researchers in cognitive science, clinical science, and neuroscience, including experimental psychologists, psychophysiologists, neuroscientists, biological psychiatrists, and clinical psychologists with research interests in psychopathology.

Michael E. Dawson is Professor of Psychology at the University of Southern California, Los Angeles.

Anne M. Schell is Professor of Psychology at Occidental College, Los Angeles, California.

Andreas H. Böhmelt is Assistant Professor at the Center for Psychobiological and Psychosomatic Research at the University of Trier, Germany.

Startle Modification

Implications for
Neuroscience,
Cognitive Science, and
Clinical Science

Edited by

Michael E. Dawson

Anne M. Schell

Andreas H. Böhmelt

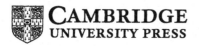

CAMBRIDGE UNIVERSITY PRESS
Cambridge, New York, Melbourne, Madrid, Cape Town, Singapore, São Paulo, Delhi

Cambridge University Press
The Edinburgh Building, Cambridge CB2 8RU, UK

Published in the United States of America by Cambridge University Press, New York

www.cambridge.org
Information on this title: www.cambridge.org/9780521580465

First published 1999
This digitally printed version 2008

A catalogue record for this publication is available from the British Library

Library of Congress Cataloguing in Publication data

Startle modification: implications for neuroscience, cognitive science, and clinical science/edited
by Michael E. Dawson, Anne M. Schell, Andreas H. Bohmelt.
    p.   cm.
    Includes bibliographical references and index.
    ISBN 0-521-58046-3 (hb)
    1. Startle reaction.   2. Cognitive neuroscience – Methodology.
I. Dawson, Michael E.   II. Schell, Anne M. (Anne McCall), 1942–
III. Bohmelt, Andreas H., 1963–   .
    [DNLM: 1. Startle Reaction.   2. Blinking.   WL 106S796 1999]
QP372.6.S73   1999
152.3'22 – dc21
DNLM/DLC
for Library of Congress   98-39368
                              CIP

ISBN 978-0-521-58046-5 hardback
ISBN 978-0-521-08789-6 paperback

To the people who fill our lives with love and make our work worthwhile

Lavina Dawson, Michael Dawson, and Christopher Dawson

Allen Chroman, Lauren Chroman, and Michael Schell

Julian Häger, Svenja Häger, Herman Böhmelt, and Inge Böhmelt

Contents

**PART III: PSYCHOLOGICAL MEDIATION OF
STARTLE MODIFICATION**

**PART IV: INDIVIDUAL DIFFERENCES AND
STARTLE MODIFICATION**

**PART V: RELATIONSHIPS WITH OTHER PARADIGMS
AND MEASURES**

Contributors

MARIE T. BALABAN
Department of Psychology
Eastern Oregon University
La Grande, Oregon 97850-2899

W. KEITH BERG
Department of Psychology
University of Florida
Gainesville, Florida 32611

TERRY D. BLUMENTHAL
Department of Psychology
Wake Forest University
Winston-Salem, North Carolina
  27109

ANDREAS H. BÖHMELT
Center for Research in Psychobiol-
  ogy and Psychosomatics
University of Trier
D-54290 Trier, Germany

MARGARET M. BRADLEY
Center for Research in Psychophysi-
  ology
University of Florida
Gainesville, Florida 32610-0165

DAVID L. BRAFF
Department of Psychiatry
University of California–San Diego
  Medical Center
San Diego, California 92103

KRISTIN S. CADENHEAD
Department of Psychiatry
University of California–San Diego
La Jolla, California 92093-0603

EDWIN W. COOK III
Department of Psychology
University of Alabama–Birmingham
Birmingham, Alabama 35294

BRUCE N. CUTHBERT
Behavioral Science Research Branch
Division of Mental Disorders, Behav-
  ioral Research, and AIDS
National Institute of Mental Health
Bethesda, Maryland 20892-8030

MICHAEL DAVIS
Department of Psychiatry
Emory University
Atlanta, Georgia 30322

MICHAEL E. DAWSON
Department of Psychology
University of Southern California
Los Angeles, California 90089-1061

DIANE L. FILION
Occupational Therapy Education
Kansas University Medical Center
Kansas City, Kansas 66160

JUDITH M. FORD
Department of Psychiatry
Stanford University
School of Medicine
Stanford, California 94305

MARK A. GEYER
Department of Psychiatry
University of California–San Diego
La Jolla, California 92093-0804

STEVEN A. HACKLEY
Department of Psychology
University of Missouri
Columbia, Missouri 65211

ERIN A. HAZLETT
Department of Psychiatry
Mount Sinai School of Medicine
New York, New York 10029-6574

HOWARD S. HOFFMAN
Department of Psychology
Bryn Mawr College
Bryn Mawr, Pennsylvania 19010-
2899

KIMBERLE A. KELLY
Aftercare Clinic
University of California–Los Angeles
Los Angeles, California 90024-6968

ALAN R. LANG
Department of Psychology
Florida State University
Tallahassee, Florida 32306-1051

PETER J. LANG
Center for Research in Psychophysi-
ology
University of Florida
Gainsville, Florida 32610-0165

YOUNGLIM LEE
Department of Psychiatry
Yale University
Connecticut Mental Health Center
New Haven, Connecticut 06508

OTTMAR V. LIPP
Department of Psychology
University of Queensland
Brisbane, Queensland 4072
Australia

EDWARD M. ORNITZ
Department of Psychiatry and Biobe-
havioral Sciences
University of California–Los Ange-
les
Los Angeles, California 90024

CHRISTOPHER J. PATRICK
Department of Psychology
Florida State University
Tallahassee, Florida 32306-1051

LOIS E. PUTNAM
Department of Psychology
Columbia University
New York, New York 10027

WALTON T. ROTH
Department of Psychiatry and
  Behavioral Sciences
Veterans Administration Medical
  Center
Stanford University
Palo Alto, California 94304

ANNE M. SCHELL
Department of Psychology
Occidental College
Los Angeles, California 90041

DAVID A. T. SIDDLE
Office of Pro-Vice-Chancellor
  (Research)
The University of Sydney
New South Wales, 2006
Australia

NEAL R. SWERDLOW
Department of Psychiatry
University of California–San Diego
School of Medicine
La Jolla, California 92093-6270

ERIC J. VANMAN
Department of Psychology
Emory University
Atlanta, Georgia 30332

DAVID L. WALKER
Department of Psychiatry
Yale University
Connecticut Mental Health Center
New Haven, Connecticut 06508

Preface

This book is the first comprehensive volume devoted to startle modification, particularly modification of the human startle eyeblink reflex. As such, it offers a unique overview of the paradigms used to study startle modification, the methods used to measure and quantify startle modification, and the physiological and psychological processes mediating and moderating the phenomena of startle modification.

Why devote an entire book to a seemingly esoteric and narrow topic such as the modification of the startle reflex? The answer is that the study of startle modification is deceptive in its appearance of being narrow and esoteric. In fact, the study of startle modification offers the potential to expose and clarify a number of important issues across diverse areas of psychology, psychiatry, and neuroscience. The startle reflex and its modification are rich with implications for neuroscience, cognitive science, and clinical science; hence, the subtitle of this book.

Beyond having implications *for* several subareas of scientific inquiry, the study of startle modification has implications for the integration *across* these areas. Startle modification in its various forms may provide a powerful integrative research tool. It is a paradigm that can bridge the methods and concepts of neuroscience, cognitive science, and clinical science. The growing interest in this paradigm attests to the emerging sense of the important integrative nature of the study of startle modification.

For cross-disciplinary integration to occur, however, researchers in different disciplines with their different terminologies and different concepts need to communicate. That is one of the primary reasons for this book. We invited distinguished investigators doing research with startle modification in different disciplines to write about how startle modification can enlighten us in their specific disciplines. In this way we can begin to see what the study of startle modification has to offer within each discipline and how this information can lead to greater integration across disciplines.

Another reason for this book is to introduce the startle modification paradigms and their immense possibilities to investigators of different disciplines who may be only vaguely familiar with them. This book will hopefully provide an introduction to those who want to learn more about the startle modification phenomena and who may be interested in adding it to their own investigation, as well as providing a thorough review for those already familiar with this versatile measure.

It is important to remember that this book is not about the startle reflex; rather, it is about *modification* of the startle reflex. That is, the focus of this book is on psychological and physiological processes initiated by nonstartling "lead stimuli" that influence subsequently elicited startle reactions. These processes include protective inhibition, sensorimotor gating, alertness and activation, attention and orienting, information processing, and affect processing in both normal and abnormal guises. The startle modification paradigms allow investigators to study the excitatory and inhibitory mechanisms underlying these processes, and to uncover their time courses, in both humans and lower animals. The startle modification paradigms permit the study of these processes and mechanisms with different lead stimuli at different times in different people. Thus, the "startle stimulus" is a convenient, nonverbal, involuntary, culture-free, and quantifiable probe of psychophysiological processes occurring at specified intervals following the "lead stimuli."

Finally, we express our great appreciation to Jonathan Wynn for his invaluable assistance with the many details necessary to put this book in its final form. Jonathan's considerable skills and good nature were put to the test with the compiling of the extensive integrated list of references, the organization of the final text and figures, and many other matters.

A Historical Note on the "Discovery" of Startle Modification

HOWARD S. HOFFMAN

The term startle modification refers to the change in the amplitude and/or the latency of a startle reaction when the startle-eliciting signal has been preceded or accompanied by another (usually weaker) stimulus. In the early 1960s my students and I discovered or, as will be seen, rediscovered these effects when we found that in rats, the startle reaction to a sudden explosive sound could be virtually eliminated if another, barely audible, sound precedes the intense sound by about a tenth of a second (Hoffman and Searle 1965). We found this effect to be so impressive that we began what has for us proven to be more than 30 years of continuing investigations of its basic features.

At the time we started that work, very little of the contemporary research involved startle, and the primary source on this reaction was a slim volume entitled *The Startle Pattern* by Carney Landis and William A. Hunt (1939). This book described an extensive series of investigations by the authors in which high-speed cinematic photographs of both animal and human startle reactions were carefully analyzed. It is significant that the book made no mention of the phenomenon of startle modification, nor had the phenomenon been noted in any of the more contemporary research literature we were examining at the time.

It was a number of years after we had "discovered" startle modification that we were to learn that James Ison at the University of Rochester had independently and almost simultaneously discovered the same phenomenon. Furthermore, Ison's subsequent historical studies revealed that the phenomenon was originally discovered by Sechenov, a Russian scientist, almost 100 years earlier (Sechenov 1863/1965). During the ensuing century, startle modification had disappeared from the literature and been rediscovered at least four times. An account of those rediscoveries and an evaluation of their role in the history of psychology is provided in Ison and Hoffman (1983).

At the time of my own rediscovery I was a new assistant professor at Pennsylvania State University, and my students and I were investigating a set of behaviors that, technically, are described as "discriminated avoidance." Our subjects were laboratory rats and we had begun to cast about for a way to assess the emotional reactions that, theoretically, were thought to motivate the avoidance response. In the experiment we were conducting, a tone ending with an electrical shock was periodically presented to a rat that was confined in a small cage with a lever protruding from one of the walls. The conditions were such that if the rat pressed the lever during a tone but prior to the onset of shock, the tone immediately terminated and the shock was avoided. If, however, the rat failed to respond prior to shock onset, both the tone and the shock stayed on until a press occurred, whereupon both tone and shock were immediately turned off.

As we considered the ways we might assess the emotional aspects of our rat's behavior, I recalled an elegant study by Judson Brown and his colleagues. They reported that after a tone ending with a brief shock had been repeatedly presented to a rat, the animal's startle reaction to a sudden intense sound was larger (i.e., it was potentiated) if the sound was presented during the tone as compared with when it was presented in the absence of the tone (Brown, Kalish, & Farber 1951). It seemed possible that we might find it useful to employ the Brown, Kalish, and Farber procedures in our own work. More specifically, we thought we might be able to track the course of emotionality during our rat's avoidance behavior by occasionally presenting an intense sound during the tone and assessing the amplitude of the ensuing reaction. As it turned out, we never pursued this, because we were diverted by the study of startle itself once we began to assess it.

As we saw it, to study startle we had to solve two problems. We had to find a convenient way to measure response amplitude and we had to find a way to reliably produce an eliciting acoustic stimulus. Brown, Kalish, and Farber had used a spring-mounted mechanical postage scale to assess startle amplitude and they used a pistol shot to elicit the reaction. We wanted to use electronic gear to accomplish both of these ends.

Our solution to the problem of assessing startle was to build a small Plexiglas chamber and to mount it on compression springs that were fastened to a rigid superstructure. An aluminum rod with a small permanent magnet at its distal end was connected to the bottom of the chamber so that the magnet rode within an electrical coil. Movements of the chamber moved the magnet in the coil and generated an electrical current that was amplified and rectified and passed to a recording milliammeter. Because the output of the system was proportional to the rate at which magnetic lines of flux crossed the coil, the device was highly sensitive to the sudden ballistic-type movements involved in startle, but it was relatively insensitive to the gross, but more or less slow, movements involved in general activity.

Our solution to the problem of eliciting startle was not so elegant. We found that the maximum acoustic signals produced by our electronic signal generators were too weak to consistently elicit startle. We also found, however, that we could reliably evoke a response by discharging a condenser through the voice coil of an inexpensive 5-inch speaker. The problem here was that the speakers were fragile and would often blow out after only two or three discharges. Fortunately, however, we also found that every now and then we would come across a speaker that was so resistant to blowout that we could deliver thousands of startle-eliciting signals with no ill effects. We cherished those speakers and used them in our subsequent experiments.

Our "discovery" of startle modification occurred as we were engaged in our initial pilot work. We had noticed that when tested in the open environment of our laboratory, the startle reactions of our rats were highly variable. In an effort to obtain better control over these reactions, we enclosed our startle apparatus within an ice chest and arranged to introduce steady noise into the chest so as to mask extraneous environmental sounds.

As expected, responses were less variable when subjects were tested in the ice chest but to our surprise response amplitude turned out to be critically dependent on the nature of the acoustic conditions at the time that startle was evoked. With the background noise turned off, the ambient acoustic level within the chamber hovered about 58 dB SPL, with occasional peaks of about 70 dB. With the noise turned on, the ambient acoustic level within the chest was a steady 85 dB.

With the background noise turned off, responses to the acoustic bursts were of moderate amplitude. When the noise was turned on, however, responses to the same bursts were much larger. It should be noted that this was exactly the opposite of what we had expected would happen. We had assumed that the background noise would, in some measure, mask the startle-eliciting signals.

As a result, responses to those signals were smaller. Even more surprising was the observation that if we pulsed the background noise (one-half second on and one-half second off), the startle responses to the intense bursts all but disappeared. Figure 1 shows the trial by trial record of an individual rat when it was exposed to a sequence of startle-eliciting acoustic bursts spaced 10 s apart.

During the first ten bursts the background noise was off. The background noise was pulsed throughout the next ten trials and then it was made steady. Since, as indicated in Figure 1, manipulation of the background noise persisted in determining overall response amplitude and since the identical effects were easily obtained with other rats, it was apparent that we had stum-

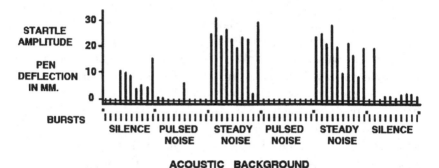

Figure 1. The effect of background acoustic stimulation on the startle reaction to an intense burst of noise. The record shows the sequence of startle reactions by a single rat that received a startle eliciting stimulus every 10 s. Throughout this session the acoustic background was changed (as indicated) shortly after every tenth startle-eliciting stimulus. (Adapted from Figure 1 in Hoffman and Fleshler, 1963. Copyright 1963 by The American Association for the Advancement of Science. Reprinted by permission.)

bled onto a robust and possibly quite important behavioral phenomenon. Accordingly, we abandoned our effort to employ startle as an index of the emotional factors in discriminated avoidance and turned our attention to the study of startle modification. In particular, we started a sequence of investigations designed to determine whether and how a single pulse of noise that was itself too weak to elicit startle might, nonetheless, influence the startle reaction to a subsequently presented intense acoustic burst.

The results of those initial investigations were reported in Hoffman and Searle (1965, 1968). It is, perhaps, of historical interest that in preparing those reports Searle and I used the term "prepulse" to describe the lead stimulus in our startle modification paradigms. Within a few years of those publications Francis Graham at the University of Wisconsin and James Ison at Rochester University independently began to publish reports of their own investigations of the startle modification effect, and it is, I suspect, also of historical interest that it was in one of those reports (Ison & Hammond, 1971) where the now popular expressions "prepulse inhibition" and "prepulse facilitation" were first used. Some of the results of the initial studies by both Graham and Ison were summarized in an early review paper (Hoffman & Ison, 1980).

As revealed in this volume, many new insights into and uses for startle modification have been developed in the decade and a half since Ison and I published our review. We ended that review with the following statement: "Clearly, the analysis of reflex modification offers an approach to a range of problems of utmost theoretical and practical importance. In some respects these preparations are comparable in their simplicity and reproducibility to the isolated systems studied by the physiologist. Yet in their appearance in the intact animal, even in the intact human animal, they are sensitive to the activity of more complex processes and offer another way to examine that activity and its determinants" (p. 187).

I can add only that it is a source of great satisfaction to me that the approaches and insights in the various chapters of the present volume are directed to the elaboration and extension of that enterprise.

CHAPTER ONE

Startle Modification: Introduction and Overview

MICHAEL E. DAWSON, ANNE M. SCHELL, AND
ANDREAS H. BÖHMELT

ABSTRACT

Startle modification refers to a set of reliable and ubiquitous phenomena. Specifically, the startle modification phenomena include the inhibition and facilitation of the startle reflex by nonstartling stimuli that accompany or precede the startle-eliciting stimulus. This chapter introduces these phenomena through historical examples drawn from both the human and nonhuman animal literature. Both the inhibition and the facilitation of the startle reflex are illustrated. The standard terms used throughout this book – "startle stimulus," "lead stimulus," and "lead interval" – are defined by reference to these prototypical examples. Potential implications of startle modification phenomena are identified for cognitive science, neuroscience, and clinical science, with special emphasis on integrative implications. Finally, the book is outlined with reference to each of the subsequent chapters.

1. Introduction and Brief History

Reflexes are often considered simple, fixed, and invariant reactions to stimuli. However, it has been known for a number of years that reflexes are not fixed; rather, they are highly modifiable by a variety of events that occur concurrent with or immediately before the elicitation of the reflex. The amplitude of the patellar tendon "knee-jerk" reflex, for example, was shown over 100 years ago to vary systematically depending upon the time at which a voluntary motor response preceded the elicitation of the reflex (Bowditch & Warren, 1890). The amplitude of the human patellar reflex was facilitated if participants voluntarily clinched their hands in response to a bell simultaneously with the blow upon the tendon, but the reflex was inhibited, sometimes disappearing entirely, if

Michael E. Dawson, Anne M. Schell, and Andreas H. Böhmelt, Eds. *Startle modification: Implications for neuroscience, cognitive science, and clinical science.* Copyright © 1999 Cambridge University Press. Printed in the United States of America. All rights reserved.

the hand clinch occurred only a few hundred milliseconds before the patellar stimulation. This early study and several others that preceded and followed it are thoroughly reviewed by Ison and Hoffman (1983).

This research in combination with others suggested that "the myth of the knee-jerk as a simple spinal reflex is shattered. . . . data have been accumulating that the knee-jerk, and perhaps all 'simple' reflexes, *cannot be regarded as isolated units of function in the intact nervous system*" (Fearing, 1930, p. 277, emphasis in original). This book provides the first contemporary and comprehensive review of the proposition that reflexes are modified by ongoing psychophysiological processes, and hence can provide a window onto those processes.

Hilgard (1933) devised a research paradigm based on the human startle eyeblink reflex to loud noise that is more relevant to present-day research than the knee-jerk paradigm employed by Bowditch and Warren. In this paradigm, simple stimuli (lights) rather than a motor response were used to modify the human startle eyeblink reflex elicited by a loud noise. The loud startling noise was preceded by a low-intensity light on some trials at various intervals, and not on other intermixed trials. When the light preceded the noise by very short intervals (e.g., 25 and 50 msec), the amplitude of the blink reflex to the noise was increased by approximately 150%; however, when the light preceded the noise by moderately short intervals (e.g., in the range of 100–300 msec), the blink reflex to the noise was inhibited to approximately half of its normal size. Thus, Hilgard concluded that "a faint stimulus, itself eliciting only minimal reflex reactions, may greatly exaggerate or depress the response to a more intense stimulus which follows it. By slight changes in the interval of time between the first and second stimulus, the reinforcing effect may be converted into an inhibitory effect" (1933, p. 86). The finding of facilitation or inhibition of the human acoustic startle eyeblink reflex by a prior occurring innocuous stimulus is an intriguing phenomenon that anticipates a large body of contemporary research.

Other historical examples of the modification of reflexes by simple stimuli preceding the elicitation of the reflex can be found in nonhuman animals. In one of the earliest and more interesting examples, Yerkes (1905) was puzzled by the fact that frogs did not respond behaviorally to sounds, and he wanted to experimentally determine whether frogs can hear. Therefore, he presented auditory stimuli (e.g., a bell) simultaneously with or shortly preceding a tactile stimulus (a tap to the head), which in turn elicited a leg withdrawal reflex. The results revealed that when the auditory stimulus occurred simultaneously with the tactile stimulus the withdrawal reflex was exaggerated, whereas on the contrary if the auditory stimulus preceded the reflex-eliciting tactile stimulus by several hundred milliseconds the reflex was partially inhibited. Yerkes concluded that "these experiments prove conclusively that sounds, although they do not call forth the reflex movement under consideration, modify in important ways the action of other stimuli" (p. 296).

Although there are obvious differences in the procedures employed by Hilgard and by Yerkes, both found that a weak innocuous stimulus has the power to significantly facilitate or inhibit an innate defensive reflex depending upon the time interval separating the two stimuli. The remarkable commonality of reflex modification effects observed across different species, different stimuli, and different response systems suggests the existence of processes of profound generalizability and importance.

Despite these early encouraging results, however, the study of reflex modification was largely ignored for several decades. Yerkes and Hilgard went on to distinguished careers, both becoming presidents of the American Psychological Association, but in research areas other than reflex modification. Ison and Hoffman (1983) suggested that the study of reflex modification was swept aside by the then burgeoning interest in classical Pavlovian conditioning (itself considered an associative reflex modification procedure) and learning theories in general.

Given the high level of interest in classical conditioning at the time, it is not surprising, therefore, that the return of research interest in reflex modification was in the context of understanding classical conditioning. Brown, Kalish, and Farber (1951), for example, classically conditioned fear in rats by pairing a neutral compound stimulus (light + buzzer) with an electric shock. In the experimental group, the onset of the light + buzzer was followed by the shock in 3 s, whereas the control group was presented the same stimuli but not in a paired arrangement. On interspersed trials during this procedure, a startle reflex was elicited by a loud noise in both groups 3 s after the onset of the light + buzzer (i.e., at the time the shock was due in the experimental group). The whole-body startle reaction (the magnitude of the jump of the rat as measured with a postage scale) was significantly larger in the experimental group than the control group. It was concluded that the pairing of the light + buzzer with the shock led to a conditioned fear state that facilitated the startle reaction to sound.

Brown et al. (1951) emphasized the importance of their findings as confirming Hull's (1943) theoretical prediction that conditioned fear has energizing properties. However, from today's perspective, the importance of the Brown et al. study is its demonstration of affective modulation of a startle reflex. Although Hullian theory has now gone the way of all grand learning theories, the affective modulation of the startle reflex has been confirmed many times in both human and nonhuman subjects and has become a commonly used paradigm with many important applications and implications.

The most recent reemergence of interest in reflex modification in the 1960s was initially motivated by an attempt to replicate the Brown et al. effect (see Prologue). Fortunately, while conducting pilot studies, Hoffman and his colleagues serendipitously noticed that the rat acoustic startle reaction was highly modifiable by mild sounds even without being paired with shock. Hoffman and Wible (1969) then systematically studied startle in rats to a loud noise (130 dB) preceded by a weaker noise (75 dB) at onset to onset intervals ranging from 100 to 6000 msec. The preceding noise was presented as a discrete 20-msec pulse or as a continuous stimulus throughout the interval. The authors observed reflex inhibition at the short lead intervals and facilitation at the long lead intervals, but the inhibition effect was strongest with the brief discrete preceding noise and the facilitation was evident only with the continuous preceding noise that was maintained throughout the entire lead interval. Hoffman and Wible suggested that two aspects of the preceding stimulus control startle amplitude. The transient *onset* of the leading stimulus can trigger a short latency, brief inhibitory effect at short lead intervals, whereas the *continuous* presence of the stimulus can have a long-lasting amplifying effect at long lead intervals. This hypothesis has been a fertile seed that has flourished and continues to bear fruit to this day, as will become clear in later chapters.

Hoffman's research influenced the independent research programs of other investigators, most notably Ison and Graham. Ison and his students soon demonstrated that the acoustic startle reflex in rats could be inhibited by stimuli in multiple sensory systems, and was not specific to an auditory refractory process (Buckland, Buckland, Jamieson, & Ison, 1969; Ison, Hammond, & Krauter, 1973), and they also examined various parametric effects with the human eyeblink reflex (e.g., Krauter, Leonard, & Ison, 1973). Graham and her students quickly followed with a systematic series of studies that demonstrated that the human acoustic startle eyeblink reflex was reliably inhibited by a mild tone presented 60–240 msec prior to the startle loud noise and was facilitated if the same mild tone was presented several seconds prior to the startling noise (Graham, 1975; Graham, Putnam, & Leavitt, 1975), and they have since gone on to study preattentive, attentive, and arousal processes with startle modification and other psychophysiological measures (Graham, 1997).

In summary, numerous studies have demonstrated that relatively small changes in environmental stimuli produce large changes in subsequently elicited reflexes, with the interval separating the stimuli being a critical determiner of the direction of the effect. The present book contains chapters that focus separately on short and long intervals precisely because the processes that modify and modulate reflexes appear to be quite different at these intervals.

In the remainder of this chapter we will describe the reflex modification paradigm and phenomena in more formal terms, suggest standard terminology to describe the reflex modification paradigm, and, most important, discuss why researchers from diverse scientific disciplines find the reflex modification phenomena worthy of renewed attention and research. We then conclude with an outline of this book, briefly indicating how each chapter contributes an important part of the story of the psychological and physiological significance of startle modification.

2. Startle Reflex Modification: Paradigms and Terminology

Rather than discuss modification of reflexes in general, one particular type of reflex is emphasized here and throughout the book, that is, the acoustic startle reflex. Many of the prototypical paradigms described above (e.g., Hilgard, 1933; Brown et al., 1951; Hoffman & Wible, 1969) measured the acoustic startle reflex and its modification. Whenever an exception to this general rule is made by reference to other reflexes, this will be made clear. Although it is empirically and theoretically important to know whether other types of reflexes are similarly modified, this is not the focus of the present book. Therefore, in the subsequent material we will refer to startle reflex modification or simply startle modification rather than the more general term reflex modification.

Given the large and rapidly growing body of startle modification research, it is impossible for one volume to adequately cover both human and nonhuman research on this topic. We chose to focus primarily but not exclusively on human research. The human acoustic startle reflex, as originally captured with high-speed motion pictures by Landis and Hunt (1939), consists of a series of involuntary muscle movements. Landis and Hunt reported that the fastest, most reliable, and most resistant to habituation component of the human startle reflex was the eyeblink reaction. For these reasons, and because it is relatively easy to measure and quantify, the eyeblink response is the most commonly used measure of startle in human research today.

In the previous section we presented prototypical examples of startle modification, some with short interstimulus intervals (e.g., in a few hundred milliseconds as in Hilgard, 1933) and others with long interstimulus intervals (e.g., several seconds as in Brown et al., 1951). Figure 1.1 depicts diagrammatically the basic procedures and results of the startle modification paradigm.

The startle modification paradigm consists of two stimuli and the interval separating their onsets. Various terms have been used in the literature to

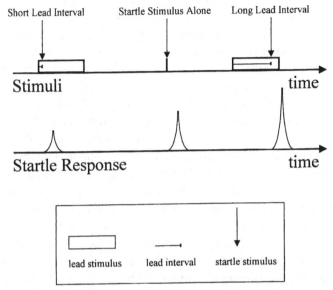

Figure 1.1. Exemplary presentation of the startle modification paradigm. (*Top*) The stimulus events; (*bottom*) a schematic startle response. To the *left*, the startle eliciting stimulus is applied shortly (e.g., 100 ms) after the onset of the lead stimulus. Startle is inhibited compared with the reference measure obtained by the following presentation of the startle stimulus alone. To the *right*, the startle stimulus is applied after a long lead interval of several seconds, in this example producing startle facilitation.

describe the stimuli used in this paradigm. The first nonstartling stimulus has been referred to as a "prestimulus," "prepulse," "conditioning stimulus," and "lead stimulus," to name just a few common terms. The most commonly used term in animal and human short lead interval startle modification studies is "prepulse" (see the Prologue for a discussion of the history of this term). The short lead interval inhibition phenomenon is consequently frequently referred to as "prepulse inhibition" (PPI) (Ison & Hammond, 1971). On the other hand, in the long lead interval startle modification paradigm the terms for the first stimulus are more heterogeneous. To have consistency across the paradigms within the present book, we have chosen "lead stimulus" as being the most descriptive term without excessive theoretical meaning to be used for both short and long lead interval research. "Lead" points to the fact that the stimulus temporally leads the elicitation of the startle response independent of the interval duration and whether the lead stimulus is continuous or discrete.

Terms to describe the critical time interval between onsets of the two stimuli have included "interstimulus interval," "stimulus onset asynchrony," and "lead interval." Again, for standardization, descriptive simplicity, and theoretical neutrality we chose "lead interval" for use in this book. Also, based on the reasoning that "lead stimulus" describes the stimulus that is in the temporal lead, the term "lead interval" points to the duration of the interval between the lead stimulus and the response-eliciting stimulus.

This second stimulus has been called an "eliciting stimulus," "pulse," and "startle probe." Whereas the term "pulse," as pointed out earlier, refers to physical characteristics of the stimulus, the term "probe" bears the conceptual meaning of startle modification as a technique to probe into neurophysiological and psychological processes. Again, for consistency, ease of description, and theoretical neutrality we have chosen the term "startle stimulus."

Figure 1.1 illustrates "short lead interval" startle inhibition and "long lead interval" facilitation. Although the use of common terms for short and long lead interval startle modification is convenient and parsimonious, the use of such standard terms for both long and short lead interval procedures is admittedly disputable. On the one hand, short and long lead interval studies investigate the same dependent variable with the only difference in the experimental paradigm being the timing of stimulus onsets ("lead interval"). On the other hand, not only do the effects between the two types of startle modification differ markedly, they may reflect distinct and independent neurophysiological and psychological processes. The distinctions between these processes will be outlined in various chapters of this volume and may suggest that a standard terminology may not necessarily suit both paradigms. One of the exciting prospects of this book is that it provides the first overview of human startle modification research across both short and long lead interval research.

3. Significance of Startle Modification Phenomena

Although early examples of the experimental modification of reflexes can be found, as documented in Section 1 of this chapter and reviewed in detail by Ison and Hoffman (1983), this phenomenon has proven to be of particular interest during the past quarter-century. Figure 1.2 illustrates the remarkable growth of research on startle modification in humans from 1970 to 1995. The exploding growth of interest in human startle modification is reminiscent of the interest in the P300 component of the evoked brain potential in the early 1960s. Startle modification research with nonhuman animals, although not included in Figure 1.2, has likewise shown dramatic growth over this same period of time. Clearly, the significance of reflex modification phenomena has been reappreciated recently, igniting intense research interest.

It is clear that researchers from different disciplines believe that the study of startle modification can be of considerable use and significance. What is

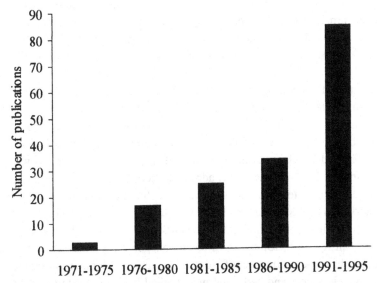

Figure 1.2. Number of publications dealing with human startle modification in five-year epochs from 1971 to 1995. The data are derived from MedLine and PsycLit database searches. (From Filion, Dawson, & Schell, 1998.)

the nature of that significance? What can startle modification tell us about psychological and physiological processes that cannot be learned from more standard experimental paradigms and techniques? What do we currently know about the stimulus factors, subject factors, psychological processes, and physiological mechanisms that affect the modification of the startle reflex? What are the current gaps in our knowledge about these processes? It is the purpose of this book to address these questions, and hopefully provide some tentative answers. In the remainder of this chapter, we will briefly outline the general implications of startle modification for neuroscience, cognitive science, and clinical science. We provide here only a general sense of the broad potential implications of startle modification. Evaluation of how well the startle modification paradigm has achieved this potential, and how well it will be able to expand upon its potential, must await reading the various lines of evidence reviewed within this book.

3.1. Neuroscience Implications

As discussed previously, early examples of startle modification at short lead intervals were demonstrated with nonhuman animals (e.g., Yerkes, 1905; see review by Ison & Hoffman, 1983). To this day, the majority of experimental investigations of startle modification at short lead intervals are conducted with nonhuman animals under the rubric of "prepulse inhibition." Computer database searches of studies of prepulse inhibition reveal approximately four times the number of publications using nonhuman participants as human participants.

Nonhuman and human startle modification research have followed different paths and asked somewhat different questions about startle modification. Most nonhuman research has to do with the neurophysiological and/or neuropharmacological mediation of short lead interval inhibition ("prepulse inhibition"). The independent variable in most of this research has to do with pharmacological interventions (e.g., administration of agonists and antagonists of neurotransmitters such as dopamine and glutamate) and the effects of lesions and electrical stimulation. Long lead interval modification, particularly dealing with affective modulation of startle, also has a clear presence in the nonhuman research, following in the footsteps of Brown et al. (1951). Here again, the current direction of work in this area is the determination of the neurophysiological and neuropharmacological basis of startle modification, particularly fear potentiation of startle. Great strides are being made; the neural circuits underlying the acoustic startle reflex and its modification are becoming relatively well understood in nonhuman participants.

The significance of the startle modification paradigm for neuroscience is that it offers a simple and well-controlled paradigm for the study of the neurophysiological basis of behaviorally relevant processes in the intact animal. Davis (1980) reviewed several reasons that the startle reflex and its modification are valuable behavioral measures for neuroscience. These include the fact that the startle reflex is clearly under stimulus control, is mediated by a simple neural circuit, can be measured easily, shows high plasticity, and can be studied comparatively across species. Thus, for the neuroscientist, the startle modification paradigm provides an attractive behavioral vehicle with which to test neurophysiological and neuropharmacological mechanisms.

3.2. Cognitive Science Implications

Cognitive science is a multidisciplinary effort to understand the component processes involved in how organisms extract information from their environments. The startle modification paradigm has the potential to shed light on the nature and the timing of the sequence of processing operations following environmental stimuli. That is, one can use the startle stimulus to "probe" into cognitive and emotional processing initiated by lead stimuli at various specific lead intervals (see Anthony, 1985, pp. 168–170 for a description of the rationale of reflex activity as a probe of ongoing cognitive processes). As detailed in subsequent chapters, changes in the startle response elicited at different lead intervals may be used to infer, for example, the time at which the significance of auditory lead stimuli is appreciated, or the time at which positive and negative affective valence has begun to be differentially processed. The startle stimulus can be used to probe the processing of stimuli in different modalities, including simple auditory or visual lead stimuli, complex pictures, semantic stimuli, or even "private" images. Even more, the startle probe technique can be used to study processing of lead stimuli in various states, such as sleep (Silverstein, Graham, & Calloway, 1980).

The startle modification paradigm has the potential to separately quantify both automatic and controlled cognitive processes following presentation of a lead stimulus. That is, startle inhibition at short lead intervals can occur automatically without subjects attending to the lead stimulus, and yet at a slightly longer lead interval, the amount of startle inhibition can be modulated by attention. Thus, one may be able to infer from the presence of startle inhibition at one short lead interval (e.g., 60 ms) whether the lead stimulus has been automatically detected and processed, and also infer from the degree of inhibition at another short lead interval (e.g., 120 ms) when controlled attentional processes are engaged.

Practically all of the methodological advantages reviewed above of using startle for neuroscience (Davis, 1980) also apply to cognitive science (and clinical science, for that matter). That is, the tight stimulus control, ease of measurement, and simplicity of underlying processes also make startle an attractive measure for cognitive science. Thus a new quantitative tool may be added to the methodological armamentarium of cognitive science. Because it is a nonverbal reflex, startle can be used in a wide number of situations where other tools such as verbal reports and/or voluntary reaction time are inappropriate.

3.3. Clinical Science Implications

A primary goal of clinical science is to identify basic underlying processes and mechanisms that mediate pathology, in this case psychopathology. Once the basic mechanisms and processes are identified, one can target both primary and preventive interventions in a more rational manner. Among the basic processes frequently hypothesized to be critical mediators of psychopathology are information processing and affective dysfunctions.

To the degree that cognitive and emotional processes are involved in psychopathology, and to the degree that startle modification is sensitive to cognitive and emotional processes, the startle modification paradigm promises to provide a useful methodology for clinical science. It can be used to test theories regarding the etiology of psychopathology in high-risk individuals, to identify subgroups within disorders, and to track changes with treatment. Moreover, startle modification holds the promise of providing new information about the basic mechanisms and processes underlying psychopathology. For example, we alluded above to the fact that startle modification in some circumstances may be used to separately evaluate automatic and controlled cognitive processes. Therefore, the startle modification paradigm may be used to determine whether cognitive dysfunctions in different psychopathologies are specific to automatic or controlled processing deficits. Moreover, startle modification may be used to assess emotional processing deficits and determine whether those deficits are specific to processing different emotional valences or are more general emotional processing deficits.

Beyond the inferences regarding cognitive and emotional processing at the theoretical conceptual level, startle modification may also have implications for testing neurophysiological and neuropharmacological mechanisms involved in psychopathology. Thus, startle modification may enlighten us about the neurobiology of psychopathology, providing information to test existing theories as well as to generate new theories.

3.4. Integrative Implications

Startle modification may provide a unique window on the central nervous system (neuroscience) and the "conceptual nervous system" (cognitive science) in both normal and abnormal states (clinical science). However, the most important implication of the startle modification paradigm and phenomena is not for neuroscience, cognitive science, or clinical science considered individually; rather, it is for the *integration* of these three branches of science. We believe that startle modification has the potential to be a model system for integrative research. It may provide a rare opportunity to study the same basic process at different levels of analyses. Attention and emotion, for example, may be studied with quantitative precision with nearly identical paradigms and stimulus parameters in normal human participants, disordered human patients, and in nonhuman animals. Thus, the same basic phenomenon can be studied from the perspectives of cognitive science, clinical science, and neuroscience.

Startle modification promises to be an important bridging paradigm. It promises to bridge human and infrahuman research; cognitive, motivational, and affective processes; and concepts drawn from neuroscience, cognitive science, and clinical science. We hope that this book will help construct a more sturdy foundation for this bridge to complete its promise, allowing it to be transversed by future generations of researchers from diverse disciplines.

4. Outline of This Book

We asked some of the most experienced and knowledgeable investigators to review the most important and the most recent findings in startle modification and to discuss their theoretical and practical implications. Contrary to many edited books, we explicitly asked contributors not only to review their own programs of research, but rather to survey their fields more broadly.

As described in Section 1 of this chapter, the magnitude and direction of the startle modification effect depends in large part on the length of the lead interval. Therefore, most chapters in this book are devoted primarily to startle modification at either short or long lead intervals. Chapters deal with short and long intervals separately because the processes that modify and modulate startle appear to be quite different at these intervals.

In Part 1 (Chapters 2–4), we begin with the basic issues surrounding the elicitation and measurement of the human startle eyeblink reflex and its modification at short and long lead intervals. In Chapter 2, Berg and Balaban discuss the characteristics of the startle stimulus necessary to reliably elicit the startle response, the methods of recording the startle eyeblink response, and the methods of scoring the startle eyeblink reflex, including computer scoring algorithms. In Chapter 3, Blumenthal discusses the effects of lead stimulus and startle stimulus parameters (intensity, change, duration, modality, etc.) on short lead interval startle modification, as well as the functional significance of short lead interval startle modification. In Chapter 4, Putnam and Vanman discuss the effects of lead stimulus parameters such as intensity, duration, and modality on long lead interval startle modification. Both diffuse and selective attentional effects on startle at long lead intervals are explored.

In Part II (Chapters 5 and 6), the neurophysiology and neuropharmacology of startle modification are presented. In Chapter 5, Davis, Walker, and Lee describe new information regarding the neural circuits underlying the basic startle circuit and the mechanisms of affective startle modification. In Chapter 6, Swerdlow and Geyer discuss the neurophysiology and neuropharmacology of short lead interval startle modification, including the role of forebrain regulation of short lead interval startle modification and its potential relevance for psychopathology.

In Part III (Chapters 7 and 8), the relevance of psychological processes in startle modification is discussed. In Chapter 7, Hackley discusses issues regarding the roles of attention, arousal, and consciousness in startle modification. In Chapter 8, Bradley, Cuthbert, and Lang deal with modification of the startle reflex by affectively valenced sensory material and images within the context of the motivational priming theory.

In Part IV (Chapters 9–12), a variety of individual differences in startle modification are examined. In Chapter 9, Cook discusses the effects of affective individual differences in both normal and abnormal populations, particularly with respect to fearfulness, using both picture-viewing and imagery paradigms. In Chapter 10, Patrick and Lang extend research with affective modification of startle to the study of psychopathy and alcohol intoxication. Evidence for a core affective disorder in psychopathy is reviewed and acute alcohol intoxication is then advanced as a model of simple antisocial deviance. In Chapter 11, Cadenhead and Braff advance the view that short lead interval startle inhibition is an index of sensorimotor gating deficits in schizophrenia and schizophrenia spectrum disorders. In Chapter 12, Ornitz discusses developmental aspects of startle modification. Habituation of the startle response is also covered, as are autonomic and neurophysiologic events (event-related potential measures) that accompany the startle response during childhood.

In Part V (Chapters 13–15), a broad view of startle modification, including its relationship to other measures obtained in other paradigms, is considered. In Chapter 13, Filion, Kelly, and Hazlett discuss the possible relationships between short lead interval startle inhibition and the attentional blink, backward masking performance, and negative priming in the Stroop task. In Chapter 14, Ford and Roth examine the parallels between the effects of lead stimuli on the startle response and the effects on event-related potential components. Brainstem responses and the component amplitudes of P50, N1-P2, Mismatch Negativity, P300, and N400 are reviewed, with each component being evaluated with respect to criteria for reflexivity, effects of attention, effects of interstimulus interval length in stimulus train paradigms, and effects of lead interval in paired stimulus paradigms. Finally, in Chapter 15, Lipp and Siddle discuss the relationships between startle modification, orienting, and Pavlovian conditioning. The usefulness of the startle response in clarifying the attentional and affective processes at work during orienting and conditioning is explored.

We wish the reader a stimulating exploration of startle modification and its implications for neuroscience, cognitive science, and clinical science.

PART I

Basic Paradigms, Methods, and Phenomena

Startle Elicitation: Stimulus Parameters, Recording Techniques, and Quantification

W. KEITH BERG AND MARIE T. BALABAN

ABSTRACT

This chapter reviews methods for eliciting, measuring, and quantifying the blink component of the startle response in humans. We begin with a brief summary of what is known about the physiological circuitry of the human startle blink. We discuss laboratory techniques for eliciting the startle blink with probe stimuli in auditory, cutaneous, or visual modalities. In a discussion of recording the human blink reflex, we focus on electromyographic (EMG) recording but consider other methods. We then address approaches for quantification of blink latency and amplitude, and also raise methodological questions that warrant further experimental investigation. This overview provides an introduction for researchers who are interested in learning how to measure startle. Issues relevant to startle modification techniques are also discussed.

1. Overview of Methodological Issues

In this chapter, we discuss methodological issues relevant to eliciting, recording, and quantifying the blink component of startle. This review is intended for new investigators because it provides a guide to methodological issues, as well as for experienced investigators, in the hope that this attempt to synthesize methodological concerns will stimulate discussion. Some aspects of startle methodology have been presented at meetings (Cook & Berg, 1995), in methodological abstracts (Balaban, Losito, Simons, & Graham, 1986a), and papers (Clarkson & Berg, 1984; Blumenthal, 1994).

There are three general topics to be addressed: How is the startle blink *elicited, recorded,* and *quantified?* We discuss startle elicited in auditory, cutaneous, and visual modalities. In the section on recording, we focus on electromyography (EMG) but briefly consider other methods. Aspects of signal processing are also addressed in this section. Issues relevant to the quan-

Michael E. Dawson, Anne M. Schell, and Andreas H. Böhmelt, Eds. *Startle modification: Implications for neuroscience, cognitive science, and clinical science.* Copyright © 1999 Cambridge University Press. Printed in the United States of America. All rights reserved.

tification of startle include the definition of response parameters and the use of computer-scoring methods. We also consider questions about quantifying reflex modification effects.

Our goal in this chapter is to describe methodological issues and options rather than to stipulate rules. Individual researchers may have different reasons for selecting stimulus parameters, recording systems, and scoring criteria. Thus, standardization in startle methodology is unlikely. Nonetheless, it is critical to compare results across laboratories that employ different methods. In an attempt to guide new investigators, we offer advice on methodology based on synthesis of current research practices and on our experience.

As with any physiological response system, to make informed methodological decisions about the blink reflex, it is important to consider characteristics of the response, including its neural control. Thus, we begin with the physiological underpinnings of the blink reflex component of human startle. This description is limited to the intrinsic blink reflex pathways and does not address extrinsic reflex modification circuits (see Chapters 5 and 6).

2. Physiology of the Human Startle Blink

Our understanding of the neural circuitry underlying the startle reflex in animals is due, in large part, to the achievements of Davis and colleagues (see Chapter 5). Although we assume that a relation exists between the neural pathways controlling the whole-body startle reaction in rats and humans, our knowledge of the neural organization specific to the human blink reflex pathway remains incomplete. The following sections review characteristics of the blink motor response and outline the putative neural pathways underlying the blink reflex to auditory, visual, and cutaneous stimulation.

The reflex blink is a motor response that can be elicited by stimulation in various sensory modalities. This description begins with the *efferent* side of the reflex pathway – the blink motor response. We then describe the *central* portion of the reflex pathway, including the brainstem startle center and other potential areas of convergence of transient sensory information. Finally, we outline the specific *afferent* portions of the reflex pathway, which differ for each sensory modality.

2.1. The Blink Motor Response

The blink reflex consists of the coordinated movements of several muscle groups, primarily contraction of the orbicularis oculi, which has fibers in the eyelid and around the eye (Fig. 2.1), and reciprocal inhibition of the levator palpebrae, which raises the eyelid. Lid closure occurs about 10–12 msec after the initial orbicularis oculi EMG activity.

Although description of muscle anatomy and innervation is beyond the scope of this chapter, an understanding of the reflex musculature is important for investigators of startle modification. For example, Jancke, Bauer, and von Giesen (1994) reported that the latency and amplitude of the electrically evoked blink reflex could be facilitated by tonic voluntary contraction of the orbicularis oculi. In some reflex modification studies, this type of change at the musculature might contribute to differences between blinks elicited during different task conditions.

2.2. Efferent and Central Startle Blink Pathways

The orbicularis oculi muscle is innervated by the facial nerve (seventh cranial nerve). Thus, the final motor pathway for the blink reflex stems from the facial motor nucleus located at the pontine level of the brain stem. Areas in the pontine tegmentum that project to the intermediate facial nucleus are presumed to be involved in the premotor control of blinking as well as in the response of the retractor bulbi eye muscle (Holstege, Van Ham, & Tan, 1986).

Questions remain about the relation between the central/premotor control of the blink reflex and whole-body startle (see Chapter 5). This relation is complicated further by recent distinctions, for auditory startle, between the blink reflexes that occur with versus without other startle flexor reactions (Brown, Rothwell, Thompson, Britton, Day, & Marsden, 1991). These authors suggest that the former responses are controlled at the bulbopontine level by the brainstem startle center whereas the latter responses are controlled at the mesencephalic level by the midbrain reticular formation and inferior colliculus. Hackley and Boelhouwer (1997) review additional evidence, based on acoustic startle, suggesting a dissociation between the blink and other components of the startle response.

In summary, differences between the underlying pathways for human blink reflexes and whole-body startle remain to be clarified. Whereas some reflex modification effects are similar across these domains (e.g., Hoffman & Ison, 1980), it is important to consider that differences in the level of organization of blink versus whole-body startle could result in different patterns of reflex modification for these responses.

2.3. Afferent Startle Blink Pathways

Because the premotor area in the pontine tegmentum projects to the area of the facial motor nucleus mediating the blink reflex, we would expect to find con-

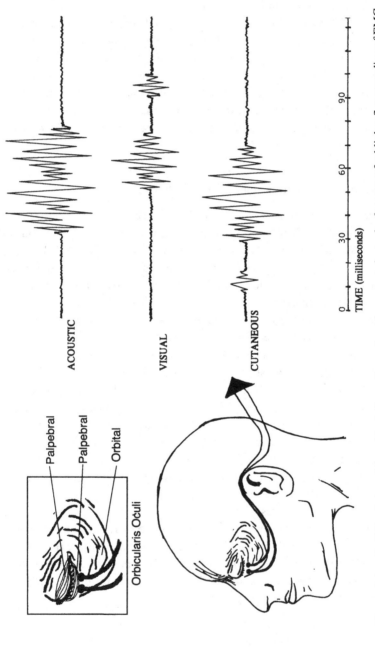

Figure 2.1. (*Left*) Depiction of the orbicularis oculi muscle and common electrode placement for blink reflex recording of EMG activity. (*Right*) Schematic illustration of EMG recordings of blinks elicited by auditory, cutaneous, and visual stimulation.

verging connections between the afferent reflex pathways for each sensory modality and this premotor area. In this section, we review available evidence on the afferent reflex pathways for acoustic, cutaneous, and visual blink reflexes.

The *acoustic* blink reflex typically consists of a burst of orbicularis oculi EMG activity at a latency of about 30–50 msec in human adults, depending on attributes of the eliciting stimulus (Fig. 2.1). The afferent pathway begins with sound transduced in the ear and transmitted along the cochlear nerve. There is debate over the intervening steps between the cochlear output and the blink premotor area. The neural circuit might include the ventral cochlear nucleus, the superior olive, the lateral lemniscus, and the inferior colliculus (Takmann, Ettlin, & Barth, 1982; Hori, Yasuhara, Naito, & Yasuhara, 1986).

The afferent pathway for the *cutaneous* blink reflex begins with the supra-orbital portion of the trigeminal nerve, which receives sensory stimulation from the upper regions of the face. The cutaneous blink occurs to mechanical stimulation rendered by a tap to the forehead, a sudden puff of air directed toward the skin, or electrical stimulation of the brow/forehead region.

The cutaneous blink reflex consists of at least two components (Fig. 2.1): an early ipsilateral component (8–12 msec with electrical stimulation) called the R1 response, and a later, bilateral component called R2 (Ongerboer de Visser & Kuypers, 1978). The latter response is associated with observable eyelid closure and occurs at latencies similar to the acoustic blink (25–50 msec). In addition, a third R3 component has sometimes been reported at longer latencies (e.g., 70–80 msec); it may be associated with nociceptive (pain) fibers (Rossi, Risaliti, & Rossi, 1989). Clinical observations of dissociations between the R1 and R2 components have helped delineate their neural pathways. The R1 pathway begins with the afferent input from the trigeminal nerve conveyed to the principal sensory trigeminal nucleus. This nucleus projects, via at least one interneuron, to the facial nucleus (Ongerboer de Visser, 1983a, b; Inagaki, Takeshita, Nakao, Shiraishi, & Oikawa, 1989). The poly-synaptic R2 pathway diverges from the R1 path as the trigeminal nerve enters the brain stem, and follows the spinal trigeminal tract in the brain stem to the spinal trigeminal nucleus. Further connections to the lateral reticular formation may provide the link to the facial nucleus (Ongerboer de Visser & Kuypers, 1978; Cruccu, Ferracuti, Leardi, Fabbri, & Manfredi, 1991).

Two components have also been described for the *visual* blink reflex to a light flash (Fig. 2.1). The initial component, with a latency of about 50–70 msec, is thought to be mediated subcortically (Tavy, van Woerkom, Bots, & Endtz, 1984). The afferent pathway begins at the optic nerve and, according to some accounts, involves a sequence of connections to the pretectal area in the midbrain and then to the facial nucleus (Itoh, Takada, Yasui, & Mizuno, 1983; Holstege et al., 1986).

A different type of blink response to visual "threat" has also been described (see Balaban, 1986, or Hackley & Boelhouwer, 1997, for further description). This response is cortically mediated and occurs, for example, to looming stimuli that approach the face.

3. Eliciting Startle

The startle response could probably be elicited from any sensory system given sufficient control over stimulus parameters. In practice, however, the critical conditions for eliciting startle are not easily produced in olfactory or gustatory stimuli. Vestibular manipulations that might produce startle would also likely result in large corrective motor responses that would not be easily separated from startle responding. Thus, the startle literature is nearly exclusively related to stimulation in auditory, cutaneous, and visual modalities. The following sections outline the critical stimulus parameters for startle in each of these sensory systems.

3.1. Eliciting Stimulus Characteristics: General Issues

There are common parameters critical to eliciting startle, regardless of modality stimulated. Foremost among these are rise time (the rapidity with which a stimulus reaches maximum intensity), intensity, and duration. These qualities are considered along with the description of parameters specific to each stimulus modality. These parameters strongly interact to dictate the threshold conditions and the amplitudes of suprathreshold responses. Many details of these interactions have not been fully explored parametrically, but the results described in the following sections demonstrate the potency of such interactions.

3.2. Auditory Startle

In humans, at least four qualities of auditory stimuli can have pronounced effects on either the threshold for startle or the amplitude of suprathreshold responding: rise time, intensity, duration, and bandwidth. In general, startle is enhanced (lower thresholds or larger responses) when the rise time is faster, the intensity is higher, the duration is longer, and the bandwidth is wider (e.g., white noise). There are, however, many limitations to these generalizations and considerable interaction among these parameters.

Rise time, for example, has clear effects at lower stimulus intensities (Blumenthal, 1988) or when assessing startle threshold (K. M. Berg, 1973). However, at higher intensities it may still affect response probability but not response amplitude (Blumenthal & Berg, 1986a). Stimulus duration effects on startle are limited to about the first 10–50 msec, with the limit depending on bandwidth and response measure. Part of this limitation is due to the fact that the onset latency of the response is about 30–50 msec (based on EMG), depending on the stimulus and response measure. Logically, durations that exceed the response latency (or at least the peak of the response) cannot influence that response. However, Fleshler (1965) argued that, for rats, the critical factor in eliciting startle was the peak intensity reached within the first 10–12 msec of stimulation. In humans, K. M. Berg (1973) found evidence for a similar critical interval of 10–12 msec in some conditions, but it was the amount of energy integrated over that period that was crucial, not the peak intensity. This energy integration view was also espoused by Marsh, Hoffman, and Stitt (1973) for rat startle. The extent of temporal integration appears to be different at startle threshold and at suprathreshold intensities (K. M. Berg, 1973), leading Blumenthal and Berg (1986b) to suggest two factors in startle elaboration, a "trigger" and an "amplifier."

The effect of bandwidth on startle has been evaluated by comparing the extremes of this dimension: the single frequency tone versus the wideband white noise. The effects of this factor strongly interact with duration and, possibly, with intensity. When testing startle threshold, short duration tones (under about 16 msec) are more effective than white noise, but tone and white noise are equally effective at longer (32 msec) durations (K. M. Berg, 1973). At suprathreshold levels, the interactive crossover appears complete, with noise consistently outperforming tone for both amplitude and probability (Blumenthal & Berg, 1986a). This latter difference can be quite pronounced, with response amplitudes as much as 2.5 times larger for noise, and probability increased by 50 percent (Blumenthal and Berg, 1986a). Thus, except with short duration, low intensity stimulation, the wide bandwidth noise is more effective than the narrow bandwidth tone.

Although the effect of stimulus intensity on startle is generally straightforward, there is some disagreement about the absolute threshold for response elicitation under optimal conditions (e.g., fast rise time, long duration, wide bandwidth). K. M. Berg (1973) provided probably the most complete evaluation of thresholds, finding that with fast rise time noise of 50 msec, thresholds using a sensitive "up-and-down" method were about 84–87 dB(A) in adults. These data were obtained by recording the actual movement of the eyelid using the potentiometric method (see Section 4.2).

More recently, Blumenthal and Goode (1991) have reported startle blinks at intensity levels as low as 50 or 60 dB(A) when recording orbicularis oculi EMG activity. These data need to be viewed cautiously, however. Responding was down to about 20 percent probability for tones at 50 or 60 dB(A), and at about 45 to 50 percent for noise at these intensities, and the study did not statistically compare these with the false alarm rates.

An additional problem arises from the use of fast rise times. The rapid voltage change produced by abrupt stimulus onsets will commonly exceed the ability of the speaker or earphone to accurately reproduce them. At onset, a brief transient is created during which the frequency spectrum is distorted and the intensity exceeds that of the remaining steady portion of the signal (Fig. 2.2). Blumenthal and Goode (1991) reported the increased onset intensity to be only 3 dB higher for tone stimuli, but transients can be more exaggerated with noise stimuli, because moment-to-moment signal amplitude varies considerably. As a result, stimulus onset can occur at one of the randomly higher peaks in the noise signal, further exaggerating the transient distortions (Fig. 2.2). Thus, intensity measurements that average over several seconds of signal (the typical sound measurement procedure) may significantly underestimate the momentary onset intensity. The measurements of such transients requires a sound level meter with a peak intensity memory function.

3.3. Cutaneous Startle

Methods of evoking cutaneous startle have been quite varied, including air-puff, electrical stimulation of the supraorbital trigeminal nerve, and taps on the face near the glabella (the flattened area between the eyebrows). These methods involve different procedures for producing and controlling the stimulus and different problems in assessing factors such as intensity, rise time and duration, and, also, each generates different practical concerns.

3.3.1. Air-Puff Elicitation of Startle

Elicitation of a reflex blink to a puff of air to the face near the eye has long been a tool in psychology; however, the literature on the basic stimulus characteristics controlling the response is quite limited.

The source of the "air" to generate the air puff is generally a tank of compressed air or some other gas. A small electrical air compressor can provide a source of compressed air, or one can purchase tanks of highly compressed gas from medical supply companies (for oxygen, for example) or dive shops (for air).

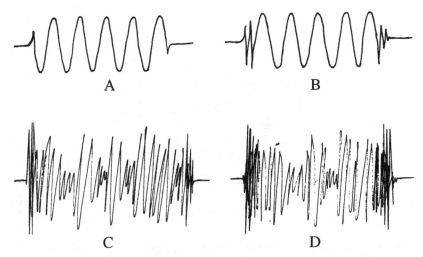

Figure 2.2. Diagram of the effect of abrupt rise time at stimulus onset and abrupt fall time at stimulus offset on acoustic tone (*A, B*) and noise (*C, D*) stimuli. Note that the effects produced by the oscillator (*A*) and noise generator (*C*) may be more pronounced at the output of the speaker (or earphone) (*B, D*).

When compressed gas is utilized, at least two critical devices must be employed for puffing near the eye (Fig. 2.3). The first is a pressure reduction valve that steps down the pressure levels, which might be several thousand pounds per square inch, to pressures safe and effective to use, commonly 0.5–5 pounds per square inch. When the tank of gas is highly compressed, it is advisable to use a two-stage pressure reduction valve. Attached to the final stage is an adjustment valve and gauge that allow fine variations in the final pressure. The second device needed is a solenoid-operated valve to release the gas by remote switch (e.g., from a computer-operated relay). The solenoid can create two kinds of noise problems: acoustic and electrical. Acoustic noise can be a problem when one wishes to avoid any auditory contamination in startle elicitation, such as in modality-specific selective attention studies. This can be solved by surrounding the solenoid with foam and placing it inside a concrete block. This, together with some ear protectors for the subject, can usually reduce the sound below a level likely to elicit acoustic startle. Electrical noise can be more difficult to eliminate. Solenoids inherently produce a large electrical artifact when they are operated, and can disrupt the blink EMG or other psychophysiological recording. Electrically shielding the subject and/or the solenoid may be necessary. It is advisable to use as small a solenoid as is practical, and locate it as far from the subject as possible.

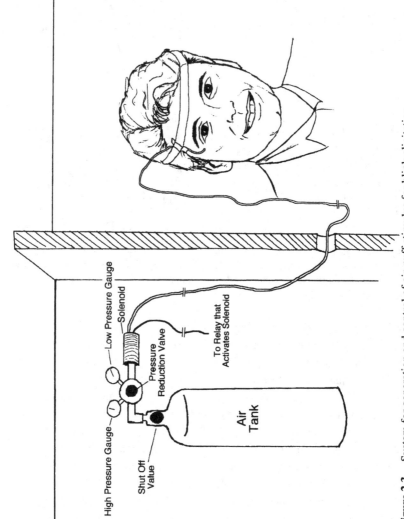

Figure 2.3. System for generation and control of air-puff stimulus for blink elicitation.

Regardless of the source of the air or gas, the final channel to bring the air to the participant is a tube, usually one made of flexible plastic. The diameter, length, and elasticity of the tube, and the tube orifice and its distance from the skin, will all substantially influence the tactile quality of the stimulation.

The tube length contributes to a puff delay of approximately 1 msec per foot. In addition, there can be a substantial delay (e.g., 20–25 msec) from the time the electrical signal is sent to the solenoid until that valve opens. For these reasons, the delay from the signaled onset of the puff to the actual arrival of a puff must be determined for individual systems, and this delay needs to be accounted for when scoring responses.

The tube orifice also will affect the amount of acoustic artifact, that is, the noise created when the puff is produced. If using ear protectors is insufficient to reduce the puff noise, another solution may be to mask the noise with continuous background sound. Shortley and Berg (1996) found that most of the acoustic artifact in the puff was in the lower frequencies, below about 600 Hz for their apparatus. By using a low frequency masking stimulus and acoustically isolating earphones, they were able to present puffs uncontaminated by audible acoustic artifact, and intermix these with acoustic probe stimuli at frequencies above the masking stimulus.

Finally, the distance from the tube orifice to the face may influence the response. As this distance increases, the area stimulated will likely increase, and the pressure per unit area decrease. In practice, a distance of about 1 cm directed 1 cm lateral to the outer canthus of the eye generally produces a reasonable response at under 1 lb/sq. in. for adults.

3.3.2. Electrical Elicitation of Startle

In the medical literature, the most popular method of eliciting startle cutaneously is with electrical stimulation of skin overlaying the supraorbital portion of the ophthalmic branch of the trigeminal nerve. This portion of the nerve emerges from the skull at the supraorbital foramen and travels upward under the skin, spreading across the forehead. Stimulation electrodes are attached to the skin surface over the nerve, one near the supraorbital foramen, which can be palpated as a small indentation in the ridge above each eye socket, and the second about 1 cm above this. However, Shahani and Young (1972, 1973) report the response can be electrically elicited from many facial areas. Few careful parametric studies exist, but our survey of studies published since 1972 indicates stimulus durations have ranged from 0.1–1 msec. With respect to intensity, many studies fail to report mean or range of threshold values, but Plant and Hammond (1989) indicated that the constant current needed to elicit three consecutive blinks, with a 0.5 msec biphasic stimulus, ranged from 1.5 to 5.2 mA, with a mean of 3.6 mA. According to Penders and Delwaide (1973), response amplitudes increased as current increased from about 3 to 6 mA, asymptoting thereafter. The use of constant current stimulators is preferred over the simpler constant voltage stimulator because current level is the more critical parameter for stimulating nerves (Brown, Maxfield, & Moraff, 1973).

3.3.3. Elicitation of Startle with Tap to Glabella

Elicitation of the blink reflex with a tap to the forehead is often referred to as the glabella reflex. However, it can be elicited from a variety of other regions of the forehead. Kugelberg (1952) proposed that the response resulted from stimulation of stretch receptors in the facial muscles, but Shahani and Young (1973) elicited responses in monkeys from a flap of skin surgically separated from the underlying muscles, thus providing convincing evidence that the response truly originates in the skin. In fact, this response appears to be closely related to the electrically elicited response, with both producing both an early EMG component (R1) and a later component (R2) associated with the visible blink. Latencies of each component are approximately the same for the two methods of elicitation, suggesting that both result from stimulation of the same orbicular branch of the trigeminal nerve (but see Snow & Frith, 1989, for possible differences in muscle involvement following tap vs. electrical stimulation).

The method of delivering taps has varied widely across studies, from handheld rods (Kugelberg, 1952) to taps with a phonograph cartridge (Shahani & Young, 1972) to a solenoid-driven tapper devised by Hoffman and colleagues (Marsh, Hoffman, & Stitt, 1979). The latter device was perhaps the best controlled because intensity could be determined by the voltage delivered to the solenoid. We are aware of no parametric studies of intensity or threshold employing the glabella reflex, and by the nature of the stimulus, studies of duration are not feasible.

3.3.4. Comparisons among Methods of Eliciting Cutaneous Startle

The investigator who wishes to employ cutaneously elicited startle is faced with decisions about the optimal stimulus for eliciting the response: air puff, electrical, or glabella tap. That decision will be determined by several factors that can differ across experiments. We offer no specific recommendation, but rather some factors that may help investigators make that choice for any given study.

In terms of control over stimulus parameters, the stimuli can be ordered from most to least readily controlled: electrical, air-puff, and tap. For both electrical and air-puff stimulation, duration and intensity are readily controlled, and for electrical stimulation rise time could be controlled with appropriate instrumentation. Intensity, but not duration, can be controlled for tap. It is unclear whether rise time could be manipulated without also changing intensity.

In terms of reliability of elicitation, all three work well, but electrical stimulation has a slight edge because it directly stimulates the nerve. One of us (W.K.B.) has found it difficult to get consistent air-puff intensity across trials, possibly because of small variations in solenoid openings. No information is available on the consistency of response amplitude with tapping devices, but it is unlikely to be as consistent as an electrical stimulus. Both air-puffers and tappers involve delays from the time the devices are activated until they actually stimulate the skin; these delays must be accounted for and could add to response variability.

With regard to the ease of producing the stimulus, electrical stimulation probably wins again because constant current stimulators are readily available from vendors. Air-puff is probably next in line because components for stimulus control and sources of pressurized air are readily available, although they require assembly by the investigator. The best tappers for eliciting the glabella reflex are handmade. Marsh and colleagues (1979) have provided details for this, and the cost is minimal, but some mechanical skill is required, and calibration is necessary.

It is probably only with electrical stimulation that contamination from acoustic events is avoided completely. Acoustic artifacts are produced by air-puff devices, and tapping devices could also produce acoustic components because vibration of the skull could stimulate the cochlea via bone conduction.

From this analysis, it would seem that electrical stimulation is the optimal choice for eliciting cutaneous startle. Indeed, surveys of the extant literature on the blink reflex, particularly the neurologically oriented literature, show the electrical stimulus to be the favorite. However, within the realm of psychological research, it has an obvious drawback: Subjects are typically very concerned about electrical stimulation. Use of electrical stimulation at near-blink elicitation threshold levels normally does not produce pain, just a "tingling" sensation of the skin. But even this can cause many subjects concern, assuming they agree to participate in the study in the first place. When it comes to perceived risk to the subject, electrical stimulation is clearly in last place. Air puffs can also cause some subjects concern because the puff is presented near the eye (Haerich, 1994). Subjects may find the glabellar tap to be most tolerable of these stimuli.

3.3.5. Is There a True Cutaneous Startle?

One final question that arises in reviewing the literature on cutaneously elicited blink responses is whether these qualify as startle responses. The medically oriented literature on these responses typically does not make reference to startle. Rather, the response is identified as a blink reflex or blink response, and often put in the same class as reflexive blinks elicited by touches to the cornea. The common element of the modes of cutaneous blink elicitation described above is that some portion of the trigeminal nerve is stimulated to produce the response. Determining whether cutaneously elicited blinks are part of a startle reflex may be important because much of the literature on blink modification involves using a loud acoustic stimulus, which almost certainly does involve startle. Studies comparing acoustically and cutaneously elicited blink responses, such as studies of selective attention, may be problematic if both the sensory system and the response type differ. Further, Bonnet, Bradley, Lang, and Requin (1995) reported that, unlike the startle response, a nondefensive reflex (the spinal tendinous reflex) is not modified by affective responses.

One desirable approach to assessing whether cutaneously elicited blinks qualify as startle responses is to determine whether the parameters of stimulation critical for eliciting acoustic startle are also found for cutaneously elicited startle. There has been scant comparative work, and none with such critical factors as stimulus rise time. Thus, it is unclear whether cutaneously elicited blinks are startle responses or whether they should be classified separately.

3.4. Visual Startle

Although abrupt light flashes can elicit the startle response, there is disagreement as to how readily this stimulus produces the response compared with auditory stimuli. Hackley and Johnson (1996, p. 243 n. 2) report that photically elicited blinks ". . . are usually quite small (e.g., 2–20 microvolts compared with 50–200 microvolts for acoustic blinks)." Conclusions of early studies (Landis & Hunt, 1939; Yates & Brown, 1981) were based on cross-modal comparisons where the stimuli were not matched psychophysically.

In contrast with auditory startle, little is known about the critical stimulus parameters that control visual startle. We know of only two parametric studies. Hopf, Bier, Breurer, and Scheerer (1973) examined the effect of several parameters of light on threshold blink responses. Using white light, they reported marked effects of both duration and exposure area: Responding reached asymptote at durations of about 16 msec, and visual angles of about 14 degrees. These factors interacted such that the effects of each could be seen only when the other factor was well below asymptotic level. The marked effect of visual angle could account for much of the disagreement between laboratories on subjects' startle sensitivity to light, because the visual angle is rarely reported.

Hopf and colleagues (1973) also found a marked effect of light wavelength by using colored filters centered at 463, 522, 580, and 655 nm. The lowest threshold was at 580 and the highest at 655 nm. Wide-band (white) light produced a threshold close to that of the most sensitive colored light. These authors reported that reflex latencies generally corresponded to threshold levels, with conditions producing higher thresholds resulting in longer latencies. However, the latency values are somewhat suspect since they are very long, between 100 and 120 msec, compared with latencies on the order of 50 msec reported elsewhere (Yates & Brown, 1981). Hopf and colleagues (1973) concluded that the blink response to light is mediated by both scotopic and photopic visual systems.

Yates and Brown (1981) examined the effects of light intensity on suprathreshold responding by comparing effects of the different intensity settings of a Grass PS22 photic stimulator. These uncalibrated light levels produced asymptotic responding at the midpoint stimulator setting of 8. Blink latencies decreased over the entire range of settings, from about 55 to 45 msec.

4. Recording Startle Blink Responses

Once investigators are able to elicit a blink response, they are faced with the problem of recording the response accurately. Many different procedures have been employed: photographic, direct lid movement, optic indicators, and assessing muscle electrical activity (EMG). Because most investigators now record blink EMG, we emphasize this method here. However, in Section 4.2, we describe some of these other measures.

4.1. EMG Measures

The orbicularis oculi muscle has orbital and palpebral portions (Fig. 2.1). The reflex blink can be recorded from electrodes located over either portion. Maximum sensitivity is obtained from recordings from the palpebral portion (Silverstein & Graham, 1978); however, recording is easier to measure over the orbital area.

4.1.1. Electrodes, Placement, and Skin Preparation

Two types of electrodes have been employed to record EMG activity: needle electrodes and skin surface electrodes. In medical settings, needle electrodes placed directly into the muscle are generally preferred because they avoid potential contaminants of skin surface recordings. For obvious reasons, psychologically oriented studies generally do not find this approach useful, and instead utilize electrodes placed on the skin surface directly over the muscle. Fridlund and Cacioppo (1986) reviewed EMG recording techniques; we focus here on factors specific to blink recording.

With a circular muscle such as orbicularis oculi, one could presumably record from any portion of the muscle circumference. Typically, however, one electrode is placed at or just below the margin of the bony orbit, centered under the eye, and a second electrode about 1 cm lateral to this (Fig. 2.1). This puts the electrodes over the orbital portion of orbicularis oculi, but still close to the more sensitive palpebral portion. Which eye is selected is a matter of convenience and preference, but should be consistent within a study and should be reported. Maintaining a constant interelectrode distance among subjects may be important because van Boxtel, Goudswaard, and Schomaker (1984) reported that variations in this distance can affect EMG levels when recording from frontalis muscles.

The preparation of skin sites near the eyes and the procedures for attachment of electrodes will differ somewhat from most other skin areas. As with all EMG recording, cleansing of the skin is advisable, but care must be taken with substances that can irritate the eye, such as isopropyl alcohol. Once cleansed, it is highly desirable to gently abrade the skin sites with a substance such as Omniprep (D.O. Weaver and Co.). Because this skin area is sensitive, little abrasion is needed. Abrasion lowers the skin resistance substantially, greatly reducing recording noise (see following sections).

As with most psychophysiological recordings, the optimal skin surface electrodes are silver/silver chloride cup electrodes. Because the orbicularis oculi muscle is small, use of smaller (e.g., 5 mm) electrodes is advisable, such as those made by Sensor Medics. These electrodes, filled with standard recording paste, can be attached just below the orbital ridge.

Silverstein and Graham (1978) designed a much smaller electrode and an application procedure that allows one to record from the upper eyelid, directly over the more sensitive palpebral portion of the muscle. Because this technique requires investigators to fabricate their own electrodes, it has not been used extensively. However, in studies where threshold levels of startle are of central interest, this procedure may be useful.

Skin resistance should be assessed with an impedance meter (e.g., Grass

Instruments) and efforts made to reduce resistance to 2000 ohms or less. With appropriate skin preparation, this is readily possible with most adult subjects.

4.1.2. Filtering EMG

The intent of filtering a signal is to eliminate all electrical potentials not of interest (the biological and 60-Hz "noise") and retain the unaltered electrical potential of interest (the "signal"), in this case the signal emanating from the orbicularis oculi. Filtering can accomplish this when the frequencies of the noise sources differ from the frequencies of the signal.

Thus, to filter appropriately it is critical to know the frequencies of both the contaminants and signal of interest. EMG frequencies span a wide spectral range. Van Boxtel, Boelhouwer, and Bos (1996) report that recordings of orbicularis oculi with skin surface electrodes span a range from about 28 to 512 Hz, with peak power at a frequency of about 78–100 Hz. If a 60-Hz "notch" filter is available, it may be used where line noise is a problem, but with good electrode application and shielding, this problem may be minimal. When it is not minimal, as is often the case, a more restricted frequency range may be considered.

Many blink studies have employed a range of 90–250 Hz as their lower and upper cutoff frequencies. These particular values come about because they are settings on a popular biological amplifier (Coulbourn Inc.). Filtering signals below 90 Hz substantially reduces the 60-Hz noise and probably reduces cross-talk from other muscle sites (Fridlund & Cacioppo, 1986); the 250-Hz upper cutoff allows the investigator to sample a signal at a slower rate without aliasing (see below). But at what loss? Dropping most of the activity below 90 Hz will reduce the signal available by about 50%. The amount of the signal above 250 Hz, however, is minimal because the signal drops off exponentially above its peak, with probably less than 5% above 250 Hz (see Fig. 3 in van Boxtel et al., 1996). Use of a higher cutoff has an important benefit when eliciting startle visually because it eliminates all or most of the serious contamination from the electroretinogram (Hackley & Johnson, 1996). Certainly, when startle is not elicited visually and noise can be eliminated at its source, the optimal choice is to include the entire EMG spectrum.

4.1.3. "Smoothing" the Signal: Rectification and Integration

Most commonly, the amplified and filtered EMG signal is not scored directly because it has numerous negative and positive peaks occurring within short intervals. Typically this raw signal is processed in two stages to make it more amenable to scoring. The first stage is to rectify the signal, which involves taking any part of the signal that falls below zero (or below the ongoing baseline), inverting it, and combining it with the positive portion of the signal (see Fig. 2.4). Once this is done, the resulting signal is then "smoothed" or "integrated" by passing the rectified signal through a low-pass filter. The intent is to produce a signal that approximately follows the outline of the rectified signal, although in reality this approximation is crude at best. How smooth the final signal becomes and how closely it follows the outline of the rectified signal depends on the signal itself and on the setting of the low-pass filter, which is ordinarily specified as a time constant. Shorter time constants indicate less filtering and result in less smoothing but a closer approximation to an abruptly changing rectified signal (Fig. 2.4). However, the less smooth the signal is, the more difficult it may become to specify the peak of the blink because, as with the raw signal, several peaks may occur. Longer time constants result in greater smoothing but also greater overall reduction in the signal (Fig. 2.4), which can become substantial (Blumenthal, 1994). Additionally, with a longer time constant the peak of the processed signal can be significantly delayed compared with the original signal. Signals processed with longer time constants do not have delayed blink onset, but onsets appear more gradual and that may make it difficult to detect a precise onset latency. The majority of studies of startle in the psychological literature have employed time constants of about 100 msec, but some have used much shorter ones (e.g., Ornitz, Guthrie, Lane, & Sugiyama, 1990). One alternative is to send the raw signal through two processing channels, one with a very short time constant used to detect smaller responses and score onset latency, and one with a longer time constant to score peak amplitudes.

4.1.4. Computer versus Hardware Rectifying and Smoothing

Rectifying and low-pass filtering can be done by either hardware or software. Most commonly both are handled by a single piece of hardware, such as Coulbourn's "contour-following integrator." These devices make it quite simple for the investigator, but have the disadvantage that once the time constant is selected and the subject tested, it cannot be changed. Also, the specified settings on the units may differ substantially from the actual values. The true time constant should be independently established by putting a long duration square wave signal into the unit, and determining the time it takes the output signal to reach 63.2 percent of its asymptotic amplitude.

The alternative to this approach is to digitally sample the raw EMG signal on-line and subsequently utilize software to rectify and smooth with a digital low-pass filter (Cook & Miller, 1992). The major advantage of this approach is its flexibility. One can easily select different time constants for different scoring purposes, or compare the data with other studies using different time

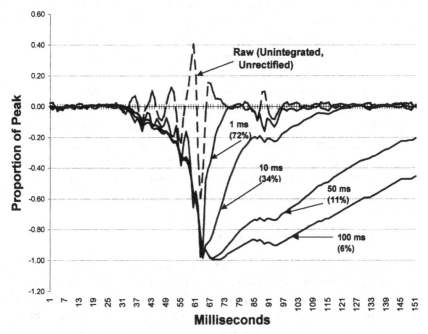

Figure 2.4. Depiction of EMG recordings in raw, rectified only, and rectified and smoothed form (short vs. long time constants)

constants. Additionally, one has the potential of detecting the small R1 response present in the raw EMG signal, but easily lost in the processed signal. The disadvantage is that raw EMG data must be sampled at a much faster rate than integrated and smoothed data, and this method involves storing data in several different formats.

4.1.5. Computer Sampling of Data

Two major questions face the investigator when dealing with computer sampling: how fast and when to sample the data. The speed of sampling is dictated in part by the frequencies that are in the signal. To avoid aliasing, a situation in which the sampling process creates activity at a different frequency from what was in the original signal, the sampling rate must be at least twice the fastest frequency in the signal being sampled, the Nyquist rate. As discussed earlier, the fastest rate in the signal will depend largely on the filtering of the original EMG. But with the upper limit of EMG at about 500 Hz, the fastest sampling rate for raw EMG should be at least 1000 Hz. When rectification and smoothing is done by hardware prior to computer sampling, sampling rates can be considerably lower. How low will depend on the time constant of the low-pass smoothing filter. This time constant can be converted into a frequency value by the formula $F_c = 1/(2 \cdot \pi \cdot t_c)$, where F_c is the cut-off frequency and t_c is the time constant in seconds. However, to attain adequate resolution of response latency, sampling rates should probably never drop below 100 Hz, and a higher rate is preferable.

The question of when to sample and for how long is somewhat simpler. It is desirable to begin sampling prior to startle stimulus onset, perhaps by as much as 0.5–1 s. This extended prestimulus recording allows one to assess the possibility of prestartle movements and blinks, and to assess the prestimulus tonic contraction of the orbicularis oculi, which might influence startle magnitude (Bradley, Cuthbert, & Lang, 1990). Following startle stimulus onset, sampling should continue for at least 250 msec with adults.

4.2. Other Measures of Startle Blink

Although recording of the electrical activity of the orbicularis oculi muscle is undoubtedly the most popular measure of the startle blink response, other effective measures have been employed. A photoelectric measure, developed principally by Hoffman (Marsh et al., 1979; Marsh & Hoffman, 1981), involves directing a tiny infrared light-emitting diode toward the eye, and detecting the light reflected from the lid by an infrared sensitive phototransistor. In another measure, one can record the movement of the eyelid electrophysiologically (as opposed to the muscles related to eyelid movement) using electrodes placed above and below the eye and amplifiers adjusted to allow slow changes in potential (Clarkson & Berg, 1984). This is the same placement that is used to record vertical eye movement (electrooculography) and these two signals are difficult to distinguish unless the participant can minimize eye movements. An associated problem is that the amplitude of the electrical signal is decreased when subjects fixate at a lower position and increased when they fixate at a higher position. A third method is to record lid movement directly by attaching one end of a small string to the margin of upper lid, and the other end to a micropotentiometer positioned just above the eye. This direct potentiometric recording of measuring blink responses was utilized extensively in the literature on eyelid conditioning (e.g., Ross & Nelson, 1973; Kadlac & Grant, 1977).

The various procedures for assessing blink responses can be grouped into two categories: Those that attempt to track the actual lid closure itself (potentiometric, electrooculographic, and the original high-speed photography of Landis and Hunt), and those that record activity more closely related with the intensity of signal sent to the muscle, regardless of how much actual lid closure occurs (orbicularis oculi EMG and photoelectric). The choice of measurement might depend in part on which type of response is of principal interest. It might seem that measurement of lid closure itself would be preferable because the response is identified as a "blink," implying actual lid movement. However, lid movement is altered by a range of mechanical alterations, such as when the fixation point moves vertically, and also may differ among racial groups whose eyelid structure and attachment differ. In addition, restricting responding to actual lid movement will make it difficult to include assessing startle responses during sleep states. Thus, despite the nomenclature of the startle "blink," the measures that may be more simply related to brain control mechanisms would be those affecting the musculature. For this reason, the EMG measure is, under most circumstances, the best choice for recording. How good an alternative the photoelectric measurement is to this cannot be determined easily until it is directly compared with EMG in a variety of circumstances.

5. Quantifying Startle

There are several general issues related to quantification and analysis of the blink reflex. Computerized scoring is essential. Some researchers use commercial systems that include scoring algorithms, whereas others develop their own scoring systems.

What characteristics of the response waveform should be scored? Although typically the measures of interest are those that describe reflex size and speed, researchers have investigated various other parameters. Also, there are concerns about discriminating signal from noise in scoring responses. Other scoring issues include how to quantify aspects of reflex modification and how to measure, or control for, between-subject differences in startle reactivity.

In the following sections, we address questions regarding quantification; however, it is important to note that in many cases there are insufficient data to recommend one scoring method over another. In addition, we do not attempt to catalog all the different scoring techniques currently in use. Instead, we describe some attributes that are important in devising an approach to scoring response characteristics. We emphasize scoring of blinks from integrated EMG recordings; other recording methods may require different scoring approaches.

5.1. Computer Scoring Methods

The typical approach is to acquire and store the physiological recordings of the blink reflex on-line during an experiment, and later analyze those responses off-line. Frances Graham and her students developed one such computer-based scoring system that was later translated into a format more accessible to other laboratories (Balaban, Losito, Simons, & Graham, 1986a, b). This program emphasized *computer-automated* scoring. That is, the investigator played a limited role in checking or overriding the computer-derived scores. Certain program parameters were adjusted depending upon the probe stimulus modality, type of recording (e.g., EMG vs. potentiometric), and age of subjects (infants vs. adults).

Other researchers have developed different algorithms to score blink reflexes. Some emphasize *computer-assisted* scoring. In some cases, this entails plotting each trial on the computer screen so that the investigator can position cursors to score various parameters, such as the response peak. In other cases, the computer may score all the trials, but investigators can inspect the computer scores and overrule and replace the scores on individual trials. The scorer should be naive to the test conditions to avoid scoring bias. In one study, Jennings, Schell, Filion, and Dawson (1996) reported interrater reliabilities of .80–.99 by comparing three different scorers.

Regardless of whether a computer-automated or -assisted method is used, one recommended strategy is to include no-stimulus "catch" trials to assess the likelihood of scoring a response when no stimulus occurred. This procedure is useful even with pronounced blinks to suprathreshold stimuli, but it is particularly recommended when blink responses are small and/or there are high levels of noise or background EMG activity.

There are also commercial systems that are equipped with capabilities to elicit, record, and quantify blink reflexes. Two such systems include both hardware and software: the Startle Response System (San Diego Instruments) and the Startle Response Analysis System (James Long Company). When considering a commercial system, request detailed descriptions from the company and investigate the merits and drawbacks of particular systems from researchers who use them.

For new investigators, the choice of what computer scoring system to use will depend on various factors, including cost, available recording and computer equipment, whether other psychophysiological measures are to be recorded, and programming expertise.

5.2. Scoring Parameters

Most studies emphasize measures of reflex size and speed; therefore, we focus on the scoring of reflex amplitude/magnitude and reflex latency. Other parameters such as area, duration, and response probability are described briefly.

5.2.1. Response Window

Because the blink reflex occurs in a background of activity that may include spontaneous blinking, eye movements, and so on, it is important to define the time window during which a response will be considered a reflex response. An onset window describes the time during which a response onset will be considered a reflex blink, and a peak response window describes the time during which the peak of the reflex blink must occur (Fig. 2.5).

Selection of these temporal parameters may vary depending upon aspects of a particular experiment, such as subject age or probe stimulus intensity or modality. For example, Anthony, Zeigler, and Graham (1987) summarized results for onset latency in acoustic and visual modalities across studies of infants and adults in several laboratories (see Anthony et al., Fig. 1). With adult EMG recording, the recommended windows for scoring onset latency were 21–120 msec for acoustic blinks and 21–145 msec for visual blinks, and the recommended peak response windows were 21–150 msec for acoustic and 21–200 msec for visual blinks (Balaban et al., 1986b). If the selected parameters define a short onset window, there is a risk of not scoring longer-latency blinks. A long window increases the likelihood of scoring spontaneous or voluntary blinks.

5.2.2. Baseline

To detect a response and define its size, an initial baseline level is typically defined. There have been numerous definitions of such a baseline, including (1) the level of prestimulus activity present during a window just prior to the probe stimulus onset, (2) the first 20 msec following probe onset, because blink reflexes (with the exception of the R1 cutaneous reflex) typically do not occur at such short latencies, or (3) the first n samples prior to the detected onset of the response.

The baseline is important for several reasons. Response size is often defined as the difference between amplitudes at baseline and at the response peak. In some methods, the baseline may be used to detect the onset of a response (see following section). In addition, measures of average baseline activity have been used to give a rough estimate of prestimulus contraction of orbicularis oculi (e.g., Bradley, Cuthbert, & Lang, 1990).

5.2.3. Response Detection

To score responses, it is necessary to determine whether a response occurred on any given trial. For response detection, scoring algorithms may use threshold parameters such as a change in slope or an increment in amplitude rela-

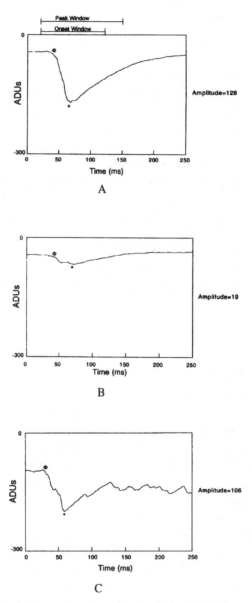

Figure 2.5. Examples of the scoring of acoustically elicited blinks from the integrated EMG of one subject, showing the approximate points where onset latency (designated by Φ) and peak latency (designated by *) were computer-scored, and indicating blink amplitude in analog-to-digital units. Stimulus onset occurred at time 0. (*A*) Large blink; (*B*) small blink; (*C*) blink occurring during period of active background muscle activity; (*D*) potential small blink that did not meet the program's amplitude criterion; (*E*) trial not scored due to baseline shift prior to blink and in prestimulus period (not shown).

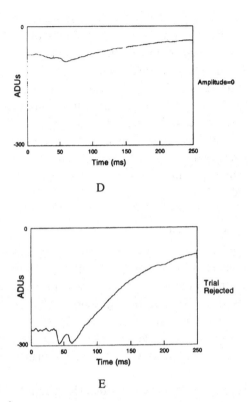

Figure 2.5. (*cont.*)

tive to the baseline (Fig. 2.5). With a slope criterion, thresholds will vary as a function of recording time constants. With measures of change from baseline (e.g., Balaban et al., 1986a, b), the sensitivity of the analog-to-digital converter may influence the threshold criterion used; ideally, it would be defined in real units (e.g., microvolts). Other algorithms for response detection use a statistical criterion, such as the point at which the activity exceeds a criterion standard deviation (Ornitz, Russell, Yuan, & Liu, 1996).

The goals are to correctly identify true reflex blinks and omit scoring other spurious deflections due to noise. This is an easy feat to accomplish, for example, when blink reflexes of normal adult subjects are elicited by suprathreshold stimuli in a paradigm that does not use inhibitory modification. In these circumstances, it is likely that the different methods of response detection, described in the preceding paragraph, would produce similar results.

However, when responses are small and/or baselines are noisy, response detection becomes more problematic. This may occur when responses are inhibited in reflex modification studies. In addition, difficulties in response detection may occur when comparing the responses between two groups of subjects that differ in signal-to-noise ratio.

If the minimum threshold for a response is too low, noise can be misidentified as a response. If the threshold is too high, trials with small responses can be scored as no-response trials. Methodological studies are needed on the effects of different response detection techniques under these conditions. As mentioned earlier, a good strategy is to check how many false-alarm responses would be scored during control trials, defined as recording intervals when no stimulus occurred.

5.2.4. Peak Amplitude/Magnitude

The description of the smoothed response over time includes a relatively rapid onset, attainment of a peak, and then return to a baseline level (Fig. 2.5). Some researchers simply define a peak response as the maximal voltage value during the response window; others may adopt a more complex definition, such as one that selects the first voltage peak after response onset, which is followed by some specified size decrement. A voltage peak here means that point at which successive changes in voltage shift from increasing to decreasing.

A recent report by Blumenthal (1995) found high correlations among measures of peak magnitude of the electrically elicited blink in (1) an integrated EMG signal, (2) a raw EMG signal, and (3) a measure of area under the integrated EMG curve. Thus, assessment of reflex size may be impervious to variations in response scoring, at least in the conditions tested in that study. Grillon and Davis (1995) also reported a high correlation between the peak magnitude scored from integrated blink reflexes and a measure of power in the EMG signal.

When reporting response amplitude, it is advisable to use real units of measurement for scoring reflex size, such as microvolts, rather than arbitrary units, such as analog-to-digital units. At the least, a conversion factor should be reported if analog-to-digital units are the selected measure. Voltage units allow more direct comparison across studies and laboratories (assuming recording parameters such as integrator time constants are reported).

Once the peak amplitudes are scored for all trials, mean response sizes have been described in two ways. If responses are averaged over all trials, including values of zero for trials without detectable responses, the mean is sometimes referred to as peak magnitude. However, if the responses are averaged for trials with nonzero responses only, the mean is sometimes referred to as peak amplitude. According to this distinction, magnitude, by definition, is influenced by both amplitude and response probability.

Blumenthal and Berg (1986b) suggested that blink amplitude and response probability are two attributes that may operate independently, at least in part (see also Humphreys, 1943; Prokasy & Kumpfer, 1973; Dawson, Schell, & Filion, 1990). There may be circumstances in which investigators choose to measure these separate attributes. However, the accuracy of probability measures is reduced when baseline noise is high or blink responses are small. With suprathreshold stimuli and consistent responding, probability is near ceiling and unlikely to provide useful information. The probability measure may be most useful when blinks are elicited near threshold, for example, in reflex modification by short lead interval stimulation. In general, we recommend that studies of blink reflexes or blink modification report blink magnitude, because this measure is commonly reported. Additional analysis of blink amplitude, or reporting the frequency of occurrence of zero-response trials, is also informative.

5.2.5. Response Latency

The relation between reflex size and speed is complex. Measurements of size and speed may be positively correlated in some circumstances; however, descriptions of the intrinsic blink reflex as well as reflex modification posit independent mechanisms that influence reflex size and speed (Graham & Murray, 1977).

Several aspects of response latency have been quantified. Latency is measured as the time between probe stimulus onset and the time of some measurable attribute of the response. Onset latency refers to the time at which the reflex response begins (Fig. 2.5). Peak latency is the time when the peak of the response was designated.

5.3. Other Scoring Issues: Multiple Responses and Excluding Trials

Occasionally, multiple peaks are evident within the integrated EMG blink response. The prevalence of this effect depends in part on the selected filtering parameters. Multiple peaks are more likely to occur with shorter time constants. Also, multiple peaks are more prevalent with cutaneous and with visual blinks, which have multiple components, than with auditory blinks. In these circumstances, the scoring system should include provisions for choosing which peak to score. These may include selecting the largest peak within the response window or selecting the peak with the latency closest to the mean peak latency for that experimental condition.

Another important aspect of response scoring is specifying the rationale for trial exclusion. For example, trials during which a voluntary or spontaneous blink occurred at or near the startle stimulus onset should be omitted from analysis, because the nonreflexive blink will interfere with accurate scoring of the reflex blink. In many circumstances, trials with excessive background noise should be eliminated. It is customary to report how many trials were excluded from analyses for these, or other, reasons. Across many studies from different laboratories, this number is typically low (e.g., 3%) for normal adults tested with suprathreshold stimuli.

In addition to trial exclusion, investigators may set criteria to exclude subjects from analysis. Subjects who habituate rapidly and stop responding and/or subjects with too few responses per experimental condition may be excluded from the main sample. As with any other measure of exclusion, it is advisable to consider whether the excluded subjects differ from the subjects included in analyses because such differences may limit the generalizability of results.

5.4. Quantifying Startle Modification

Studies of blink reflex modification compare, within subjects, conditions in which the startle response is modified, for example, by a lead stimulus or by task instructions, and a control condition in which the subject's blink reflex reactivity is measured. In some cases, unmodulated probe stimuli are also presented during the intertrial intervals, to allow scaling of responses between subjects.

Following Hoffman and Ison's (1980) observation that short lead interval stimulation subtracted a constant amount from small or large startle responses, some early studies reported blink reflex modification as difference scores from the control condition (e.g., Graham, 1975). Other investigators have used proportional measures. For example, Boelhouwer, Teurlings, and Brunia (1991) elicited blink reflexes during intertrial intervals and used the size of these responses as the control value. For each subject, the responses elicited during the reflex modification conditions were expressed as percentages of this control value. Recent reports demonstrated the advantage of this type of measure. Jennings et al. (1996) reported high correlations between absolute sizes of blink reflexes in a control condition and modified blinks and between the control condition; and modified blinks expressed as difference scores from the control condition; however, correlations were low between the control condition and percent change scores from the control condition. Thus, with percent change scores, the effects of reflex modification were less confounded by individual differences in response to the control startle stimulus (see also Schell, Dawson, Hazlett, & Filion, 1995).

Ison and Pinckney (1990) used a different type of relative response measure. For each subject, the sum of response means in all conditions was set to 100 and then the response for each condition expressed proportionately to that sum. The disadvantage of this approach, relative to a percentage change from control score, is that the magnitude in a given condition is not easily translated between experiments with different numbers of conditions.

5.5. Individual and Group Differences

When the comparisons of interest are among conditions in a within-subject design, individual variation in overall response amplitude may be relegated to noise. In some circumstances, however, methodological decisions arise concerning how to study, or how to correct for, individual and group differences. For example, individual differences in sensory and/or response thresholds might interact with the amount of reflex modification that a subject demonstrates. Or group differences in overall response level, for example, between female and male subjects, might cause difficulties in comparing the degree of reflex modification that each group evinces.

One way of correcting for individual and group differences is to scale the blink reflex responses. For example, Ornitz and colleagues (1996) noted that the amplitude of blink reflexes across subjects varied almost 30-fold in a sample of 7- to 11-year-old subjects. They used a log transformation of the blink amplitude scores to reduce this response range. Other researchers have scaled blink amplitudes within subjects when testing differences between conditions that were varied within subjects. For example, Cuthbert, Bradley, and Lang (1996) standardized blink magnitude scores for each subject. Typically, investigators report similar findings when such standardized measures are compared with untransformed measures of reflex size (e.g., Grillon & Davis, 1995; Bradley, Cuthbert, & Lang, 1996).

6. Conclusions

Given the current variation in recording equipment and computer-scoring techniques, standardization of startle blink methods across laboratories is unlikely. To foster comparison or results across laboratories, published descriptions of reflex blink studies should contain all relevant attributes of the stimulus, recording, and scoring characteristics. More detailed descriptions of scoring algorithms should be available to other researchers for comparison purposes.

   In this chapter, we delineated basic approaches to eliciting, recording, and scoring blink reflexes, and, in addition, we introduced some of the critical issues regarding blink circuitry and methodology that remain to be resolved. We hope that this information is useful as a guide to new investigators. In addition, we believe that the field of psychophysiological research on startle will benefit if some of the open questions regarding methodology are addressed empirically.

ACKNOWLEDGMENTS

Preparation of this chapter was supported in part by grants to W.K.B. from the National Institutes of Mental Health (NIMH) (5R01MH46568) and from the University of Florida Division of Sponsored Research and by NIMH grant R03MH51131 to M.T.B. We thank Tam Nguyen for assistance with figure preparation.

CHAPTER THREE

Short Lead Interval Startle Modification

TERRY D. BLUMENTHAL

ABSTRACT

This chapter deals with the modification of startle caused by a lead stimulus presented at a lead interval of less than 1 s. This modification of startle can be affected by a variety of parameters of the lead stimulus, such as duration, intensity, and lead interval. Startle modification at short lead intervals can also be affected by the intensity of the startle stimulus itself. The modification of startle decreases as a testing session progresses, and this is due either to habituation of the inhibitory mechanism or to a decrease in control startle reactivity. In some cases, lead stimuli can facilitate the startle response at short lead intervals, usually when the lead and startle stimuli are presented in different sensory systems. Short lead interval modification of startle may serve to protect the processing of the lead stimulus from interruption, but this reflex modification also illustrates automatic sensory gating and the influences of attentional mechanisms early in stimulus processing.

1. Introduction

The startle reflex can be elicited by sufficiently sudden and intense stimuli in several sensory modalities, and this reflex has been studied in a wide variety of animals, including humans, across the life span (see Chapter 2). Graham (1975) suggested that the modification of the startle reflex could be useful in identifying the neural mechanisms, at several levels of the central nervous system, that underlie a variety of information-processing functions (see Chapter 1). This chapter will focus on the effects of lead stimulus presentation or change on startle responding, when those lead stimuli are presented within a few hundred milliseconds of the startle stimulus. Unless otherwise stated, all findings described in this chapter are based on measures of the eyeblink component of the adult human startle response, specifically, the elec-

Michael E. Dawson, Anne M. Schell, and Andreas H. Böhmelt, Eds. *Startle modification: Implications for neuroscience, cognitive science, and clinical science.* Copyright © 1999 Cambridge University Press. Printed in the United States of America. All rights reserved.

51

tromyographic (EMG) activity of the orbicularis oculi muscle. This blink reflex is usually elicited with either a sudden acoustic stimulus or an electrical pulse to the forehead. This electrical stimulus activates an eyeblink reflex that usually has two reliable components, an ipsilateral R1 with a latency of approximately 15 msec, and a bilateral R2 with a latency of approximately 40 msec. This R2 component is believed to be analogous in many ways to the blink elicited by an acoustic startle stimulus (see Chapter 2).

Startle modification involves the presentation of trials in at least two stimulus conditions, one being a control condition in which a startle stimulus is presented alone, and the other being a lead stimulus condition in which a lead stimulus is presented shortly before the startle stimulus. The degree to which startle responding differs on control and lead stimulus trials is taken as the extent of modification of startle. This modification can be quantified as an amount of change caused by the lead stimulus (the difference between the control and lead stimulus conditions), as a proportional effect (finding the difference between control and lead stimulus conditions and then dividing this difference by the control value), or in a variety of other ways (see Chapter 2). Lead stimuli can be any change in the stimulus environment (onset, offset, or change in some parameter) that can either inhibit or facilitate startle reactivity, with the nature and timing of the lead stimulus affecting the degree and direction of startle modification.

Previous reviews (Graham, 1975, 1980; Hoffman & Ison, 1980; Anthony, 1985; Hackley & Boelhouwer, 1997) summarize studies that show that: (1) inhibition of startle is present on the first pairing of the lead stimulus and the startle stimulus, so the effect is not dependent upon conditioning (Graham, Putnam, & Leavitt, 1975); (2) this inhibition is not a function of sensory masking, refractoriness, or middle-ear protective muscle activity generated by the lead stimulus, since lead stimuli at very low intensities or in sensory modalities other than that of the startle stimulus can modify startle (Reiter & Ison, 1977; Ison, Reiter, & Warren, 1979; Blumenthal & Gescheider, 1987); (3) short lead interval modification is considered to be automatic, not under attentional control (Filion, Dawson, & Schell, 1993). In fact, this eyeblink modification has been demonstrated in subjects while they were asleep (Silverstein, Graham, & Calloway, 1980) or while the subject is reading a book or watching television (although the attentional factors involved might influence this modification; see Chapter 7). The size of this startle inhibition effect is impressive, in that the startle response to a very intense stimulus can, in some cases, be prevented altogether by a lead stimulus (Blumenthal, 1996). This means that the lead stimulus does not simply decrease the magnitude of the startle response; it can decrease that magnitude to zero in some cases.

Startle modification is a useful and reliable tool for evaluating information processing at different levels of the central nervous system in a variety of situations. In fact, reflex modification has been the "North America" of experimental psychology, always there and continually being "rediscovered" (see Prologue; Ison & Hoffman, 1983). Short lead interval modification of startle is a response measure that has several obvious advantages, including: (1) availability of animal models, leading to an understanding of the neurological mechanisms underlying the effect; (2) availability of developmental models; (3) minimal compliance and motivation required of the subject; (4) sensitivity to manipulations of the sensory, cognitive, social, and pharmacological environment; (5) an effect size that is great enough that even rather large changes in methodology cannot obscure this effect; (6) functional significance in the life of the organism. What more can we ask of a response measure?

2. Effects of Variations of the Lead Stimulus

The term "lead stimulus" can refer to the onset or offset of a stimulus, or a change in an ongoing stimulus, each of which represents a stimulus event. Under optimal laboratory conditions, we can reduce extraneous stimuli, but, since lead stimuli can be in any modality, anything short of complete sensory deprivation (including internal senses) will fall short of guaranteeing a pure control condition. Therefore, a control condition is not really a "no lead stimulus" condition; it is instead a condition in which the extra lead stimulus that we are adding in other conditions is not presented. A "lead stimulus condition" is one in which one more stimulus is added to the attenuated cacophony of the laboratory environment.

2.1. Stimulus Presentation

The most common way of modifying the startle response is by presenting a lead stimulus some time before the startle stimulus.

2.1.1. Lead Interval

Varying the lead interval involves changing the interval between two sensory events. The first of these is the lead stimulus, which initiates a sequence of neural activation that is initially specific to one sensory system, and then diverges in both ascending and descending pathways (Perlstein, Fiorito, Simons, & Graham, 1993). The second stimulus event is the startle stimulus. The fact that a lead stimulus can modify the response to a startle stimulus proves that the neural signals activated by the two stimuli converge at some point. The dependence of startle modification on lead interval has helped to identify the neural mechanisms underlying startle elicitation and modification (see Chapter 5 and 6).

The range of lead intervals at which startle inhibition is found, for acoustic lead stimuli and acoustic startle stimuli, has traditionally been considered to be 15–400 msec (Hoffman & Wible, 1969, 1970; Anthony, 1985), with maximal inhibition at approximately 100–150 msec (Graham et al., 1975). The amount of inhibition decreases at lead intervals below or above this range (Graham, 1975; Graham & Murray, 1977; Blumenthal & Creps, 1994; Norris & Blumenthal, 1996) (see Fig. 3.1).

When acoustic startle stimuli are preceded by vibrotactile lead stimuli presented to the hand, startle inhibition is maximal at lead intervals of 150–250 msec (Blumenthal & Tolomeo, 1989), although vibrotactile lead stimuli can inhibit acoustic startle at lead intervals of 100–800 msec, longer than lead intervals at which acoustic lead stimuli are effective (Norris & Blumenthal, 1996). Visual lead stimuli can inhibit acoustic startle at lead intervals of 60–240 msec (Boehmelt, Dawson, Vanman, & Schell, 1996) and the electrically elicited blink reflex at lead intervals of 60–110 msec (Boelhouwer, Frints, & Westerkamp, 1989). Inhibition of the electrically elicited blink reflex is more pronounced as the intensity of the visual lead stimulus increases (Sarno, Blumenthal, & Boelhouwer, 1996). Eyeblinks that are elicited by a glabellar tap can be inhibited by an acoustic lead stimulus at lead intervals of 75–600 msec (Hoffman, Cohen, & English, 1985).

By investigating the impact of varying lead intervals, researchers can estimate the temporal parameters involved in the convergence of lead stimulus and startle stimulus effects, which can help in the identification of the neurological mechanisms underlying stimulus processing in various sensory systems.

2.1.2. Lead Stimulus Duration

Graham and Murray (1977) put forth the hypothesis that both elicitation and short interval inhibition of startle are due to activation of neurons in the auditory pathway that are preferentially sensitive to transient stimulus aspects, such as stimulus onset, based on the work of Gersuni (1971). Transient and sustained neurons were thought to function in the service of stimulus detection and stimulus identification, respectively (Berg, 1985). Gersuni (1971) found that short time constant neurons are sensitive to changes in stimulus energy that occur within a window of up to 20 msec, demonstrating the ability of this system to show rapid temporal summation. The distinction between

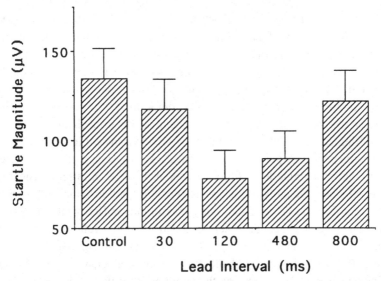

Figure 3.1. Startle magnitude as a function of lead interval. (Reprinted from C. M. Norris & T. D. Blumenthal, (1996), A relationship between inhibition of the acoustic startle response and the protection of prepulse processing, *Psychobiology, 24,* 160–168; copyright The Psychonomic Society. Reprinted with permission.)

short and long time constant neurons generated a great deal of research in the 1970s and 1980s, and an analogous distinction between transient and sustained systems was identified in the visual (Schwartz & Loop, 1984) and tactile systems (Gescheider, Hoffman, Harrison, Travis, & Bolanowski, 1994). Graham (1992) expressed the distinction between transient and sustained systems as one of low- versus high-pass filtered processing. Startle elicitation is a function of a high-pass filtered system, whereas orienting and defensive responses are functions of a low-pass filtered system (Graham, 1992).

Temporal summation refers to the process of integrating stimulus energy over time, with response magnitude increasing as stimulus duration or rate increases (Zwislocki, 1969; Gelfland, 1990). The time window in which this summation occurs can be identified as the point at which the response increment as a function of stimulus duration or rate reaches asymptote. Temporal summation is a characteristic of all sensory systems and, indeed, of neural integration at the most basic level. Evaluation of temporal summation can be used to quantify hearing loss (Stephens, 1976; Florentine, Fastl, & Buus, 1988) and to assist in identifying the mechanisms underlying information processing (Zwislocki, 1969, 1983).

The amount of startle inhibition increases as lead stimulus duration increases, with this function reaching asymptote at 20–50 msec (Dykman & Ison, 1979; Harbin & Berg, 1983; Mansbach & Geyer, 1991; Blumenthal, 1995) (see Fig. 3.2). When two brief lead stimuli (3-msec duration) are presented on the same trial, the temporal summation window is the same as that found with single lead stimuli varying in duration (Blumenthal, 1995). Furthermore, a single lead stimulus contains an onset, offset, and steady-state portion, whereas a pair of lead stimuli constitute two onsets, if the duration of the clicks is below the temporal resolution ability of the peripheral sensory mechanism (Green, 1973). Blumenthal (1995) showed that the second transient in a pair adds as much to the inhibitory power of that pair as the steady-state portion and offset adds to that of a single lead stimulus. This means that an onset transient is processed more efficiently, or makes a greater contribution to the inhibition of startle, than does the 47-msec-long body of a stimulus and its offset. This "transient advantage" has also been demonstrated for startle reflex elicitation in human adults (Blumenthal & Berg, 1986), neonates (Blumenthal, Avendano, & Berg, 1987), and 16-week-old infants (Anthony, Zeigler, & Graham, 1987).

The effects of either increasing the duration of single lead stimuli or presenting multiple transient pulses as lead stimuli suggest that startle modification can be used to evaluate the ability of a sensory system to integrate information over time, as a test of temporal summation.

2.1.3. Lead Stimulus Intensity

There are two main reasons for interest in the effects of lead stimulus intensity on startle modification. The first has to do with an attempt to evaluate the extent to which the neural mechanisms underlying startle modification are sensitive to an increase in stimulus energy. This is similar in some ways to the evaluation of the impact of temporal summation on startle inhibition described in the previous section. Startle inhibition is generally more pronounced for more intense lead stimuli (Graham & Murray, 1977; Blumenthal, 1995). Schwarzkopf, McCoy, Smith, and Boutros (1993) showed that inhibition of startle to 116-dB noise bursts increased as lead stimulus intensity increased from 75 to 80 to 85 dB. Blumenthal and Creps (1994) showed that increasing lead stimulus intensity from 55 to 70 dB resulted in more pronounced inhibition of startle to 100-dB noise bursts. Blumenthal (1995) showed that increasing lead stimulus intensity from 40 to 50 to 60 dB resulted in progressively more pronounced inhibition of startle to an 85-dB noise burst (see Fig. 3.2).

This lead stimulus intensity effect is present even when the two stimuli are in different sensory modalities. For example, Blumenthal and Gescheider (1987) presented acoustic startle stimuli, preceded on some trials by a brief vibrotactile lead stimulus to the hand, and found that the amount of inhibition

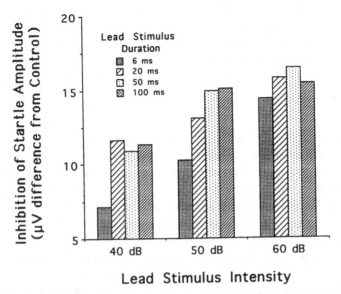

Figure 3.2. Inhibition of startle as a function of lead stimulus duration and intensity. (Reprinted from T. D. Blumenthal (1995), Prepulse inhibition of the startle eyeblink as an indicator of temporal summation, *Perception and Psychophysics, 57,* 487–494; copyright The Psychonomic Society. Reprinted with permission.)

caused by the vibrotactile lead stimulus increased as the intensity of the vibration increased.

When dealing with lead stimulus intensity, one must be aware of the fact that, at a sufficiently high intensity, the lead stimulus itself can activate the startle response (Graham & Murray, 1977; Blumenthal & Goode, 1991). The lead stimulus then has two separate effects, activating both the inhibitory mechanism and the startle response itself. Some researchers ignore this divergence of activation, whereas others try to minimize the extent to which the lead stimulus activates a startle reflex by increasing the rise time of the lead stimulus (see Chapter 2).

A second reason to be interested in lead stimulus intensity is the potential application of this methodology to the assessment of sensory thresholds, by identifying the lead stimulus intensity below which no inhibitory effect is seen. For example, Reiter and Ison (1977) showed that the air-puff-elicited blink reflex in humans was inhibited by acoustic lead stimuli at and slightly below the psychophysical detection threshold. This reflex inhibition audiometry has also been demonstrated by Marsh, Hoffman, and Stitt (1978) and Reiter, Goetzinger, and Press (1981), and has been reviewed by Hoffman (1984).

An interesting application of reflex inhibition audiometry is found in the evaluation of toxins that impair sensory functioning. Crofton and Sheets (1989) review a number of studies in which drugs that normally result in acoustic sensory dysfunction also lead to a decrease in startle inhibition by acoustic lead stimuli (Fechter & Young, 1983; Young & Fechter, 1983). This suggests that the startle inhibition procedure may be valuable in identifying sensory dysfunction.

2.1.4. Lead Stimulus Frequency (Hz)

The measurement of startle modification while using acoustic lead stimuli of different frequencies (Hz) may be a valuable tool in the audiological assessment of difficult-to-test subjects, such as young infants and handicapped or noncompliant adults. Acocella and Blumenthal (1990) compared the amount of startle inhibition caused by 60-dB lead stimuli that were either 1000 or 2000 Hz tones, or broadband noise bursts, preceding 90-dB blink-eliciting noise bursts. No differences in startle inhibition were found for these three lead stimuli. Reiter (1977, 1981) also found no difference in startle inhibition as a function of lead stimulus frequency, across a range of 250–8000 Hz. From the perspective of audiological assessment, this absence of a frequency effect is an advantage in favor of this technique. That is, reflex inhibition audiometry may be equivalently applicable across a wide range of frequencies (Reiter, 1981). In fact, this conclusion has led to the application of startle inhibition as an audiological measure following exposure to drugs that cause hearing loss in animals. By testing for startle inhibition with lead stimuli at a variety of frequencies, researchers can identify the frequency region that is affected by a given ototoxic agent (Wecker, Ison, & Foss, 1985; Jaspers, Muijser, Lammers, & Kulig, 1993).

2.1.5. Lead Stimulus Rise Time

In an effort to differentially activate the transient system in a startle inhibition situation, Blumenthal and Levey (1989) preceded a 95-dB startle noise burst with a noise lead stimulus, at rise times of 0.1–150 msec. Lead stimuli reliably inhibited startle, but no effect of rise time was found. Ison (1978) found that changing the rise time of lead stimuli also had no effect on the startle response in rats.

2.1.6. Discrete versus Continuous Lead Stimuli

One way to investigate the relative contributions of transient and sustained stimulus properties to startle modification is to present lead stimuli that are either discrete or continuous. A discrete lead stimulus is one that begins and ends before the startle stimulus begins, so that there is a gap between the two stimuli. A continuous lead stimulus begins before the startle stimulus, but ends either at or after startle stimulus onset. Therefore, a discrete lead stimulus includes an onset transient, a sustained portion, and an offset transient. A continuous lead stimulus includes an onset transient and a sustained portion, with this sustained portion being longer than that of a discrete lead stimulus. If the degree of startle inhibition is not significantly different for these two types of lead stimuli, then the onset of the lead stimulus dominates in determining startle inhibition. This supports the hypothesis that startle inhibition is based on transient system activation (Graham, 1979). Graham and Murray (1977) showed that discrete (20-msec duration) and continuous lead stimuli, at lead intervals of 30–240 msec, did not differ in their effectiveness as startle inhibitors.

2.2. Stimulus Removal

2.2.1. Gaps as Stimuli

The definition of "lead stimulus" is not restricted to the presentation of a stimulus, but includes any informational event in the environment. One can also think of this in terms of "transients," in that both stimulus onset and offset are transient events, or changes. If a background noise is interrupted shortly before the onset of a startle stimulus, that interruption can act as a lead stimulus. In this context, a background stimulus that is terminated and is then turned on again before startle stimulus onset is said to contain a gap, with an "offset" and an "onset," whereas a background stimulus that is turned off and not turned on again before startle stimulus onset constitutes an offset only. Lane, Ornitz, and Guthrie (1991) showed that a 1000-Hz tone with a 25-msec gap beginning 120 msec before the onset of a 104-dB noise burst resulted in startle inhibition. Cranney and Cohen (1985) measured eyeblinks with a photocell, eliciting the blinks with a tap to the glabella. They presented a 4-msec gap in a 70-dB, 1000-Hz tone, with the gap beginning 154 msec before tap presentation, and found that this gap inhibited the response to the glabellar tap. Krauter (1987) measured the elctrooculogram to a 112-dB tone in adults, with a visual lead stimulus interrupted for 20 msec before the startle-eliciting tone. Krauter found facilitation of startle when the onset of this gap preceded the startle stimulus by a lead interval of 40 msec, no effect at a lead interval of 80 msec, and inhibition of startle at lead intervals of 120–360 msec. At a lead interval of 200 msec, the effectiveness of the gap in the visual stimulus increased as the duration of the gap increased from 8 to 20 msec. This is similar to the finding of Harbin and Berg (1983), who measured the electrooculogram to air-puff stimuli, and found that the inhibition caused by a gap in a background tone increased as the duration of the gap increased from 10 to 40 msec. Harbin and Berg suggested that startle inhibition increased as the two transients (gap onset and offset) became more separated in time, another demonstration of temporal summation in startle modification.

2.2.2. Offsets as Stimuli

A situation in which a background stimulus is terminated, but not turned on again, before startle stimulus onset might be thought of as an offset alone. Lane et al. (1991) found that a tone offset presented 100 msec before a startle-eliciting noise resulted in startle inhibition, and this inhibition was not significantly different from that produced by a gap in a continuous tone. However, the presentation of a discrete lead stimulus was more effective at inhibiting startle than was either a gap or an offset of a lead stimulus. These data suggest that startle can be inhibited by any transient change in stimulation, either a stimulus onset or a stimulus offset, but that stimulus onsets are more effective than offsets as startle inhibitors.

2.3. Stimulus Change

As stated above, any unit of information in the sensory environment can act as a lead stimulus. Cranney and Cohen (1985) measured eyeblinks with a photocell, eliciting the blinks with a tap to the glabella. They changed the frequency of a 70-dB tone from 1750 to 1000 Hz, with this linear frequency change taking 24 msec and beginning 164 msec before tap presentation. This frequency shift inhibited the response to the glabellar tap as effectively as did a gap in a background tone. Both a gap and a frequency shift became more effective inhibitors as the intensity of the lead stimulus was increased (Cranney & Cohen, 1985). Also, both a gap and a frequency shift were as effective as a discrete tone lead stimulus in inhibiting the blink reflex. This points to the fact that startle inhibition can result from any change in the stimulus environment at an appropriate lead interval.

3. Effect of Variations of the Startle Stimulus

Hoffman and Ison (1992) state that the amount of startle inhibition (that is, the difference between responding on control and lead stimulus trials) is independent of the intensity of the startle stimulus, and they refer to this independence as the "First Law of Reflex Modification." Other researchers have found that increasing the intensity of the startle stimulus can result in more pronounced startle inhibition, without changing the lead stimulus (Perlstein et al., 1993; Blumenthal & Creps, 1994; Blumenthal, Schicatano, Chapman, Norris, & Ergenzinger, 1996).

Blumenthal (1996) specifically tested the "First Law of Reflex Modification" as stated by Hoffman and Ison (1992), and found that increasing acoustic startle stimulus intensity from 85 to 95 dB resulted in more pronounced inhibition caused by either a 60- or a 70-dB acoustic lead stimulus. This has important implications for the hypothesized flow of information through the neural mechanisms underlying startle elicitation and inhibition, since these data suggest that the inhibitory input to the startle center is in place before the startle stimulus is presented (see Blumenthal, 1996, for a more complete description of this "latent inhibition").

As the impact of the startle stimulus increases, the ability of the lead stimulus to inhibit the response may reach asymptote. Blumenthal (1996) found that increasing startle stimulus intensity beyond 95 dB showed no greater effect for inhibition of startle response amplitude. Therefore, the "First Law" appeared to hold at high startle stimulus intensities, but not at lower intensities. All of the preceding statements are based on the absolute difference between responding in the control and lead stimulus conditions. However, again contrary to the predictions of Hoffman and Ison (1992), Blumenthal (1996) showed that the proportion of startle inhibition (difference between control and lead stimulus conditions, divided by the control value) was not affected by startle stimulus intensity. These data suggest that the startle stimulus has its effect after the inhibitory input to the startle center has been activated (see Hoffman & Ison, 1992, p. 93). These data also show that the measure of startle inhibition that is used, either absolute difference or proportional difference, can influence the conclusions that will be reached.

4. Habituation of Short Lead Interval Inhibition

The amount of inhibition of startle caused by a given lead stimulus (difference between control and lead stimulus conditions) has been shown to decrease as a testing session progresses (Graham et al., 1975; Graham & Murray, 1977; Lipp, Arnold, Siddle, & Dawson, 1994; Blumenthal, 1996; Norris & Blumenthal, 1996). This decrease may be due to one of two mechanisms: (1) habituation of either the sensory input to the lead stimulus inhibition center or the neural signal projecting from that inhibition center to the startle center or (2) a decrease in the magnitude of the startle response itself. The extent to which a lead stimulus can inhibit startle might be partially determined by the magnitude of the startle response itself. This is supported by the finding that the extent to which a lead stimulus can inhibit startle increases as startle stimulus intensity increases (Blumenthal, 1996), as described in Section 3 above.

Therefore, decreased startle inhibition across trial blocks might be explained by a relationship analogous to the Law of Dynamic Range (Berntson, Cacioppo, & Quigley, 1991), which implies that a decrease in startle reactivity on control trials will be paired with a decrease in the amount of startle inhibition. That is, as the startle response habituates, the amount of startle inhibition decreases as well, because the response being measured is approaching its lower limit.

Blumenthal (1997) attempted to determine whether a decrease in short lead interval inhibition of startle across trials is a function of habituation of the lead stimulus or a decrease in control startle responding. Blumenthal presented 60- or 70-dB tones as lead stimuli, preceding a 95-dB noise startle stimulus on some trials. Subjects were assigned to one of three groups, in which the first 18 trials of the testing session included: (1) lead stimuli alone, with no startle stimuli; (2) startle stimuli alone, with no lead stimuli; (3) lead stimuli and startle stimuli paired on some trials. After this, all subjects received 18 more trials, involving lead stimuli and startle stimuli paired on some trials. By comparing the amount of startle inhibition present at the beginning of this second set of trials, Blumenthal (1997) evaluated the impact of repeated presentations of either lead or startle stimuli on inhibition. The response to the startle stimulus on control trials decreased as trial blocks progressed, demonstrating habituation of the startle response (see Fig. 3.3). The amount of inhibition caused by the lead stimuli also decreased as trial blocks progressed. The repeated presentation of a number of lead stimuli before the first lead stimulus–startle stimulus pairing had no effect on the ability of those lead stimuli to subsequently inhibit startle. That is, prior exposure to lead stimuli did not influence the ability of subsequent lead stimuli to inhibit startle. A similar result has been shown in humans (Lipp, Krinitzky, & Siddle, 1996; Wynn, Schell, & Dawson, 1996) and in rats (Hoffman, Cohen, & Corso, 1984; Wu, Kreuger, lson, & Gerrard, 1984). Gewirtz and Davis (1995) summarized several rat studies and concluded that inhibition caused by a lead stimulus does not decrease across trials if startle habituation is prevented, and if the lead stimulus is easily detectable. Blumenthal (1997) showed that lead stimulus inhibition only decreases across trials if startle reactivity is habituating across the same trials. Therefore, this decrease in inhibition is not an example of "habituation of the lead stimulus effect"; it is instead due to a change in the startle reactivity on which the lead stimulus has its effect, and on which the calculation of inhibition is based. This conclusion is supported by the finding that the proportion of startle inhibition did not change across trials in Blumenthal's study (1997).

These data help to answer an interesting question that arises concerning

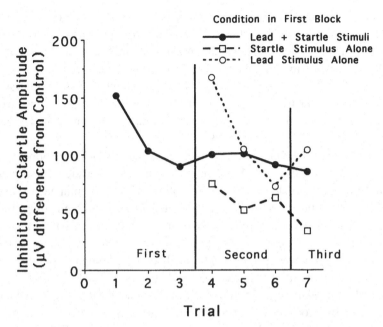

Figure 3.3. Inhibition of startle as a function of trial, in subjects who received an initial trial block with lead stimuli alone, startle stimuli alone, or lead stimuli paired with startle stimuli on some trials. (Reprinted from T. D. Blumenthal (1997), Prepulse inhibition decreases as startle reactivity habituates, *Psychophysiology, 34,* 446–450; copyright Cambridge University Press. Reprinted with permission.)

short lead interval startle inhibition. If a wide variety of stimuli can act as lead stimuli, inhibiting startle, and if we are constantly being presented with stimuli in the sensory environment, then a repetitive stimulus may be expected to have less of an effect as an inhibitor of startle, due to habituation of that stimulus. The data of Lipp et al. (1996), Wynn et al. (1996), and Blumenthal (1997) show that this is not the case, since simple repetition of the lead stimulus does not affect the amount of startle inhibition. A reduction of startle inhibition is seen only after repeated *pairing* of the lead stimulus and the startle stimulus. Therefore, repetitive stimuli retain their ability to inhibit startle when this pairing finally occurs.

5. Startle Facilitation at Short Positive and Negative Lead Intervals

The probability of obtaining startle inhibition generally increases as the lead interval increases to 100–150 msec, and then generally decreases as the lead interval increases beyond 150 msec. However, at lead intervals of 50 msec or less, some researchers have shown that lead stimuli can actually facilitate the startle response, when the lead stimulus and the startle stimulus are in different sensory modalities (Graham, 1980; Sanes, 1984; Boelhouwer et al., 1989; Aitken, Siddle, & Lipp, 1995; Burke & Hackley, 1997). This facilitation is independent of the inhibition seen at longer lead intervals, and the two effects can compensate for each other if two lead stimuli are presented on the same trial (Blumenthal & Tolomeo, 1989).

Boelhouwer, Teurlings, and Brunia (1991) and Nakashima, Shimoyama, Yokoyama, and Takahashi (1993) found that a weak acoustic lead stimulus could facilitate the electrically elicited blink reflex (R2 component), even when the acoustic lead stimulus was presented *after* the blink-eliciting stimulus. Schmolesky, Boelhouwer, and Blumenthal (1996) found that the amount of facilitation increases as the intensity of the acoustic stimulus increases (see Fig. 3.4). Boelhouwer et al. (1989) found that the R2 component of the electrically elicited blink reflex could be facilitated by a visual stimulus at lead intervals of 0–30 msec, and Sarno et al. (1996) found that the interval at which this facilitation occurred decreased as the intensity of the visual stimulus increased. That is, a visual lead stimulus facilitated the blink reflex at a shorter lead interval for strong visual pulses than for weak visual pulses.

Boelhouwer et al. (1991) explain this facilitation of the blink reflex by a simultaneous or following "lead" stimulus in terms of temporal summation, with an interesting caveat. When we present stimuli in different sensory systems, the time between the onsets of the two stimuli is less important than is the time window within which neural energy reaches some common site (Rimpel, Geyer, & Hopf, 1982). Temporal summation at that common site will be determined by both the time of stimulus presentation and the speed of transmission of information in a sensory pathway. If one pathway conducts information more rapidly than another, the timing of stimulus presentation need not be simultaneous for the neural impact of the two stimuli to combine. In this context, short lead interval facilitation of startle may be useful in determining not just the convergence of sensory pathways, but the conduction velocities within those pathways.

6. The Function of Short Lead Interval Inhibition of Startle

The phylogenetic ubiquity of short lead interval startle inhibition has led researchers to speculate on the functional significance of this effect. Of course, this phenomenon may have more than one function, so alternative explanations are not necessarily contradictory, exhaustive, or mutually exclu-

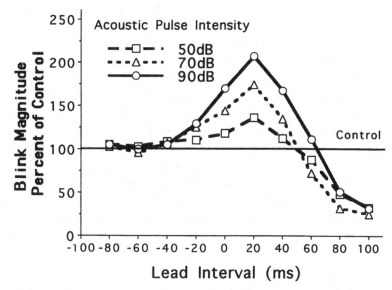

Figure 3.4. Startle magnitude as a function of lead stimulus intensity and lead interval (negative lead intervals involved the "lead stimulus" being presented after the blink-eliciting electrical pulse). (Reprinted from M. T. Schmolesky, A. J. W. Boelhouwer, & T. D. Blumenthal (1996), The effect of acoustic pulse intensity upon the electrically elicited blink reflex at positive and negative stimulus onset asynchrocies, *Biological Psychology, 44,* 69-84; with kind permission of Elsevier Science- NL, Sara Burgerhartstraat 25, 1055 KV Amsterdam, The Netherlands.)

sive. Three functional hypotheses have been proposed, and these explanations share many characteristics but differ from each other in important ways.

6.1. Sensory Gating

Startle inhibition has been explained in terms of sensory gating, or perceptual filtering (Braff, Grillon, & Geyer, 1992), the reduction of processing of and distraction by irrelevant or repetitive stimuli. Geyer and Braff (1987) review a number of studies that suggest that sensory gating is deficient in schizophrenics, leading to their high distractibility, sensory overload, and reduced habituation. Also, short lead interval startle inhibition is less pronounced in schizophrenics than in control subjects (Braff et al., 1992). This deficiency of startle modification occurs without any difference between schizophrenic and control subjects in startle reactivity on control trials. Startle inhibition is also deficient in adults with obsessive–compulsive disorder (Swerdlow, Auerbach, Monroe, Hartston, Geyer, & Braff, 1993) or Huntington's disease (Swerdlow,

Caine, Braff, & Geyer, 1992), and in children with Tourette's syndrome (Castellanos, Fine, Kaysen, Marsh, Rapoport, & Hallett, 1996), all of which are characterized by an impaired ability to inhibit irrelevant information. This sensory gating is automatic and preattentive at very short lead intervals (60 msec), but may involve controlled processing at longer lead intervals (see next section). The inability to successfully inhibit irrelevant sensory information may have significant behavioral and cognitive implications, and may also reveal some degree of commonality in the mechanisms underlying these various disorders (Swerdlow et al., 1992). In fact, deficits in startle inhibition can be produced in animal models by the administration of dopamine agonists, and dopamine receptor blockers can reverse this impairment (Davis, Mansbach, Swerdlow, Campeau, Braff, & Geyer, 1990; Swerdlow et al., 1992; Hoffman & Donovan, 1994). This has resulted in startle modification becoming a powerful tool in testing the clinical effectiveness of a variety of drugs (Braff et al. 1992) (see Chapter 6).

6.2. Protection of Preattentive Processing

Graham's (1975, 1980, 1992) protection theory is similar in many ways to the sensory gating theory described above, but Graham goes one step further, to predict differential processing of the lead stimulus as a function of startle inhibition. In Graham's theory, the onset of a lead stimulus initiates two automatic processes, one serving to identify the lead stimulus, and the other serving to protect the processing of the lead stimulus from interruption by the startle stimulus and/or response. The degree to which this protective mechanism is activated largely determines the extent of startle inhibition. This protective mechanism is activated by lead stimulus onset, builds to a maximum level of effectiveness, then decays, as shown by the variation of inhibition across lead intervals. Lead stimuli that are more intense or longer in duration activate the protective mechanism more strongly, reflecting greater neural activation.

Inherent in this explanation of startle modification is the conceptualization of the startle stimulus as a probe that is used to evaluate the activation of the protective mechanism and, by inference, the protected processing of the lead stimulus. That is, if startle is more strongly inhibited, the protective mechanism is assumed to be more strongly activated, and the lead stimulus is, therefore, assumed to be more fully processed. Most studies that conclude that the processing of the lead stimulus has been protected base this conclusion on the extent to which the startle response is inhibited. However, a more direct assessment of this protection is possible, by actually measuring the processing of the lead stimulus itself.

Perlstein et al. (1993) asked subjects to judge the magnitude of the lead stimulus in the presence or absence of a startle stimulus. This procedure adds a different sort of control condition to the methodology, that of the lead stimulus presented alone. Estimates of the magnitude of the lead stimuli were increased on trials on which the startle stimulus followed the lead stimulus by 500 msec, relative to lead-stimulus-alone trials. Whether this demonstrates protection of preattentive processing is unclear, however, since this increased magnitude estimation may have been due to loudness assimilation, a situation in which the loudness of both members of a pair of sounds shifts toward the loudness of the other sound in the pair (Zwislocki & Sokolich, 1974; Elmasian, Galambos, & Bernheim, 1980). Filion and Ciranni (1994) also found loudness assimilation at both 120- and 500-msec lead intervals. However, in the 120-msec lead interval condition, the amount of startle inhibition was negatively correlated (between subjects) with loudness assimilation. That is, subjects who showed more inhibition of startle showed less loudness assimilation, suggesting that the processing of the lead stimulus was interfered with less in subjects who had more pronounced startle inhibition.

Norris and Blumenthal (1996) assessed the protection of preattentive processing in a different way, requiring the subject to decide whether a lead stimulus was a low- or high-frequency tone. Startle was inhibited at lead intervals of 30–480 msec. The accuracy of identifying the lead stimulus (low- or high-frequency) was significantly higher on trials on which startle was inhibited compared with trials on which startle was not inhibited, at lead intervals of 30–800 msec (see Fig. 3.5). In a second experiment, Norris and Blumenthal (1996) avoided any impact of loudness assimilation by using a lead stimulus and startle stimulus that were in different sensory modalities (Massaro & Kahn, 1973), preceding a noise startle stimulus with a vibrotactile lead stimulus presented to the hand (50- or 200-Hz vibration) on some trials. Again, lead stimulus identification accuracy was higher on trials on which startle was inhibited, compared with noninhibited trials, at lead intervals of 50–800 msec. These data show that inhibition of startle by a lead stimulus and higher accuracy of lead stimulus identification occur together, providing support for Graham's hypothesis of protection of preattentive processing in a way different from that of previous research. Mussat-Whitlow and Blumenthal (1997) have demonstrated essentially the same effect with a matching task, using acoustic startle stimuli and either acoustic or vibrotactile lead stimuli.

Graham's hypothesis of startle inhibition reflecting protection of preattentive processing can be seen as a conceptual extension of the sensory gating hypothesis, in that Graham's hypothesis proposes that the lead stimulus activates a perceptual filter, but also makes a specific prediction as to the effect of this perceptual filter on processing of the lead stimulus.

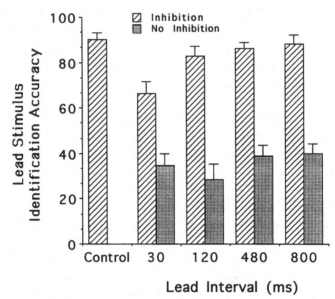

Figure 3.5. Lead stimulus identification accuracy as a function of lead interval and whether or not startle was inhibited. (Reprinted from C. M. Norris & T. D. Blumenthal (1996), A relationship between inhibition of the acoustic response and the protection of prepulse processing, *Psychobiology, 24,* 160-168; copyright The Psychonomic Society. Reprinted with permission.)

6.3. Attentional and Automatic Processing

Dawson, Schell, Swerdlow, and Filion (1997) take Graham's protection hypothesis one step further, by separately evaluating the automatic and controlled aspects of startle inhibition. These researchers, along with others (DelPezzo & Hoffman, 1980; Hackley & Graham, 1987) have shown that short lead interval startle inhibition can be more pronounced if the subject is told to attend to the lead stimulus. For example, Filion, Dawson, and Schell (1993) and Dawson, Hazlett, Filion, Nuechterlein, and Schell (1993) found that the amount of inhibition at a 120-ms lead interval was significantly more pronounced for attended than ignored lead stimuli, although attention had no effect on startle inhibition at lead intervals of 60 or 240 msec (see Fig. 3.6). This suggests that, although startle modification at short lead intervals is an automatic process, it can also be affected by controlled attentional processing.

Filion et al. (1993) explain the effects of attention on short lead interval startle inhibition as an extension of Graham's (1980) explanation of the function of startle inhibition, by stating the following: "short lead interval SEM may reflect not only the nonselective protection of preattentive processing,

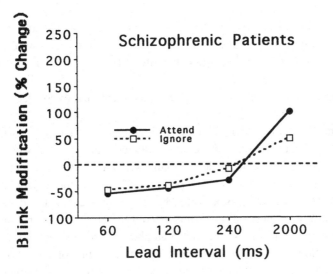

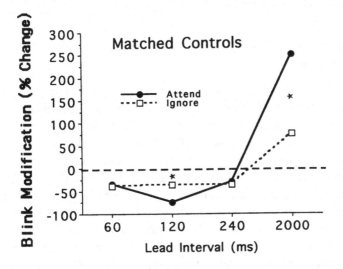

Figure 3.6. Startle blink modification as a function of lead interval and attention condition in schizophrenic patients (A) and matched controls (B). (Reprinted from M. E. Dawson, E. A. Hazlett, D. L. Filion, K. N. Nuechterlein, & A. M. Schell (1993), Attention and schizophrenia: Impaired modulation of the startle reflex, *Journal of Abnormal Psychology, 102,* 633-641; copyright 1993 by the American Psychological Association. Adapted with permission.)

but also the outcome of preattentive processing in terms of an early evaluation of the significance of the lead stimulus" (p. 197). By making the lead
stimulus a target of directed attention, the inferred activation of the protective
mechanism is increased.

In an intersection of the sensory gating and attentional hypotheses, Dawson et al. (1993) showed that attentional manipulations affected startle inhibition in normal subjects but not in schizophrenic subjects (see Fig. 3.6). Furthermore, the schizophrenic and control subjects only differed when they
were instructed to attend to the lead stimuli, with an attentional effect found
for control subjects but not for schizophrenics. Therefore, the schizophrenics
showed normal automatic processing, but were deficient in the degree to
which controlled attentional mechanisms could contribute to startle inhibition. Dawson et al. (1997) summarize a number of studies dealing with startle modification in clinical subjects, and find that the nature of the testing procedure, and the extent to which the patient is actively psychotic, are important
in determining whether attentional instructions have an impact on startle inhibition at short lead intervals.

6.4. Comparing the Sensory Gating, Protection, and Attentional Hypotheses

All three of the theories describing the function of short lead interval inhibition of startle include the statement that the lead stimulus activates some
mechanism that decreases the interruption caused by the startle stimulus or
response. The protection (Graham, 1992) and attentional (Filion et al., 1993)
hypotheses state that this inhibition of startle will result in the interruption of
the processing of the lead stimulus being reduced (inhibition of response
amplitude) or prevented (inhibition of response probability) (see Blumenthal,
1996, p. 100, for a description of the impact of startle inhibition as reflected
by these response measures). In the sensory gating hypothesis (Geyer &
Braff, 1987), the main focus is on "gating" of the startle stimulus, and the
extent to which the lead stimulus is processed is of secondary interest. In the
attention hypothesis, startle inhibition is used to distinguish between automatic and controlled processing. In research based on this hypothesis,
directed attention instructions have been used to enhance lead stimulus processing, but the processing of the lead stimulus has generally been assumed
but not assessed. In the protection hypothesis, the processing of the lead stimulus is the critical aspect, and variations in the amount of this processing were
inferred but not measured until recently (Norris & Blumenthal, 1996). Comparing the three hypotheses, the processing of the lead stimulus is least impor-

tant under the sensory gating hypothesis; this processing is important and manipulated under the attentional hypothesis; and lead stimulus processing is important and measurable under the protection hypothesis.

The sensory gating hypothesis is mainly applied in comparing clinical populations with control subjects, or in animal models of human psychiatric disorders. The protection hypothesis applies most directly to automatic processing of stimuli, whereas the attentional hypothesis includes this protection, but also adds a level of controlled processing. This reflects the focus of the sensory gating, protection, and attentional hypotheses in clinical science, neuroscience, and cognitive science, respectively, although each hypothesis can be applied in any of these areas. Both the sensory gating hypothesis and the automatic portion of the attentional hypothesis can be subsumed under Graham's (1992) protection of preattentive processing hypothesis.

7. Conclusion

Startle modification by lead stimuli at short lead intervals remains one of the most reliable, robust, and informative phenomena in all of psychophysiology. The ubiquity of this effect is demonstrated by the fact that this startle modification is being studied in dozens of laboratories all over the world, with a wide range of subject populations and stimulus parameters. Each researcher looks at this phenomenon in a slightly different way, and all arrive at similar basic conclusions. This is not to say that all aspects of short lead interval modification of startle have been sufficiently investigated. Instead, the reliability of the effect allows researchers to use this modification in a wide variety of research questions.

CHAPTER FOUR

Long Lead Interval Startle Modification

LOIS E. PUTNAM AND ERIC J. VANMAN

ABSTRACT

In this chapter we review typical paradigms employed in investigations of startle modification at long lead intervals. We also summarize some of the basic phenomena associated with long lead interval startle modification. Such phenomena include the facilitation or inhibition of startle magnitude as a function of lead stimulus intensity and duration, cardiac deceleration, the modalities of the lead stimulus and the startle probe, whether participants are instructed to attend to or ignore the lead stimulus, and the emotional valence and arousal of the lead stimulus. Both relevant animal and human studies are reviewed, some of which have appeared previously only in doctoral dissertations. In addition, we discuss some of the conceptual issues that have driven much of this research, highlighting particular controversies that have received more attention, such as whether the relationship between lead stimulus intensity and startle amplitude is actually an inverted-U function, and what are the relative contributions of attentional and emotional processes in long lead startle modification.

1. Introduction

A burst of sound punctures the empty silence. Though brief, the noise burst is sufficiently intense to startle the hearer, producing a reflex blink. Now imagine that instead of being superimposed on silence, the noise burst follows a prior stimulus of several seconds duration – what we will refer to in this chapter as a "long lead stimulus." What effect will that lead stimulus have on the hearer's startle blink to the subsequent noise burst? Will it mask the noise burst and thus attenuate the startle response? Will it summate with the noise burst and thus facilitate the reflex blink? Will it arouse and alert the listener, enhancing the reflex? How would these masking and alerting effects change

Michael E. Dawson, Anne M. Schell, and Andreas H. Böhmelt, Eds. *Startle modification: Implications for neuroscience, cognitive science, and clinical science.* Copyright © 1999 Cambridge University Press. Printed in the United States of America. All rights reserved.

with variation in lead stimulus modality, intensity, or duration? If the lead stimulus engenders positive affect, or if it directed our listener's attention away from the auditory sense modality, will the reflex be diminished?

This chapter summarizes the basic paradigms and phenomena associated with startle modification at long lead intervals (i.e., generally 800 msec or more), beginning with a description of the effects that lead stimulus intensity and duration – and the lead interval itself – have on the startle response. As noted in previous chapters in this volume, many of these phenomena were first demonstrated in rats, pigeons, and/or rabbits, but later also in humans. Observing a relationship between cardiac deceleration and startle facilitation, Graham and her students added attentional mechanisms and manipulations to the growing inventory of long lead interval phenomena and paradigms. More recently, Davis, Lang, and their colleagues highlighted the role of affective processes in the modulation of startle at long lead intervals. This chapter reviews some of the relevant stimulus paradigms, findings, and conceptual issues relevant to long lead interval startle modification; more details regarding attentional and affective modulation of startle are provided in Chapters 7 and 8.

2. Effects of Lead Stimulus Intensity

2.1. Animal Studies

Hoffman and Fleshler (1963) were among the first to demonstrate that, contrary to its expected masking effect, background noise[1] can actually increase rather than decrease acoustic startle. They found that continuous 85-dB noise, in comparison to a "silent" background, facilitated rat whole-body startle, whereas pulsatile noise had an inhibitory effect. Hoffman and Searle (1968) then demonstrated that the magnitude of startle grew as background noise intensity increased from 50 to 90 dB and that both white-noise and tonal background stimuli could produce a facilitatory effect that was relatively unaffected by variations in background bandwidth or frequency.

Hoffman and his colleagues proposed two different mechanisms to account for these findings. Initially, they hypothesized that background-

---

[1] A note on terminology: In the early work, "effects of background" could refer to effects of continuous noise that had sounded a full 6 hours, as in Hoffman, Marsh, & Stein (1969), or to effects of a lead stimulus presented for as little as 100 msec prior to startle evocation, as in Hoffman & Wible (1969). In this chapter we reserve the term "lead stimulus" for a stimulus that is presented on individual trials and use the term "background stimulus" to indicate stimuli continuously present over a series of trials.

produced facilitation was an indirect effect of removal of prepulse inhibition. Although the inhibitory effect of lead stimuli at short lead intervals (see Chapter 3) was far from completely specified, they had noticed such inhibition in their own studies. Hoffman and his co-workers had also observed that ambient noise during "silent" background conditions could be quite variable. They thus speculated that continuous background noise masked punctiform acoustic stimulation in ambient or physiological noise, which would otherwise partially activate the startle center, thereby rendering it refractory (Hoffman & Fleshler, 1963; Hoffman & Searle, 1968). However, Hoffman and his colleagues later posited a more direct facilitatory role for background stimulation, when they suggested that the presence of acoustic input at the time of startle evocation can, through some unspecified mechanism, facilitate startle (Hoffman & Wible, 1969; Stitt, Hoffman, Marsh, & Boskoff, 1974).

When these findings were extrapolated to a different species, stimulus modality, and reflex response, Ison and Leonard (1971) discovered an important effect of high-intensity lead stimulation. Measuring the rabbit's nictitating membrane response to an electrotactile stimulus, two intensities of continuous auditory lead stimuli were presented at lead intervals ranging from 20 to 1280 msec. The lead stimulus produced significant greater responsivity at 94 than at 82 dB, particularly at the longer lead intervals. Thus, while demonstrating the effect of lead stimulus intensity on startle modification, this experiment also showed that an auditory lead stimulus could facilitate the reflex response to a nonacoustic stimulus.

In yet another demonstration of crossmodal effects of lead stimuli, this time on rat whole-body startle to tone bursts, Ison and Hammond (1971, Experiment 3) demonstrated that acoustic startle was significantly enhanced by visual as well as by auditory lead stimuli at lead intervals of 2500 msec. Paralleling findings from Hoffman's lab using intramodal (acoustic–acoustic) stimuli, Ison and Hammond showed that the magnitude of the crossmodal (visual–acoustic) facilitation increased directly with the intensity of the 2500-msec visual lead stimulus (1971, Experiment 4). Interestingly, a second intramodal condition of the same experiment failed to replicate the Hoffman lab studies' background noise effect. In this condition, acoustic startle was evoked 2500 msec after the onset of a continuous *auditory* lead stimulus that was presented at three different intensities (75, 84, and 93 dB). Instead of the expected facilitatory effect, startle amplitude was inversely related to lead stimulus intensity, with the strongest lead stimulus producing no facilitation at all.

This unexpected finding of *decreasing* startle amplitude with increasing lead stimulus intensity suggested to Ison and his colleagues that startle amplitude might be a nonmonotonic function of background stimulus intensity. Pursuing this hypothesis, they extended the range of stimulus intensities and were able to show that acoustic startle magnitude was indeed an inverted-U function of background noise intensity (Ison & Hammond, 1971; Ison, McAdam, & Hammond, 1973). It should be noted that both of these studies abandoned the use of "explicit" lead stimuli in favor of a constant background noise level presented for at least 1 min prior to any startle stimuli. In Ison and Hammond (1971, Experiment 6), background white noise was presented at a constant intensity for 5 min prior to, as well as throughout, a series of five startle stimuli. Noise levels ranged from 65 to 90 dB, and the amplitude of rat whole-body startle to a 20-msec tone burst (9 kHz, 119 dB, 5 msec rise/fall time) was greatest following the 75-dB noise. A somewhat different procedure was followed in Ison et al. (1973, Experiment 2) but with similar results; again the amplitude of rat whole-body startle was a nonmonotonic function of prior noise intensity (60–90 dB) with an inflection point at 75 dB.

Ison and Hammond (1971) observed that this inverted-U effect was consistent with the notion of an optimal arousal level (e.g., Yerkes & Dodson, 1908; Lindsley, 1951; Hebb, 1955; Duffy, 1957; Malmo, 1958), and that the decline in startle responsivity at high background noise levels could be attributable to the degrading consequences of overarousal. However, an optimal arousal hypothesis would predict an inverted-U effect even when background and startle stimuli were in different modalities, yet such a relation had not been demonstrated. Lacking evidence for a crossmodal inverted U-effect, lson and his colleagues favored a dual-process account, whereby a monotonically increasing facilitatory process such as "arousal" combines at high background intensities with a high-threshold inhibitory process specific to the auditory system (Ison & Hammond, 1971; Ison et al., 1973). Davis (1974b) also favored such an explanation, citing facilitatory effects on startle of such arousal-like states as fear (Brown, Kalish, & Farber, 1951) and frustration (Wagner, 1963).

In sum, by the mid-1970s numerous studies of infrahuman species had shown increasing facilitation of startle with increasing intensities of lead or background stimuli, and several studies had shown that this facilitation occurs even when background and startle stimuli are in different modalities. Two mechanisms were proposed to account for these facilitatory effects: nonspecific arousal and masking of inhibitory processes. Some studies had observed an inhibitory downturn at high background intensities, but only when both background and startle stimuli were acoustic, leading Ison and his colleagues to propose that peripheral auditory mechanisms such as masking and/or the acoustic reflex were responsible for the inhibition.

2.2. Human Studies

In the early 1970s, Frances Graham's laboratory began to study the human startle eyeblink response. The first startle study in Graham's lab, initiated in the spring of 1970, had succeeded in finding both the short lead interval inhibitory and long lead interval facilitatory effects on human startle blink that had earlier been demonstrated for rat whole-body startle (Hoffman & Wible, 1969). Putnam (1975), for her dissertation research, then carried out a series of experiments in Graham's laboratory to determine whether human startle blink would show effects of background stimulus intensity similar to those demonstrated in previous animal studies and to identify more clearly the contribution of modality dependent and independent mechanisms to these effects.

Putnam was particularly interested in the mechanism(s) underlying the descending wing of the inverted-U function. While both auditory masking and the middle-ear muscle ("acoustic") reflex are potentially capable of attenuating the impact of an acoustic startle stimulus, as suggested by Ison and colleagues, Putnam noted that they would do so only under specific intensity and frequency conditions of background and startle stimuli. It was not clear that these conditions had been met in the Ison and Hammond (1971) and Ison et al. (1973) studies. If they had not, then the inhibitory effect observed at high background intensities might require a modality-nonspecific explanation, such as the degrading consequences of overarousal.

To assess the relative contributions of modality-specific and -nonspecific effects, Putnam employed acoustic lead stimuli along with either acoustic or tactile (air-puff) startle stimuli. Two experiments were conducted in which the intensity of the auditory stimulus was varied within subjects while the modality of the startle stimulus was varied between subjects (Tone vs. Puff groups). In both experiments, continuous lead stimuli were initiated 2.6 s prior to startle stimulus onset (following Ison & Hammond, 1971) and consisted of narrow-band (730–1270 Hz) white noise. Four levels of lead stimulus intensity, in addition to a no-lead stimulus control condition, were presented within each block of five trials, and subjects received a total of 50 trials each.

Within the Tone groups, stimulus parameters were chosen to maximize auditory-specific inhibitory effects – masking and the acoustic reflex – in the first experiment but to minimize them in the second. Thus, the 1000-Hz tone burst used in Experiment 1 was purposely centered on the narrow-band noise so that, at a lead stimulus intensity of 95 dB, the band pressure level in its critical band would be sufficiently high for some masking to occur (Sharf, 1970). On the other hand, the 3500-Hz tone burst used in Experiment 2 was designed to be sufficiently above its masked threshold to be released from masking altogether,[2] both by virtue of its increased intensity (119 dB in Experiment 2 vs. 109 dB in Experiment 1) and because of its spectral distance from the narrow-band lead stimulus (Carter & Kryter, 1962). Unlike the 1000-Hz tone, the 3500-Hz tone was also unlikely to be attenuated by the acoustic reflex.[3] As with masking, effects of the acoustic reflex on sound transmission are frequency-dependent. In humans, transmission loss due to the reflex is negligible for test stimuli above 2000 Hz but may be as great as 20 dB for frequencies below 1000 Hz (Simmons, 1959; Jepsen, 1963). Likewise, considerable care was taken to construct a tactile stimulus for the Puff groups that would not have an audible acoustic component.

Experiment 1 employed lead stimulus intensities of 65, 75, 85, and 95 dB. As can be seen in Figure 4.1 (left panel), both Tone and Puff groups showed the expected facilitation of startle blink amplitude at the lower background intensities relative to the no-lead control condition. Whether evoked by tone or puff, startle was significantly enhanced by the 65-dB lead stimulus and declined with increases in intensity above 85 dB. The decrement in startle responsivity from 85 to 95 dB was significant in both groups, although considerably larger for Tone than for Puff. The Tone data thus replicated previous animal studies showing an inhibitory effect of high-intensity acoustic lead stimuli on acoustic startle, but the Puff data provided the first demonstration that the inhibitory effect is not limited to the auditory system or to intramodal stimulus arrangements.

As described above, Experiment 2 again employed both tone and puff startle stimuli, but raised the frequency of the startle tone to 3500 Hz to eliminate any attenuation due to masking or the acoustic reflex. The same narrow-band lead stimulus was used, but its intensity was varied over a wider range (35–95 dB) to observe the ascending wing of the inverted-U function. The 35-dB stimulus was just audible above the continuous white-noise masking stimu-

---

[2] A masking stimulus does not produce a uniform degree of attenuation of a test stimulus across all intensities of the latter. Rather, as the intensity of a test stimulus is increased above its masked threshold, the Intensity × Loudness function is abnormally steep until the point where the stimulus is "released from masking," that is, experienced at normal loudness (see Steinberg & Gardner, 1937; Small & Thurlow, 1954).

[3] The acoustic reflex consists of a contraction of muscles in the middle ear, with resultant stiffening of the ossicular chain and reduced transmission of sound-produced vibration to the inner ear. Features of reflex elicitation, and consequences for sound transmission, vary considerably across mammalian species (see van den Berge, Kingma, Lluge, & Marres, 1990). In humans, the function relating eliciting stimulus frequency to acoustic reflex threshold roughly parallels that for hearing threshold, with acoustic reflex thresholds approximately 65–70 dB above hearing thresholds.

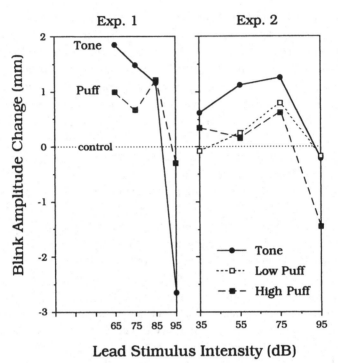

Figure 4.1. Startle blink amplitude change (measured in mm at the eye using potentiometric method) from the no-lead-stimulus control condition as a function of intensity of the narrow-band acoustic lead stimulus in Putnam (1975). In Experiment 1 (*left*), the startle stimulus was a 109-dB 1000-Hz tone burst in the Tone group and a 3-psi puff of air to the right cheek in the Puff group. Mean control amplitudes were 5.1 mm (Tone) and 5.5 mm (Puff). In Experiment 2 (*right*), startle stimuli were a 118-dB 3500-Hz tone burst in the Tone group, a 1.5-psi puff of air in the Low-Puff group, and a 3-psi puff of air in the High-Puff group. Control amplitudes were 3.8 mm (Tone), 3.3 mm (Low Puff), and 5.7 mm (High Puff).

lus. After the Tone and Puff groups were completed, it became clear that the 3500-Hz tone produced a much weaker startle response than did the 3-psi puff. Since tone intensity could not be increased, a new "Low Puff" group was completed using a 1.5-psi air puff that evoked blink amplitudes comparable to those in the Tone group.

The right panel of Figure 4.1 shows effects of lead stimulus intensity on blink change scores in all three groups. Although High-Puff data are included, only Tone and Low-Puff groups were statistically compared. Tone and Low-Puff groups showed similar nonmonotonic effects of lead stimulus intensity, reflected in significant quadratic trends. In contrast to Experiment 1, the Tone group no longer showed the pronounced inhibitory effect at 95 dB, suggesting that the inhibitory effect observed in Experiment 1 was associated with frequency-specific masking. Only the High-Puff group showed a linear trend over intensities, reflecting the pronounced drop at 95 dB in that group.

Taken together, Putnam's (1975) first two experiments demonstrate (1) that an auditory lead stimulus can have both facilitatory and inhibitory effects on startle responsivity at long lead intervals; (2) that, over a 60-dB range of lead stimulus intensities, startle responsivity can be seen to vary both linearly (as in the High-Puff group) and curvilinearly (as in Low-Puff and Tone groups) with stimulus intensity; (3) that under appropriate conditions auditory-specific mechanisms such as masking and the acoustic reflex can contribute to the inhibitory effect on acoustic startle at high lead stimulus intensities; and (4) that both wings of the curvilinear function can be obtained under inter- as well as intramodal stimulus conditions, thus requiring a modality nonspecific mechanism. Whereas most of these findings replicated animal work, some noteworthy differences are discussed below.

For instance, the patterns of intensity effects in Putnam's crossmodal (High- and Low-Puff) groups are somewhat at odds with the intramodal findings of Davis (1974b) concerning the inflection point of the inverted-U curve. In experiments on rat acoustic startle, Davis showed that the louder the startle tone, the greater the background noise level required to produce an inhibitory downturn in the nonmonotonic function relating background intensity to startle responsivity. In Experiment 2, Davis found that the inflection point always occurred at a signal-to-noise ratio of 50 dB – that is, at a difference of 50 dB between startle and background stimulus intensities. He interpreted this as support for the dual process theory of Ison and his colleagues, with arousal responsible for the ascending wing but a decreasing signal-to-noise ratio producing the descending wing. Interestingly, the inflection point shifted downward not only with decreasing startle stimulus intensity but also with habituation to the startle stimulus.

Davis and Gendelman (1977) reported similar results, and also found that decerebrate rats showed only an inhibitory effect of increasing lead stimulus intensity, leading them to conclude that the facilitatory effect of background noise requires brain areas above the midbrain.

A second departure from the Davis (1974b) finding that the inflection point of the inverted-U function is positively related to startle stimulus potency occurred in Putnam's (1975) High- and Low-Puff groups. The High-Puff group did not show a later inflection point, in spite of the stronger startle stimulus and larger blink amplitudes. Presumably, Davis's intramodal findings can be accounted for by assuming that auditory masking was primarily responsible for the decremental wing, a finding consistent with the close relationship between inflection point and signal-to-noise ratio. When masking and other intramodal inhibitory effects are eliminated, as in a crossmodal design, the terminal descending wing still obtains but is no longer attributable to a decreasing signal-to-noise ratio.

3. Temporal Factors: Effects of Lead Interval and Lead Stimulus Duration

We have seen that lead stimuli of moderate intensity facilitate the amplitude of a subsequent startle response. To what extent does this facilitatory effect vary with the temporal interval between lead and startle stimulus onsets? Are there minimum and maximum lead intervals outside of which facilitation does not occur? Another important temporal factor concerns lead stimulus duration: To what extent does the facilitatory effect of lead stimulation require a continuous, as opposed to a discrete, lead stimulus?

3.1. Animal Studies

Hoffman and Wible (1969) investigated the temporal parameters of the lead stimulus facilitation effect by presenting both discrete (20-msec) and continuous 75-dB lead stimuli at seven lead intervals, ranging from 100 to 6400 msec. Because continuous lead stimuli produced significant and asymptotic facilitation by 1600 msec, Hoffman and Wible concluded that "no more than 2000 msec of exposure to the background is adequate to generate a full facilitation effect" (p. 9). Their discrete lead stimuli produced a parallel interval by amplitude function, characterized by significant inhibition at the shortest lead intervals (100, 200, 400, and 800 msec) that dissipated by 3200 msec. Because the difference between startle amplitude following continuous versus discrete lead stimuli was essentially constant across lead intervals, Hoffman and Wible speculated that as little as 100 msec of lead stimulation prior to an intense stimulus was sufficient for the full facilitation effect. In other words, "short lead" interval prepulse inhibition and "long lead" interval facilitation co-occur over a relatively wide range of lead intervals, with the net result depending on the relative strengths of the two processes. Hoffman argued that what appears to be a growth over time in the facilitation effect is actually the result of dissipation of the short lead interval inhibitory effect.

3.2. Human Studies

As already noted, research in Graham's lab in the early 1970s aimed to replicate Hoffman and Wible's (1969) results in humans. In one of these studies (Graham, Putnam, & Leavitt, 1975), discrete (20-msec) and continuous lead stimuli were presented at lead intervals of 200, 800, 1400, and 2000 msec. The startle reflex elicited by an auditory stimulus was inhibited for the 200-msec condition, but blinks elicited in the 800-msec condition did not differ from those in control (i.e., no lead stimulus) trials. However, facilitation was observed with lead times of 1400 and 2000 msec. This facilitation was more pronounced for the continuous lead stimuli, but did occur for discrete lead stimuli as well – the only result that differed from the previous animal findings. The fact that anticipatory heart rate (HR) deceleration preceded the startle stimuli at long lead intervals in both discrete and continuous conditions suggested that an attention/orienting process contributed to the facilitated startle response in humans. Graham et al. proposed that the greater facilitation in the continuous condition reflected the combined attentional and sustained lead stimulus effects.

Several studies conducted in Graham's lab (reported in Graham, 1975) attempted to shed light on the factors responsible for facilitation following discrete lead stimuli. These studies suggested that when discrete lead stimuli do produce startle facilitation, the paradigm usually involves temporal or event uncertainty, or a specific task demand, that leads to an anticipatory attentional response, as reflected in HR deceleration.

In the Putnam (1975) Tone and Puff studies described earlier, anticipatory HR deceleration was frequently seen during the 2.6-s lead interval. Although the magnitude of this deceleration did not appear systematically related to the pattern of blink effects, its presence suggested that anticipatory attentional processes might have been a contributing factor. Putnam hypothesized that the temporal proximity of lead and startle stimulus onsets contributed to the signal quality of the lead stimulus and thus to its facilitory effect seen in Experiments 1 and 2. Of course, it was already clear from animal studies that the facilitatory effect of background noise did not require an explicit lead stimulus (i.e., one that could serve as a signal for the upcoming startle stimulus). Hoffman, Marsh, and Stein (1969), for instance, had demonstrated startle facilitation after six hours of prior background noise, and Davis (1974a) had shown that sensitization effects on startle can continue to build after more than 30 min of exposure to background noise.

Beyond the dynamogenic effects of the continuous lead stimulus, however, one aspect of Putnam's results suggested that the signal quality of lead stimulus onset may have contributed to the startle facilitation. The 35-dB lead stimulus in Experiment 2 produced significant facilitation of tone startle, even though it afforded only a negligible increase in overall sound energy above the continuous white-noise background. It seemed unlikely that the arousal increment occasioned by the small intensity increase per se could have produced this facilitation. A more plausible hypothesis was that the clearly audible onset of the 35-dB stimulus initiated a facilitatory process by virtue of its signal quality. If so, then large increases in the time interval between lead and startle stimulus onsets should reduce this facilitatory effect by reducing the signal value of lead stimulus onset. At the same time, any anticipatory component in Experiment 2 HR should become apparent when contrasted with HR responses to physically identical lead stimuli with little or no signal value.

Putnam's third experiment was identical to the Tone group of Experiment 2, except that the interval between lead and startle stimulus onsets was increased from a constant 2.6 s to a variable 15–25 s. This change was expected to reduce the signal value of lead stimulus onset, and an examination of HR responses during the lead interval suggests that it did. The two experiments showed similar decelerations during the initial second of lead stimulation, but Experiment 3 showed a subsequent acceleration that contrasted sharply with the continued deceleration in Experiment 2. Furthermore, Experiment 3 HR responses showed no evidence of anticipatory deceleration late in the 15- to 25-s lead interval, suggesting that lead stimuli in that experiment lacked the signal value they possessed in the earlier experiments and did not give rise to the same preparatory processes.

Figure 4.2 depicts blink change data for the Tone groups of Experiments 2 and 3. Although startle blink in both groups showed similar curvilinear functions, blink change scores in Experiment 3 were significantly depressed relative to those in Experiment 2. Thus although physical parameters of lead stimuli in the two groups were identical during this period, their meaning or "signal significance" differed. The additional facilitatory effect seen in the Experiment 2 Tone group may be attributable to the signal value of lead stimulus onset which, in turn, was affected by the lead interval. The moderate (2.6 s) lead intervals in Experiments 1 and 2 may have led subjects to notice the S1–S2 contingency, and to anticipate onset of the startle stimulus, to a much greater extent than did the long and variable (15–25 s) lead intervals of Experiment 3. The resulting difference in preparation, or in expectancy, was reflected in significant anticipatory deceleration and greater startle facilitation in the first two experiments than in the third.

4. Attentional Effects

4.1. Cardiac Deceleration and Long Lead Interval Effects

By 1975, numerous studies from Graham's laboratory, including Putnam's (1975), supported a link between anticipatory attention, reflected in HR

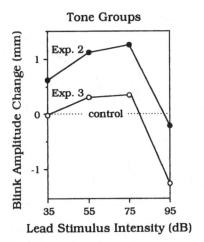

Figure 4.2. Startle blink amplitude change in the Tone groups of Experiments 2 and 3 (Putnam, 1975) as a function of intensity of the narrow-band acoustic lead stimulus. The lead interval was a constant 2.6 s in Experiment 2 but a variable 15–25 s in Experiment 3. Startle stimuli were 118-dB 3500-Hz tone bursts.

deceleration, and startle facilitation. And whereas short lead interval inhibition in human subjects appeared to follow the same pattern in lower animals (see Chapter 3), long lead interval facilitation effects in humans appeared to reflect a different process from infrahumans. Graham (1975), in summarizing research from her laboratory, suggested that an orienting response, indicated by HR deceleration, was necessary to produce startle facilitation. Viewing startle and orienting as mutually inhibitory response systems, she reasoned that "the termination of orienting [by startle stimulus onset] results in a rapid rebound of physiological effects which leads to blink facilitation" (p. 246).

To further investigate the link between cardiac deceleration and startle facilitation, Putnam and her students conducted four experiments at Columbia University in which the lead interval was varied within subjects over a relatively wide range (Putnam, Butler, & Anthony, 1978; see also Anthony, 1985, and Putnam, 1990). Lead interval predictability (varied or fixed within blocks), lead stimulus duration (continuous or discrete), and lead stimulus intensity (loud or soft, i.e., 75 or 50 dB) were varied between groups. Experiment VCL (Variable Continuous Loud) served as the comparison group for the others. Startling tone bursts (2000 Hz, 20 msec, 113 dB) were presented without warning on the ten control trials, but preceded by a "continuous loud" (75 dB) auditory stimulus of 2-, 4-, 8-, or 16-s duration on the 40 lead stimulation trials. Narrow-band white noise with gradual (100 msec) rise/fall times

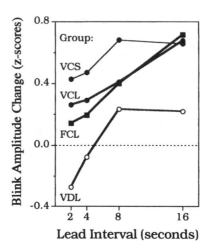

Figure 4.3. Differences from control in z-scored blink amplitudes at four lead intervals in each of the four experiments in which the timing (variable vs. fixed), intensity (loud vs. soft), and duration (continuous vs. discrete) of lead stimuli were varied. Lead stimuli in the four groups were either variable continuous soft (VCS), variable continuous loud (VCL), fixed continuous loud (FCL), or variable discrete loud (VDL).

served as the lead stimulus. Lead interval duration was varied from trial to trial, so that subjects could not predict precisely when the burst would occur. As seen in Figure 4.3, startle amplitude change in Experiment VCL increased linearly with lead interval. HR data showed significant deceleration by 6 s into the longer warning intervals, and this deceleration was maintained until a tone burst occurred. Furthermore, this deceleration in HR was associated with facilitation of eyeblink startle so that the longer the warning interval, the larger the deceleration and the larger the startle blink (see Putnam, 1990, Fig. 8.3).

Experiments FCL (Fixed Continuous Loud), VCS (Variable Continuous Soft), and VDL (Variable Discrete Loud) each varied one feature of the first experiment to determine effects of the timing (variable vs. fixed), intensity (loud vs. soft), and duration (continuous vs. discrete) of lead stimuli on anticipatory HR changes and startle blink. These studies were aimed at charting the growth of startle facilitation, and accompanying HR deceleration, with increasing lead interval and at comparing facilitation effects of lead stimuli differing in intensity and in duration to assess both dynamogenic and associative (trace-delay) effects of lead stimuli. Thus, the goal of these studies was to trace the growth of attentional effects on blink, reflected in HR deceleration, as they combined with the facilitatory effect of the long duration, continuous lead stimulus.

As seen in Figure 4.3, all four experiments showed increased startle blink amplitudes with increasing lead intervals, except in the case of the softer lead stimulus (VCS). These increases in reflex strength cannot be ascribed solely to the dynamogenic properties of the lead stimuli, given the significant effects of lead interval with a discrete lead stimulus (VDL). However, blink amplitude continued to grow as lead interval was increased from 8 to 16 s only in the two groups receiving continuous loud lead stimuli (VCL and FCL). This difference between continuous and discrete lead stimuli, and the overall depression of change scores in VDL, may reflect both dynamogenic effects of the sustained lead stimuli and weaker signal value of the discrete (trace) lead stimulus.

Recently, Sollers and Hackley (1997) reported effects of fixed and variable foreperiods – 1.5, 3, and 6 s – similar to those obtained in the four Putnam lab experiments. Using only discrete (200 msec) visual lead stimuli, Sollers and Hackley had subjects in one experiment silently count rare auditory target stimuli that were embedded in acoustic startle stimuli on 20 percent of trials. In a second experiment, subjects responded with a rapid hand-grip response to startle stimulus onset. Both experiments employed discrete (200 msec) visual lead stimuli, and as in Experiment VDL above, found increasing blink magnitude with increasing lead interval. Sollers and Hackley proposed a new "need to blink" mechanism to account for their effects of lead interval on forewarned startle. Briefly, their hypothesis states that subjects withhold blinking during the lead interval, producing a need to blink with the potential for facilitating startle blink; the longer the lead interval, the longer the suppression of blinking and the greater the need to blink.

The Sollers and Hackley need-to-blink hypothesis is reminiscent of the earlier rebound hypothesis offered by Graham (1975). However, while agreeing with Graham that lead stimuli can engage orienting-attentional processes, Anthony (1985) and Putnam (1990) interpreted the startle facilitation they had observed at the end of long lead (expectant-attentional) intervals not as the result of rebound from just-terminated orienting, but as a result of facilitation of sensory processing during orienting that was maintained. Bohlin and Graham (1977) tested the rebound hypothesis in two experiments where subjects were required to judge startle stimulus duration in a forewarned startle paradigm. This manipulation was intended to prevent the termination of anticipatory orienting at onset of the startle stimulus. Because blink facilitation still occurred under these conditions, Bohlin and Graham rejected the rebound hypothesis. It is not clear from their HR data, however, that the judgment task did prolong orienting, leaving open the possibility that rebound from orienting was responsible for the observed facilitation of startle. It therefore remained to be demonstrated whether startle facilitation was possible during an interval in which orienting was clearly maintained beyond the point of startle evocation. The startle probe paradigm described in the next section addressed this issue.

4.2. Selective Attention Effects

Anthony, Butler, and Putnam (1978) devised a new probe paradigm to more closely examine the modification of startle reflexes evoked during long lead intervals accompanied by anticipatory HR deceleration. Altogether, seven different probe experiments were completed using a 6-s continuous lead stimulus within which acoustic startle probes were presented at 2, 3, 4, 5, or 5.5 s following onset, or at a control point between trials (see Putnam, 1990, Fig. 8.4). The first five studies employed paradigms in which anticipatory deceleration was known to occur – either forewarned reaction time tasks (Experiments 1–3 and 5) or the forewarned startle paradigm (Experiment 4). Preparatory intervals of 6 s allowed examination of the anticipatory HR response independent of any deceleration evoked by the lead stimulus. By eliciting startle during periods of anticipatory deceleration, the probe procedure provided a means of comparing the time course of startle blink effects during the lead interval with that of the cardiac response. In addition, the probe procedure provided another test of Graham's rebound hypothesis.

A major question addressed by these experiments was whether the process reflected in anticipatory HR deceleration is a unitary one with uniform effects on startle blink. The Laceys proposed that HR deceleration reflects motivated attention directed toward external events (e.g., Lacey, Kagan, Lacey, & Moss, 1963). If their interpretation of anticipatory deceleration is correct, then does this HR response signify a unitary process of expectant attention whose effects on startle are always facilitatory? Alternatively, might not the preparatory process accompanying cardiac deceleration be characterized by varying degrees of afferent tuning, depending on task demands and subject motivation and attentional mobility? If so, might it sometimes be focused on a particular input channel, in which case might not startle be inhibited if the reflex-eliciting stimulus is outside of the attended channel?

To address these questions, effects of selective attention on startle modulation were assessed in tasks demanding discrimination or detection in a sensory modality congruent with (Experiments 4 and 7) or orthogonal to (Experiments 1–3, 5, and 6) that of the acoustic startle stimulus. Startle blink results are summarized in Figure 4.4 (adapted from Putnam, 1990). The four experiments on the left panel involved either a voluntary (RT) or involuntary (startle) behavioral response at the end of the 6-s warning interval, whereas those

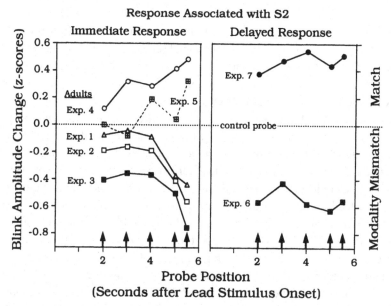

Figure 4.4. Blink amplitude change to startle probes in six adult and one child experiment. Arrows mark the positions at which acoustic startle probes (20 msec, 113 dBA, 2000 Hz tone bursts) were presented within 6-s lead intervals. Experiments involved immediate (*left*) or delayed (*right*) behavioral responses to events (S2) that terminated the lead interval and that either matched or mismatched the modality of the acoustic startle probe. In Experiments 1, 2, 3, and 5, subjects performed a speeded reaction time task that required attending to the offset of a continuous 6-s lead stimulus that was either visual (Experiment 1) or vibrotactile (Experiments 2, 3, and 5). In Experiment 4, the vibrotactile lead stimulus was followed after 6 s by an acoustic startle stimulus (50 msec, 1250 Hz, 108 dBA) more salient than the probes. Experiments 6 and 7 required a difficult vibrotactile or auditory discrimination, respectively. In the six adult experiments, probe startle was facilitated (positive change scores) when probe and S2 modalities matched, but was inhibited when they did not. However, children (Experiment 5) showed facilitated startle even though probe and S2 modalities did not match.

on the right required a difficult perceptual discrimination after 6 s, with a verbal response 6 s later. In both immediate and delayed response tasks, adult studies showed that when the salient anticipated event was not in the same modality as the acoustic startle stimulus, probe startle was inhibited rather than facilitated. These findings suggest that selective attention effects can override continuous lead stimulus facilitative effects.

Interestingly, 5-year-old children did not show any inhibitory effect of modality mismatch (Anthony & Putnam, 1985). Performing the same speeded RT task as did adults in Experiment 3, children showed increasing facilitation toward the end of the lead interval. Anthony and Putnam interpreted these data as evidence that attentional set was more diffuse in the child than in the adult subjects. Conceivably, more favorable testing conditions could lead to a more selective attentional set in children, and less favorable ones could lead to a more diffuse set in adults.

Modality match/mismatch effects on startle modification have been demonstrated in several other studies as well, indicating facilitation of startle magnitude when a lead stimulus is in the same modality as the startle stimulus (Bohlin & Graham, 1977; Bohlin, Graham, Silverstein, & Hackley, 1981; Hackley & Graham, 1983), and more attenuation when attention is directed toward a lead stimulus in a different modality from that of the startle stimulus (Silverstein, Graham, & Bohlin, 1981; Anthony, 1985). In addition, Anthony and Graham (1983, 1985) found support for their hypothesis that these effects are enhanced when the lead stimuli are highly interesting. "Interesting" lead stimuli included slides of faces of smiling young adults and recorded segments of music box tines, whereas the "dull" lead stimuli consisted of blank slides and the repetition of a 1000-Hz tone. Visual or acoustic startle probes were presented using 4000-ms lead intervals. As expected, blink magnitude was greater when the modality of the lead and startle stimuli matched than when they mismatched, but more matched modality facilitation and more mismatched modality attenuation occurred for the interesting stimuli. These effects were found for both adults and infants.

More recently, Filion, Dawson, and Schell (1993) used a paradigm that does not involve modality matching/mismatching to manipulate attention in studies of startle modification. Employing a modified version of the selective attention-orienting task of Dawson, Filion, and Schell (1989), subjects were instructed to attend high- or low-pitched tones by counting them, but to ignore low- or high-pitched tones. These to-be-attended and to-be-ignored tones thus served as the lead stimuli for acoustic startle stimuli presented at short and long lead intervals. Especially relevant to this chapter, Filion et al. found that the instruction to attend to the lead stimulus resulted in significant facilitation of blink magnitude at a lead interval of 2000 ms. This finding was subsequently replicated in another startle modification study (Filion, Dawson, & Schell, 1994), which included secondary reaction time to also index attentional processing. In that study, the attended tones were associated with greater blink facilitation at the 2000-ms lead interval, but also larger skin conductance responses (an indicator of orienting) and greater reaction time slowing, demonstrating convergent validity for the attentional manipulation. Interestingly, schizophrenic patients do not evidence this attentional modification of startle at long lead intervals, even for that subgroup of patients who perform the task as well as matched controls (Dawson, Hazlett, Filion, Nuechterlein, & Schell, 1993).

5. Affective Modification of Startle and Its Relation to Attention

Much of this chapter has been concerned with attentional effects on startle modification, but in the last two decades investigations of the affective modification of startle, especially at long lead intervals, have become especially prominent. We merely highlight some of this research here, but refer the reader to Chapter 8 for a more comprehensive review.

5.1. Fear Conditioning

When a lead stimulus that has been previously paired with shock is followed by a startle probe, blink magnitude is facilitated in rats (Brown et al., 1951). This effect has been replicated many times, including with human participants (e.g., Spence & Runquist, 1958; Ross, 1961; Davis & Astrachan, 1978; Davis, 1986). Moreover, fear-potentiated startle has been demonstrated even while human subjects simply anticipate aversive stimuli (Grillon, Ameli, Woods, Merikangas, & Davis, 1991; Grillon & Davis, 1995; Hamm, Greenwald, Bradley, & Lang, 1993).

For example, Grillon and Davis (1995), in an investigation of the laterality effects of startle stimuli, presented one of two lights at the beginning of a 60-s period that signaled either that shocks were about to be administered (threat condition) or that no shock would be (safe condition). In actuality, no shocks were ever presented. Startle probes were delivered every 17–23 s, and were presented either monaurally to the left or right ear or binaurally. As predicted, startle magnitude was greater and onset latency was decreased in the threat conditions than during the safe conditions. Moreover, the startle response to the right ear stimulation was particularly enhanced by threat. Grillon and Davis suggested that this lateralization effect might result from a greater involvement of the left hemisphere, and particularly the left amygdala, during shock anticipation (see Chapter 5 for a review of the neural circuitry involved in the affective modification of startle). Research also indicates that some phobics show similar fear potentiation of startle at long lead intervals when they view their feared objects (de Jong, Merckelbach, & Arntz, 1991; Vrana, Constantine, & Westman, 1992; Hamm, Cuthbert, Globisch, & Vaitl, 1997).

5.2. Affective Modification of Startle

In several studies Lang and his colleagues have demonstrated that the effects of conditioned fear modification of startle can be more broadly conceptualized in terms of the affective valence of lead stimuli (Lang, Bradley, & Cuthbert, 1990; Lang, 1995; see also Chapter 8). For example, while subjects view affect-laden pictures (e.g., an attractive nude, a gunshot victim), startle probes are presented at varying lead intervals. Perhaps the most robust finding is that the amplitudes of blinks elicited during affectively negative lead stimuli are greater than when they are neutral or positive, especially at long lead intervals (Vrana, Spence, & Lang, 1988; Bradley, Cuthbert, & Lang, 1993; Vanman, Boehmelt, Dawson, & Schell, 1996). This startle modification effect is said to reflect an "affect match," in which a reflex with a negative valence is enhanced during a negatively valenced lead stimulus, but diminished during a positively valenced one (Lang, 1995). Such affective modification, however, may occur only when the lead stimulus is sufficiently arousing (Cuthbert, Bradley, & Lang, 1996).

Further, this affective modification of startle is not believed to be determined by simple attention or probe modality effects (Lang et al., 1990). Bradley, Cuthbert and Lang (1990) tested this notion by using long lead intervals (2500–5500 msec) while subjects viewed positive, neutral, or negative slides. The startle stimulus either matched the lead stimulus modality (i.e., visual) or did not (i.e., acoustic). Again, the previously demonstrated effects of affect occurred, but the modality-specific effects, which might be hypothesized based on the studies reviewed in Section 4.1, did not. Bradley et al. concluded that the primary determinant of startle modification at long lead intervals is the emotional valence of the lead stimulus. Subsequently, Bradley et al. (1993) utilized the picture-viewing paradigm with acoustic startle stimuli to explicate further the time course of attention and affect effects on startle, and the results appeared to support their hypothesis that, at least in that context (viewing affect-laden pictures), attentional effects are secondary to emotional modification of startle at long (greater than 800 msec) lead intervals.

5.3. Affective versus Attentional Modification of Startle

The conclusions of Bradley et al. (1990) and Bradley et al. (1993) appeared to be inconsistent with what was already established as early as the 1970s: that attentional modification of startle can occur at long lead intervals. Vanman et al. (1996) reasoned that Bradley et al.'s (1993) failure to find an attentional effect might be due to the way they defined attention in terms of the intrinsic attention-attracting properties of the slides (the positive and negative ones had been previously rated similarly high in arousal, whereas the neutral slides had been rated low). Vanman et al. attempted to reconcile this apparent inconsistency with the attention-modification literature by combining the picture-viewing methodology with the attentional instructional manipulation used by Filion et al. (1993). In Experiment 1, subjects viewed many of the same affectively positive or negative pictures used by Bradley et al. (1993), but were instructed via a warning cue to attend to the duration of half of the slides, and to ignore the other half. Startle probes were presented at lead intervals of 250, 750, 2450, and 4450 msec. Affective modification of blink occurred (i.e., more facilitation for the negative slides) for the two long lead interval conditions, but attentional modification also occurred (i.e., more facilitation for the to-be-attended slides). However, in Experiment 2, when subjects were explicitly instructed to attend to the *valence* of the slide (e.g., "attend to the duration of the positive pictures, and ignore the negative ones"), only affective modification of startle occurred at the long lead interval. Thus, Vanman et al. concluded that, during the picture-viewing paradigm, both affective and attentional modification of startle can occur at long lead intervals, but the effects depend on the specific task requirements.

Similarly, Lipp and Siddle (see Chapter 15) have attempted to disentangle attentional and emotional effects on startle modification as well. Lipp, Siddle, and Dall (1997, Experiment 1) manipulated the modality of the lead stimulus (acoustic vs. visual) and used acoustic startle probes in aversive differential conditioning. The reinforced conditioned stimulus (CS+; a tone or picture) predicted the occurrence of an aversive unconditioned stimulus (shock), whereas the nonreinforced conditioned stimulus (CS−; a different tone or picture) predicted its absence. During the presentation of the lead stimuli, startle probes were presented at 3.5- or 7-s lead intervals. Greater blink magnitude facilitation during CS+ than during CS− was found only if the CSs were visual, a finding inconsistent with modality-specific attentional accounts of startle modification, which would predict greater facilitation when the modalities of lead and probe stimuli match. However, in Experiment 2, when the attentional instruction manipulation of Filion et al. (1993) was used with the same lead stimuli as Experiment 1, startle probes during the presentation of to-be-attended stimuli elicited more magnitude facilitation than did the to-be-ignored stimuli, regardless of modality. A follow-up set of studies (Lipp, Siddle, & Dall, 1998) replicated and extended these findings by demonstrating that, regardless of stimulus modality (acoustic, visual, and tactile), startle magnitude facilitation and latency shortening were greater for the CS+ (i.e., signaling shock) than for the CS− lead stimuli. Further, in separate studies these same lead stimuli also served as to-be-attended or to-be-ignored stimuli in a nonaversive discrimination task. Replicating previous results (i.e., Filion et al., 1993), to-be-attended visual and auditory lead stimuli produced greater startle facilitation than did to-be-ignored lead stimuli, for both stimulus modalities.

On the basis of this series of studies, Lipp et al. (1998) concluded that, whereas a modality-specific account of attention effects on startle was not supported by their results, neither was an emotion-based account. That is, similar results were obtained whether an identical lead stimulus signaled the presence or absence of shock (as in a fear conditioning study), or was merely a stimulus to be attended or ignored (as in the Filion et al., 1993, study). It is thus difficult to explain the latter result using the emotion account given for fear-potentiated startle. Lipp et al. argued that the development of a modality-nonspecific attentional account of startle modification would offer a more parsimonious explanation of both aversive differential (i.e., fear) conditioning and discrimination (i.e., attentional instruction) task effects.

6. Conclusion

In this chapter we have reviewed a few of the many paradigms, variables, and theoretical issues that have been, and will continue to be, important to research on the effects of lead stimuli at long lead intervals on startle modification. It is clear, for example, that the issue about the relative roles of attention and affect at long lead intervals needs more clarification. Perhaps this and other "controversies" will be aided by a greater understanding of the underlying neuronal circuits involved in long (and short) lead startle modification. However, at this time, it also seems just as important (if not more so) to develop a comprehensive theory of startle modification that fully accounts for the effects of lead stimulus parameters (duration, intensity, etc.), attention, modality, arousal, and emotion.

PART II

Physiological Mediation of Startle Modification

CHAPTER FIVE

Neurophysiology and Neuropharmacology of Startle and Its Affective Modulation

MICHAEL DAVIS, DAVID L. WALKER, AND
YOUNGLIM LEE

ABSTRACT

This chapter describes the neural pathways involved in the acoustic startle reflex itself and those involved in modification of startle by fear and stress. In the rat, the primary acoustic startle pathway probably involves three synapses onto (1) cochlear root neurons, (2) neurons in the nucleus reticularis pontis caudalis, and (3) motoneurons in the facial motor nucleus (pinna reflex) or spinal cord (whole body startle). The excitatory amino acid glutamate may well mediate startle at each of the three central synapses along the acoustic startle pathway. Startle can be potentiated by eliciting the reflex in the presence of a cue that has previously been paired with shock. This effect is blocked by chemical lesions or chemical inactivation of the amygdala. Very high levels of fear may fail to lead to increased startle because of activation of a brain area (the periacqueductal gray) which produces active escape behavior incompatible with startle. Startle also can be increased by sustained exposure to bright light or intraventricular administration of the stress peptide corticotropin-releasing hormone. These effects depend on a brain area called the bed nucleus of the stria terminalis. These results suggest that different brain areas may be involved in short-term increases in startle, akin to stimulus-specific fear, versus longer-lasting increases in startle, akin to anxiety.

1. Introduction

A major advantage of using the acoustic startle reflex to study behavior is that the startle reflex itself has an extraordinarily short latency (e.g., in rats, 8 msec measured electromyographically in the hind leg). This means that it must be mediated by a simple neural pathway. If one could determine the neural path-

Michael E. Dawson, Anne M. Schell, and Andreas H. Böhmelt, Eds. *Startle modification: Implications for neuroscience, cognitive science, and clinical science.* Copyright © 1999 Cambridge University Press. Printed in the United States of America. All rights reserved.

way that actually mediated the acoustic startle response, this would provide an anatomical framework for understanding how this behavior could be modified by a variety of treatments. Hence, we felt that it was critical to try to determine what this pathway was.

2. The Primary Acoustic Pathway

In 1982, our laboratory proposed that acoustic startle was mediated by four synapses, three in the brain stem (the ventral cochlear nucleus, an area just medial and ventral to the ventral nucleus of the lateral lemniscus, and the nucleus reticularis pontis caudalis) and one synapse onto motoneurons in the spinal cord (Davis, Gendelman, Tischler, & Gendelman, 1982). Electrolytic lesions of these nuclei eliminated acoustic startle and single pulse electrical stimulation of these nuclei elicited startle-like responses with a progressively shorter latency as the electrode was moved farther down the startle pathway.

2.1. New Evidence Concerning the Role of the Area around the Ventral Nucleus of the Lateral Lemniscus in Acoustic Startle

Because electrolytic lesions of the area just medial and ventral to the ventral nucleus of the lateral lemniscus eliminated the acoustic startle reflex, we concluded that this area must be part of a primary acoustic startle pathway (Davis et al., 1982). When we did the initial lesion work on this project, techniques were not yet available to selectively destroy cells versus cells plus fibers passing through the area of the lesion. Using newly developed techniques to accomplish this, we found that N-methyl-D-aspartate (NMDA)-induced lesions of the ventral nucleus of the lateral lemniscus or the area just ventral and medial to it did not affect startle (Lee, Lopez, Meloni, & Davis, 1996), whereas NMDA-induced lesions of cell bodies in the nucleus reticularis pontis caudalis completely eliminated startle.

2.2. A Direct Projection from Cochlear Root Neurons to the Nucleus Reticularis Pontis Caudalis

These new data questioned the importance of the area around the ventral nucleus of the lateral lemniscus in mediating the acoustic startle reflex, even though this area is known to receive direct auditory input. On the other hand, all data still supported the critical importance of the nucleus reticularis pontis caudalis in the acoustic startle reflex. However, until very recently, it has been unclear how auditory information gets to this traditionally nonauditory part of the brain stem. In 1962, Harrison and Warr described a small group (about 20 on each side) of very large cells (35 μm in diameter) embedded in the cochlear nerve in rodents, later termed "cochlear root neurons" (Merchan, Collia, Lopez, & Saldana, 1988). These neurons receive direct input from the cochlea (Lopez, Merchan, Bajo, & Saldana, 1993) and send thick axons through the trapezoid body directly to an area just medial and ventral to the lateral lemniscus and continue on up to the deep layers of the superior colliculus. However, they give off thick axon collaterals that terminate directly in the nucleus reticularis pontis caudalis (Lopez et al., 1993; Lingenhohl & Friauf, 1994) onto cells that then project to motoneurons in the spinal cord (Lingenhohl & Friauf, 1994) and brain stem (Meloni & Davis, 1992).

2.3. Effects of Kainic Acid-Induced Lesions of Cochlear Root Neurons on Acoustic Startle

Bilateral kainic acid-induced lesions of the cochlear root neurons essentially eliminated both whole-body acoustic startle and the pinna reflex in rats (Lee et al., 1996). In animals with only unilateral cochlear root neuron damage there was a preferential loss of the ipsilateral pinna reflex, and a partial decrease in whole-body startle. Although damage to the auditory root, where the cochlear root neurons reside, has not been fully ruled out, other tests indicated that these animals could clearly orient to auditory stimuli (e.g., suppression of licking) and had normal compound action potentials recorded from the cochlear nucleus (Lee et al., 1996).

2.4. Inputs to the Facial Motor Nucleus from the Nucleus Reticularis Pontis Caudalis: Implications for Pinna and Eyeblink Reflexes

Previous studies showed that the pinna component of the startle reflex in the rat (a rapid backward movement of the pinna, analogous to the eyeblink component of startle in humans) showed plasticity similar to that of whole-body startle (Cassella & Davis, 1986). The motor component of the pinna reflex is mediated by the interscultularis muscle, which is innervated by the posterior auricular branch of the facial motor nerve (Semba & Egger, 1986), the motoneurons of which are located exclusively in the ventral medial division of the facial motor nucleus. These neurons were found to be innervated by three major contralateral areas: (1) the ventral part of the nucleus reticularis pontis caudalis, (2) the ventrolateral tegmental nucleus, and (3) the intermediate nucleus of the lateral lemniscus and paralemniscal zone (Meloni & Davis, 1992). However, only electrolytic lesions of either the ventral medial division of the facial motor nucleus or the nucleus reticularis pontis caudalis eliminated the pinna reflex.

Hence, we now believe that the acoustic startle pathway may be simpler than we had originally thought (Fig. 5.1), consisting of only three synapses onto (1) cochlear root neurons, (2) neurons in the nucleus reticularis pontis caudalis, and (3) motoneurons in the facial motor nucleus (pinna reflex) or spinal cord (whole body startle).

3. Transmitters of the Primary Startle Pathway

3.1. Auditory Nerve to Cochlear Root Neuron Synapse

At the present time we do not have any direct data on the identity of the neurotransmitter that may mediate startle at this level. Preliminary experiments suggest it may be glutamate acting on non-NMDA receptors because local infusion of non-NMDA antagonists in the vicinity of the cochlear root neurons depressed startle whereas local infusion of NMDA antagonists did not (Miserendino & Davis, 1988).

3.2. Cochlear Root Neuron to Reticulospinal Neuron Synapse

Glutamate acting on both NMDA and non-NMDA receptors may well be the neurotransmitter that mediates startle at the level of the nucleus reticularis pontis caudalis. Local infusion in rats chronically implanted with bilateral cannulas aimed at the nucleus reticularis pontis caudalis of either NMDA and non-NMDA antagonists significantly reduced startle amplitude by as much as 70–80% (Miserendino & Davis, 1993). Although high doses of NMDA and non-NMDA antagonists did not completely eliminate startle, as would be expected if excitatory amino acids actually mediated startle at the nucleus reticularis pontis caudalis, this is probably because the infusions were restricted to the part of the nucleus reticularis pontis caudalis involved in the hindlimb components of startle, thus sparing forelimb and neck movements that we know also contribute to cage displacement. Further studies using electromyographic (EMG) recordings in the hind legs will be necessary to evaluate this possibility.

3.3. Reticulospinal Neurons to Motor Neuron Synapse

Infusion into the subarachnoid space of the spinal cord to allow drugs to diffuse in the vicinity of spinal motoneurons (intrathecal infusion) of NMDA and non-NMDA antagonists each reduced the amplitude of the whole-body startle reflex in a dose-dependent manner (Boulis, Kehne, Miserendino, & Davis, 1990). Over the dose ranges employed, both drugs were roughly equipotent

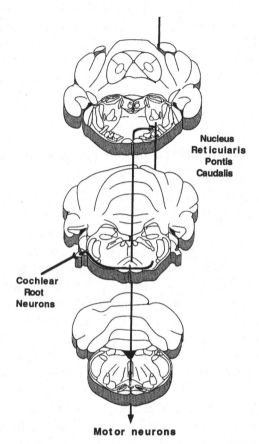

Figure 5.1. Schematic diagram of a primary acoustic startle pathway. Auditory nerve fibers synapse onto cochlear root neurons embedded in the auditory nerve. Axons from these cells project through the ventral acoustic stria and send projections to the nucleus reticularis pontis caudalis (PnC). Projections of cells in the PnC form the reticulospinal tract, which make monosynaptic and polysynaptic synapses in the spinal cord. Although not shown, these cells also project to the facial motor nucleus in areas critical for the pinna component of startle in rats and probably the eyeblink component of startle in humans. Lesions of cochlear root neurons, the ventral acoustic stria, the PnC, or reticulospinal tract eliminate the acoustic startle response. (From Lee et al., 1996.)

in depressing whole-body startle even though neither drug completely eliminated startle after intrathecal infusion into the lumbar spinal cord. However, when EMG activity in the hindlimbs was used to define startle, intrathecal administration of a combination of NMDA and non-NMDA antagonists completely eliminated all EMG components of the startle response, consistent with the hypothesis that excitatory amino acids actually mediate startle at the spinal level. Moreover, when the EMG components of the startle reflex were separated into early or late components, the non-NMDA antagonist preferentially eliminated the early components (mean latency = 8.29 msec), whereas the NMDA antagonist preferentially eliminated the later components (mean latency = 14.57 msec or longer). We have also found that local infusion of non-NMDA antagonists into the facial motor nucleus completely eliminates the pinna reflex (Meloni & Davis, unpublished observations).

4. Neural Pathways Involved in the Modification of Startle by Fear and Anxiety

Acoustic startle amplitude can be modified by exposure to a brief light previously paired with shock (fear-potentiated startle: Brown, Kalish, & Farber, 1951; Davis & Astrachan, 1978), by sustained presentation of the same light even without prior light-shock pairings (light-enhanced startle: Walker & Davis, 1997), or by intraventricular administration of the stress-related peptide corticotropin-releasing hormone (corticotropin-releasing hormone-enhanced startle: Swerdlow, Geyer, Vale, & Koob, 1986; Liang, Melia, Miserendino, Falls, Campeau, & Davis, 1992). In each case, the increase in startle amplitude can be reduced by drugs that decrease fear and anxiety in humans, suggesting that each treatment increases startle via anxiogenic actions. Recently, we have found that the central nucleus of the amygdala is critically involved in fear-potentiated startle, but not in either light-enhanced startle or corticotropin-releasing hormone-enhanced startle. Conversely, a limbic area closely related to the central nucleus of the amygdala called the bed nucleus of the stria terminalis is critically involved in light-enhanced and corticotropin-releasing hormone-enhanced startle, but not in fear-potentiated startle (Lee & Davis, 1996; Walker & Davis, 1996). We believe that the differential roles of these two structures in startle modification may have implications for understanding brain systems involved in stimulus-specific fear versus anxiety.

4.1. The Role of the Amygdala in Fear-Potentiated Startle

4.1.1. The Fear-Potentiated Startle Effect

The amplitude of the eyeblink component of startle in humans can be increased when subjects are expecting a shock, viewing unpleasant slides, or even just imagining unpleasant events (Chapters 8, 9, and 15). Like humans, rats also show an elevation of startle when they are anticipating a painful shock. In this paradigm rats are first trained to be fearful of a weak neutral stimulus, such as a visual or auditory stimulus (conditioned stimulus; CS), by consistently pairing it with an aversive stimulus, such as a footshock. Typically we use 10–20 conditioned stimulus (CS)–unconditioned stimulus (US) pairings using a 3.7-s CS and a 0.5-s US that terminate together. Following this training session, the startle reflex is elicited by a loud noise burst in the presence or the absence of the CS. Fear-potentiated startle is said to occur if startle is larger in amplitude when elicited in the presence versus the absence of the CS.

4.1.2. Relationship between Short Lead Interval Modification and Fear-Potentiated Startle

Like lead interval modification, fear-potentiated startle is tested by eliciting the startle reflex after presentation of a continuous lead stimulus. However, the lead intervals in fear-potentiated startle experiments are typically rather long (e.g., 3.5 s) and the lead stimulus needs to be paired with shock to obtain startle facilitation (Davis & Astrachan, 1978).

However, when very short lead intervals are used, short lead interval modification and fear-potentiated startle appear to summate in a reasonably straightforward manner (Davis, Schlesinger, & Sorenson, 1989). In this experiment, two groups of rats received 30 light-shock pairings, using a 200-msec light-shock interval in one group and a 51,200-msec interval in the other group. The third group had lights and shocks presented in a random relationship to each other. Several days later, all groups were tested identically by presenting startle stimuli at different lead intervals after light onset.

Figure 5.2A shows the mean startle amplitude at each of the various lead intervals for animals trained with the 200- and 51,200-msec light-shock intervals and with a random relationship between lights and shocks. Figure 5.2B shows these same data transformed in the following way. First, the startle level on the probe-alone trials was subtracted from the startle level on each of the lead-stimulus trials for every animal, allowing startle at each lead interval to be expressed in relation to the individual probe-alone baseline in that group (±SE). Next, using these difference scores, the data from the random group at each lead interval were subtracted from the data of each group at each lead interval.

The results showed that short lead interval modification and fear-potentiated startle display algebraic summation, and that when unconditioned lead interval effects are subtracted, the magnitude of fear-potentiated startle is relatively specific to the CS–US interval used in training. Hence, the group trained with a 200-msec light-shock interval had maximum potentiation 200 msec after light onset, whereas the group trained with the 51,200-msec light-

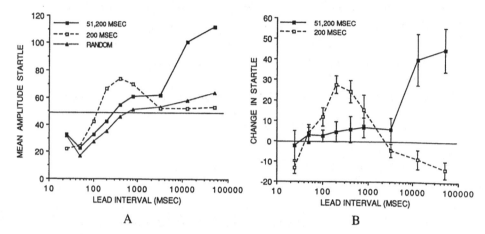

A   B

Figure 5.2. Mean amplitude startle and change in startle at each of the various lead intervals used in testing. (*A*) Raw data for the mean amplitude startle response at each of the various lead intervals (25, 50, 100, 200, 400, 800, 3,200, 12,800, or 52,200 msec plotted on a log scale) for animals trained with a 200-msec light-shock interval (open squares), 51,200-msec light-shock interval (solid squares), or a random relationship between light and shocks (solid triangles). The solid horizontal line represents the average values of the probe-alone trials for the three groups, which did not differ significantly from each other. (*B*) These same data transformed as described in the text. (From Davis et al., 1989.)

shock interval had maximum potentiation 51,200 msec after light onset. These data suggest, therefore, that fear-potentiated startle was maximal at the time when the animal was anticipating receipt of shock, making it a sensitive measure of anticipatory fear or anxiety.

4.1.3. Effects of Amygdala Lesions on Fear-Potentiated Startle

Lesions of the central nucleus of the amygdala block the expression of fear-potentiated startle using either a visual (Hitchcock & Davis, 1986) or auditory conditioned stimulus (Hitchcock & Davis, 1987; Campeau & Davis, 1995). The central nucleus of the amygdala projects directly to the nucleus reticularis pontis caudalis (Rosen, Hitchcock, Sananes, Miserendino, & Davis, 1991) and lesions at several points along this pathway blocked the expression of fear-potentiated startle (Hitchcock & Davis, 1991). Both conditioned fear and sensitization of startle by footshocks appear to ultimately modulate startle at the level of the nucleus reticularis pontis caudalis (Berg & Davis, 1985; Boulis & Davis, 1989; Krase, Koch, & Schnitzler, 1994). Selective destruction of cell bodies via local infusion of neurotoxic doses of NMDA into the lateral and basolateral nuclei, which receive sensory input and project to the central nucleus of the amygdala, caused a complete blockade of fear-potentiated startle when the lesions were made either before or after training (Sananes & Davis, 1992). This blockade of fear-potentiated startle did not seem to result from a disruption of vision, and other studies found that NMDA-induced lesions of these amygdaloid nuclei also blocked fear-potentiated startle using an auditory conditioned stimulus (Campeau & Davis, 1995). These results are consistent with other work that indicates that the lateral nucleus of the amygdala provides a critical link for relaying auditory information involved in fear conditioning to the amygdala (LeDoux, Cicchetti, Xagoraris, & Romanski, 1990).

Based on the anatomical and lesion data described above, we suggested that the direct pathway from the amygdala to the startle circuit may mediate both fear-potentiated startle and sensitization of startle produced by prior footshocks (Hitchcock, Sananes, & Davis, 1989; Hitchcock & Davis, 1991). However, those studies only used electrolytic lesions of the amygdalofugal pathway at several levels including the ventrolateral central gray, so that obligatory synapses at points along this pathway could not be ruled out (Hitchcock & Davis, 1991). Recent data now suggest that a synapse between the amygdala and central gray may be required for both fear-potentiated startle and shock sensitization because fiber-sparing chemical lesions in the vicinity of the central gray have been reported to block both phenomena (Fendt, Koch, & Schnitzler, 1994a; Yeomans & Franklin, 1994).

4.1.4. The Role of Excitatory Amino Acids in the Amygdala in the Acquisition and Expression of Fear-Potentiated Startle

Because several studies have shown that NMDA antagonists block long-term potentiation both in vitro and in vivo, as well as learning in several behavioral tasks, we tested whether local infusion of an NMDA antagonist into the amygdala would block the acquisition of fear-potentiated startle. Intra-amygdala infusion of an NMDA antagonist caused a dose-dependent blockade of fear-potentiated startle using either a visual (Miserendino, Sananes, Melia, & Davis, 1990) or an auditory conditioned stimulus (Campeau, Miserendino, & Davis, 1992). This effect did not seem to be due to a decrease in sensitivity to footshock, neurotoxic damage to the amygdala, or a decrease in visual processing. Moreover, the same NMDA antagonist did not block the expression of fear-potentiated startle using either a visual (Miserendino et al., 1990) or an auditory (Campeau et al., 1992) conditioned stimulus when infused immediately prior to testing in rats previously trained in the absence of the drug.

On the other hand, pre-test infusion of non-NMDA antagonists did block the expression of fear-potentiated startle in a dose-dependent manner (Kim, Campeau, Falls & Davis, 1993). This suggests that the conditioned stimulus ultimately results in a release of glutamate in the amygdala, which activates non-NMDA receptors for the expression of conditioned fear.

In humans, removal of the amygdala has been associated with an impairment of memory for faces (Jacobson, 1986; Tranel & Hyman, 1990; Aggleton, 1992; Young, Aggleton, Hellawell, Johnson, Broks, & Hanley, 1995) and deficits in recognition of emotion in people's faces and interpretation of gaze angle (Young et al., 1995). In a very rare case involving bilateral calcification confined to the amygdala (Urbach–Wiethe disease), the patient could not identify the emotion of fear in pictures of human faces and could not draw a fearful face, even though other emotions such as happy, sad, angry, and disgusted were identified and drawn within the normal range. Furthermore, she had no difficulty in identifying the names of familiar faces (Adolphs, Tranel, Damasio, & Damasio, 1994, 1995). The deficit in recognizing facial expressions of fear seemed to occur only after bilateral amygdala damage, whereas several patients with unilateral lesions had difficulty in naming familiar faces (Adolphs et al., 1995). Patients with unilateral (LeBar, LeDoux, Spencer, & Phelps, 1995) or bilateral (Bechara, Tranel, Damasio, Adolphs, Rockland, & Damasio, 1995) lesions of the amygdala also have been reported to have deficits in classical fear conditioning using the skin conductance response as a measure.

4.1.5. The Visual Pathway Involved in Fear-Potentiated Startle Using a Visual Conditioned Stimulus

Visual input critical for fear-potentiated startle using a visual conditioned stimulus may enter the amygdala via projections from the perirhinal cortex to the lateral and/or basolateral nuclei, which then project to the central nucleus, which in turn projects to the startle pathway. McDonald and Jackson (1987) find heavy reciprocal projections between the perirhinal cortex, which receives multimodal input (Loe & Benevento, 1969; Fallon & Genevento, 1977; Robinson & Burton, 1980; Deacon, Eichenbaum, Rosenberg, & Ecknamm, 1983; Guldin & Markowitsch, 1983) and the basolateral, basomedial, and especially the lateral nucleus of the amygdala. Relatively small lesions of the perirhinal cortex completely blocked fear-potentiated startle, provided the lesion included an area of perirhinal cortex both dorsal and ventral to the rhinal sulcus (Rosen, Hitchcock, Miserendino, Falls, Campeau, & Davis, 1992; Campeau & Davis, 1995).

Recently we have found a direct projection from the lateral posterior nucleus of the thalamus to the perirhinal cortex (Shi & Davis, 1996). Lesions of the lateral posterior nucleus of the thalamus, combined with lesions of the dorsal and ventral nuclei of the lateral geniculate, completely block fear-potentiated startle using a visual conditioned stimulus, but not using an auditory conditioned stimulus (Shi & Davis, 1996). We do not think that destruction of the dorsal nucleus of the lateral geniculate contributed to the blockade, because post-training lesions of the visual cortex, to which the dorsal nucleus of the lateral geniculate projects, do not affect fear-potentiated startle at all (Rosen et al., 1992; Falls & Davis, 1994). Currently, we are testing the effects of lesions of the ventral nucleus of the lateral geniculate alone or in combination with lesions of the lateral posterior nucleus. Figure 5.3 shows our current working hypothesis of the pathways involved in fear-potentiated startle using a visual conditioned stimulus.

4.2. The Role of the Dorsal Periacqueductal Gray in Fear-Potentiated Startle

4.2.1. Nonmonotonic Relationship between Fear-Potentiated Startle and Shock Intensity in Training: Learning or Performance?

Within a given range, fear-potentiated startle is directly related to the intensity of footshock during training. Surprisingly, however, when trained at higher intensities, rats show relatively poor potentiated startle.

Although this could reflect a learning deficit resulting from stress-induced analgesia, several experimental observations failed to support such an account (Walker & Davis, 1995). Instead, the loss of potentiated startle as training intensity increases appears to reflect a performance rather than a learning deficit.

4.2.2. Effects of Lesions or Stimulation of the Dorsal Periacqueductal Gray in Fear-Potentiated Startle

Several investigators have implicated the dorsolateral periacqueductal gray in active responses to threatening stimuli and the ventral periacqueductal gray in more passive responses (Depaulis, Keay, & Bandler, 1992, 1994). Based on these and other data (Fanselow, 1994), we hypothesized that stimuli previously paired with high footshocks may preferentially activate the dorsolateral periacqueductal gray, thereby switching animals into an active defense mode incompatible with fear-potentiated startle.

Consistent with this interpretation, animals with axon-sparing NMDA lesions of the dorsolateral periacqueductal gray showed a monotonic relationship between footshock intensity and fear-potentiated startle (Walker,

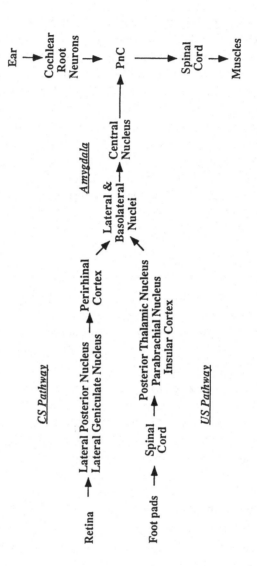

Figure 5.3. Working hypothesis of the pathways involved in fear-potentiated startle using a visual conditioned stimulus and a footshock unconditioned stimulus.

Cassella, Lee, de Lima, & Davis, 1997). Moreover, chemical activation of the dorsolateral periacqueductal gray interfered with the expression of fear-potentiated startle in animals trained with a moderate shock intensity even though it had no effect on baseline startle. Together with the lesion data, these results suggest that conditioned stimuli previously paired with highly aversive stimuli activate the dorsolateral periacqueductal gray, and that this activation interferes with fear-potentiated startle. More generally, this may reflect a transition from passive to active defense sets as threat levels increase (Fanselow, 1994).

4.3. The Role of the Bed Nucleus of the Stria Terminalis in Startle

4.3.1. The Role of the Bed Nucleus of the Stria Terminalis and the Amygdala in Contextual Conditioning or Long-Term Sensitization of the Startle Reflex

Recently, we have been testing a new hypothesis that suggests that the bed nucleus of the stria terminalis may be involved in contextual conditioning but not explicit cue conditioning, whereas the amygdala is involved in both (Davis, Gewirtz, & McNish, 1995). In one experiment, different groups of rats each were given electrolytic or sham lesions of either the central nucleus of the amygdala or the bed nucleus of the stria terminalis. One week later, rats were presented with ten startle stimuli every day for 22 days. These stimuli were followed by either two light-shock pairings and six fear-potentiated test trials or six fear-potentiated test trials followed by two light-shock pairings.

As expected, there was a gradual development of fear-potentiated startle in the sham-lesioned groups over the 22 days. Fear-potentiated startle was completely blocked by lesions of the amygdala, but not by lesions of the bed nucleus of the stria terminalis. In the sham rats, there was also a gradual increase in startle amplitude elicited by the initial ten startle stimuli, before any lights or shocks were presented. In this case, lesions of either the amygdala or the bed nucleus of the stria terminalis blocked this increase in startle. We believe that this slowly developing increase in startle may represent either contextual conditioning or long-term sensitization and that the bed nucleus of the stria terminalis may be involved in this form of startle facilitation rather than fear-potentiated startle.

4.3.2. The Role of the Bed Nucleus of the Stria Terminalis and the Amygdala in Light-Enhanced Startle

4.3.2.1. *The Light-Enhanced Startle Effect.* Although fear-potentiated startle offers several advantages as an animal model of fear and anxiety, one disadvantage, common to all procedures which rely upon conditioning, is that treatment effects cannot unambiguously be attributed to effects on fear versus memory. It is difficult to say, for example, whether a given drug that reduces fear-potentiated startle does so because the drug is anxiolytic or because the drug has a more general effect on memory retrieval. Consequently, we have developed a procedure that preserves the benefits of fear-potentiated startle, but which relies on the unconditioned aversive properties of exposure to bright light in rodents (cf. Walker & Davis, 1997).

In this test, each animal was tested on two separate days. On one day, startle was measured in the dark during phase I and in the light during phase II using either an 8-, 70-, or 700-footlambert light source in different groups of animals. On a second day, the light remained off during both phases. During each phase startle stimuli were presented every 30 s 5 min after the rats were placed in the test chambers over a 20-min test session.

Figure 5.4 shows that in both phases, startle responses habituated over the course of testing. Superimposed on this habituation was a general increase in startle amplitude that was directly related to light intensity and that remained relatively stable for the duration of the 20-min test. These results indicate that high levels of sustained illumination produce an increase in the amplitude of the acoustic startle response, which persists for at least 20 min. Other studies showed that this could not be attributed to dishabituation because when illumination levels were decreased between phase I and phase II, startle amplitude also decreased. Finally, the anxiolytic drug buspirone blocked light-enhanced startle, suggesting that light may be anxiogenic in this paradigm (Walker & Davis, 1997).

4.3.2.2. *Effects of Glutamate Antagonists Infused into the Bed Nucleus of the Stria Terminalis versus the Amygdala on Light-Enhanced Startle.* Because local infusion of glutamate antagonists into the central nucleus of the amygdala completely blocks the expression of fear-potentiated startle (Kim et al., 1993), we wondered whether this treatment would also block light-enhanced startle. However, we were also interested in testing the effects of inactivation of the bed nucleus of the stria terminalis on light-enhanced startle as well. Ongoing studies in our laboratory, outlined earlier, suggested that the bed nucleus of the stria terminalis is involved in elevations of startle that are more long-lasting than explicit cue conditioning. Such lesions also blocked the excitatory effect on startle of the peptide corticotropin-releasing hormone (Lee & Davis, 1996, and see below). The bed nucleus of the stria terminalis is considered to be part of the extended amygdala because it is highly similar to the central nucleus of the amygdala in terms of its transmitter content, cell morphology, and efferent connections (Alheid, deOlmos, & Beltramino, 1995). However, lesions of this area failed to block either fear-potentiated startle (Hitchcock & Davis, 1991) or conditioned freezing using

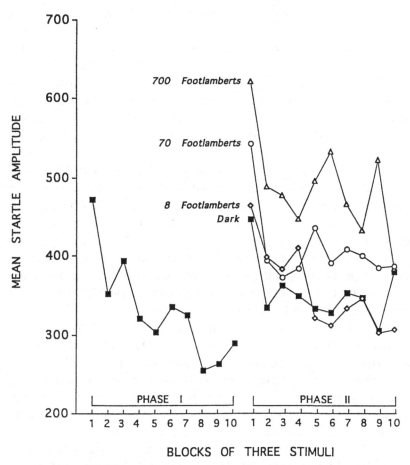

Figure 5.4. Mean startle amplitude over successive blocks of three stimuli during phase I, combined across all groups, and during phase II shown separately for the different groups that were tested in phase II in the dark or with 8, 70, or 700 footlamberts of light in phase II. (From Walker and Davis, 1997.)

an explicit cue (LeDoux, Iwata, Cicchetti, & Reis, 1988), suggesting that it may not be involved in explicit cue conditioning.

For these experiments, animals were implanted with bilateral cannulas in either the bed nucleus of the stria terminalis, the basolateral complex of the amygdala (i.e., the lateral and basolateral nuclei), or the central nucleus of the amygdala. One week later, animals were tested for light-enhanced startle using the procedures described above with the exception that half of the animals were infused with a non-NMDA antagonist and the other half with the vehicle immediately prior to being placed into the chamber during phase I.

Two days later these procedures were repeated except animals previously infused with the non-NMDA antagonist were now infused with the vehicle and vice versa.

Infusion of the non-NMDA antagonist into the central nucleus of the amygdala had no effect on light-enhanced startle. On the other hand, infusion of the non-NMDA antagonist into either the basolateral amygdala complex or the bed nucleus of the stria terminalis significantly decreased light-enhanced startle. These data indicate an important role for both the basolateral amygdala and the bed nucleus of the stria terminalis in light-enhanced startle.

4.3.2.3. *Effects of Glutamate Antagonists Infused into the Bed Nucleus of the Stria Terminalis versus the Amygdala on Fear-Potentiated Startle.* To determine the specificity of these effects, the rats used in the light-enhanced startle experiment were trained for potentiated startle. Twenty minutes prior to testing, half the animals were infused with the non-NMDA antagonist into either the amygdala or bed nucleus of the stria terminalis. The other half were infused with phosphate-buffered saline. Two days later these test procedures were repeated except rats previously infused with the non-NMDA antagonist were now infused with the vehicle and vice versa.

Consistent with previous results (Kim et al., 1993), infusion of the non-NMDA antagonist into the central nucleus or the basolateral nucleus of the amygdala completely blocked the expression of fear-potentiated startle. In contrast, infusion of the non-NMDA antagonist into the bed nucleus of the stria terminalis had no effect on fear-potentiated startle. Hence, the ineffectiveness of the non-NMDA antagonist infused into the central nucleus of the amygdala to block light-enhanced startle cannot be attributed to misplaced cannulas, an inadequate dose, or an incorrect pretreatment interval, because fear-potentiated startle testing took place at the same time as phase II testing in the light-enhanced startle paradigm after the non-NMDA antagonist infusion. Overall, these data show a double dissociation between inactivation of glutamate receptors in the central nucleus of the amygdala versus the bed nucleus of the stria terminalis with respect to fear-potentiated versus light-enhanced startle.

4.3.3. The Role of the Bed Nucleus of the Stria Terminalis and the Central Nucleus of the Amygdala in Startle Enhanced by Intraventricular Administration of Corticotropin-Releasing Hormone (Corticotropin-Releasing Hormone-Enhanced Startle)

A large number of studies in animals have shown that intraventricular administration of the peptide corticotropin-releasing hormone produces a constellation of behavioral effects similar to those produced by stress or conditioned fear (Dunn & Berridge, 1990), and that intraventricular administration of corticotropin-releasing hormone antagonists block many of the behavioral and neuroendocrine responses produced by natural stressors (Dunn & Berridge, 1990). Intraventricular infusion of corticotropin-releasing hormone (0.1–1.0 μg) produces a pronounced, dose-dependent enhancement of the acoustic startle reflex (Swerdlow et al., 1986; Liang, Melia, Campeau, Falls, Miserendino, & Davis, 1992; Liang et al., 1992) (corticotropin-releasing hormone-enhanced startle) that was not blocked by lesions of the paraventricular nucleus of the hypothalamus. Bilateral electrolytic lesions of the central nucleus of the amygdala significantly attenuated corticotropin-releasing hormone-enhanced startle although direct infusion of corticotropin-releasing hormone into the amygdala did not significantly elevate startle. These data suggested that the amygdala was part of the neural circuitry required for corticotropin-releasing hormone to elevate startle, but not the primary receptor area where corticotropin-releasing hormone acts.

However, it is possible that the ability of electrolytic lesions of the amygdala to block corticotropin-releasing hormone-enhanced startle was due to destruction of fibers passing through the amygdala rather than to destruction of cell bodies. To test this, other groups of rats were given chemical lesions of either the central nucleus of the amygdala, the basolateral nucleus of the amygdala, or the bed nucleus of the stria terminalis combined with implantation of intraventricular cannulas. Two weeks later they were tested for startle before and after intraventricular infusion of corticotropin-releasing hormone. Remarkably, chemical lesions of the amygdala failed to block corticotropin-releasing hormone-enhanced startle (Lee & Davis, 1996). On the other hand, NMDA-induced lesions of the bed nucleus of the stria terminalis completely blocked corticotropin-releasing hormone-enhanced startle. In other animals we found that local infusion of very low doses of corticotropin-releasing hormone directly into the bed nucleus of the stria terminalis produced a rapid and large increase in startle amplitude. Moreover, local infusion into the bed nucleus of the stria terminalis of the corticotropin-releasing hormone antagonist, alpha-helical corticotropin-releasing hormone$_{9-41}$, blocked the excitatory effect on startle normally seen after intraventricular administration of corticotropin-releasing hormone, whereas local infusion into the amygdala had no effect. These data provide compelling evidence that the bed nucleus of the stria terminalis, and not the amygdala, is the primary receptor site mediating the startle-enhancing effects of corticotropin-releasing hormone given intraventricularly. The ability of large electrolytic lesions of the amygdala to block corticotropin-releasing hormone-enhanced startle probably results

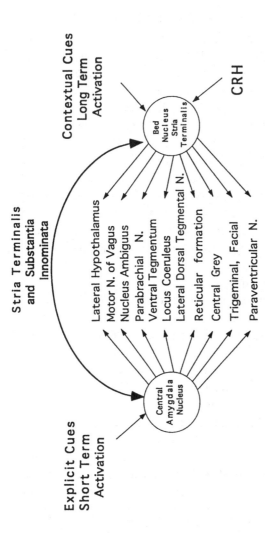

Figure 5.5. Hypothetical schematic suggesting that the central nucleus of the amygdala and the bed nucleus of the stria terminalis may be differentially involved in fear vs. anxiety, respectively. Both brain areas have highly similar hypothalamic and brainstem targets known to be involved in specific signs and symptoms of fear and anxiety. However, the stress peptide corticotropin-releasing hormone appears to act on receptors in the bed nucleus of the stria terminalis rather than the amygdala, at least in terms of an increase in the startle reflex. Furthermore, the bed nucleus of the stria terminalis seems to be involved in the anxiogenic effects of a very bright light presented for a long period of time but not when that very same light has previously been paired with a shock. Just the opposite is the case for the central nucleus of the amygdala, which is critical for fear conditioning using explicit cues such as a light or tone paired with aversive stimulation (i.e., conditioned fear).

from destruction of fibers projecting from the bed nucleus of the stria terminalis to the startle pathway.

4.3.4. Differential Roles of the Bed Nucleus of the Stria Terminalis and the Central Nucleus of the Amygdala in Fear versus Anxiety

We have found a clear distinction between the central nucleus of the amygdala and the bed nucleus of the stria terminalis in relationship to fear-potentiated startle versus corticotropin-releasing hormone-enhanced and light-enhanced startle. Lesions or chemical inactivation of the central nucleus of the amygdala completely block the expression of fear-potentiated startle but have no effect whatsoever on either light-enhanced startle or corticotropin-releasing hormone-enhanced startle. Conversely, lesions or chemical inactivation of the bed nucleus of the stria terminalis significantly attenuated either light-enhanced startle or corticotropin-releasing hormone-enhanced startle without having any effect whatsoever on fear-potentiated startle.

We suggest that the bed nucleus of the stria terminalis may be a system that responds to signals more akin to anxiety than those akin to fear, whereas the central nucleus of the amygdala is clearly involved in fear and perhaps not as much in anxiety (Fig. 5.5). Both these structures have very similar efferent connections to various hypothalamic and brain-stem target areas known to be involved in specific signs and symptoms of fear and anxiety (cf. Davis, 1992). Both receive highly processed sensory information from the basolateral nucleus of the amygdala and hence are in a position to respond to emotionally significant stimuli. Corticotropin-releasing hormone is known to be released during periods of stress or anxiety, some of which may come from corticotropin-releasing hormone-containing neurons in the amygdala which project to and act on receptors in the bed nucleus of the stria terminalis. Thus, phasic activation of the amygdala by certain stressors could lead to a long-term activation of the bed nucleus of the stria terminalis via corticotropin-releasing hormone. Assuming that phasic activation is like fear, whereas sustained activation of similar structures is like anxiety, this would suggest differential roles of the amygdala versus the bed nucleus of the stria terminalis in fear versus anxiety, respectively. Because of the potential clinical implications of this distinction, further investigation of these possibilities is currently under way.

CHAPTER SIX

Neurophysiology and Neuropharmacology of Short Lead Interval Startle Modification

NEAL R. SWERDLOW AND MARK A. GEYER

ABSTRACT

Studies of the neural basis of short lead interval startle modification have been one extension of the anatomical and behavioral "mapping" of the "primary startle circuit." The neural substrates of prepulse inhibition (PPI) – an operational measure of sensorimotor gating – are studied partly because several neuropsychiatric disorders are characterized both by deficits in PPI and by clinical evidence of impaired inhibition of cognitive, sensory, or motor information. Brain regions implicated in the pathophysiology of these disorders – limbic cortex, ventral striatum, pallidum, and pontine tegmentum – critically regulate PPI. The neurochemistry of PPI includes neurotransmitters that subserve this circuitry, particularly dopamine, glutamate, serotonin, acetylcholine, and gamma-amino-butyric acid; specific neuropeptides also appear to regulate PPI. These neural substrates have been studied via traditional neuropharmacological techniques in laboratory rats, via studies of PPI in specific patient populations, and via developmental and genetic manipulations. Collectively, these studies may identify perturbations of brain function in this circuitry that lead to deficits in PPI – such as those observed in schizophrenia and other disorders – and, conversely, what interventions might act at each level of the circuitry to enhance or restore normal levels of sensorimotor gating.

1. Overview: Temporal Relationships in the Phasic and Tonic Regulation of Startle

Startle response modification by short lead stimuli has been studied systematically, drawing on the tremendous strengths of startle as a quantifiable, parametrically sensitive behavior. This work has important implications for understanding fundamental principles of information processing and for examining

Michael E. Dawson, Anne M. Schell, and Andreas H. Böhmelt, Eds. *Startle modification: Implications for neuroscience, cognitive science, and clinical science.* Copyright © 1999 Cambridge University Press. Printed in the United States of America. All rights reserved.

the biological basis of specific time-linked information-processing deficits in neuropsychiatric disorders.

In humans, studies typically measure the blink component of the startle response, using electromyography of orbicularis oculi. In rats, a stabilimeter chamber is used to measure whole-body flinch elicited by stimuli that are similar to those used in humans. The startle reflex demonstrates important forms of plasticity – including habituation (Hoffman & Searle, 1968) and fear potentiation (Davis, 1984) – that are regulated by forebrain circuitry (see below) and appear to exhibit striking similarities across species (Geyer & Braff, 1987; Grillon, Falls, Ameli, & Davis, 1994). One form of startle plasticity related to short lead intervals is prepulse inhibition (PPI; alternatively described as lead stimulus inhibition), the normal suppression of the startle reflex when the intense startling stimulus is preceded 30–500 msec by a weak lead stimulus (Ison, McAdam, & Hammond, 1973; Graham, 1975; see Chapter 3) (Fig. 6.1, top).

In PPI, a weak lead stimulus inhibits a reflex response to a powerful sensory stimulus. PPI occurs when the lead stimulus and startling stimuli are in the same or different sensory modalities. Virtually all mammals and primates exhibit PPI. While the inhibitory effect of the lead stimulus on startle reactivity is undoubtedly exerted in the pons (Davis & Gendelman, 1977), studies have described the descending limbic cortico–striato–pallido–pontine influences that regulate inhibitory "tone" within the pons, and determine the degree to which the lead stimulus inhibits the reflex (see below). PPI thus appears to reflect the activation of ubiquitous "hard-wired" behavioral gating processes that are regulated by forebrain neural circuitry.

Sensorimotor modulation can also result in the potentiation of the startle reflex. Startle magnitude is *increased* when the startling stimulus is preceded at very short (less than 20 msec) or long (greater than 1000 msec) intervals by lead stimuli (Hoffman & Searle, 1968). Prepulse facilitation (alternatively described as lead stimulus facilitation) is most evident with weak lead stimuli (Fig. 6.1, bottom). Lead stimulus modulation changes from facilitation to inhibition with increasing lead interval and lead stimulus intensity, although in humans (but generally not in rodents, except with very weak prepulses), prepulse facilitation "re-emerges" at longer lead intervals. Prepulse facilitation and PPI may be opposing forms of sensorimotor modulation that result from activity within either a single brain system or two separable substrates (Schwarzkopf, Ison, Taylor, & Barlow, 1992).

While PPI and prepulse facilitation are examples of lead stimulus-induced changes in startle *magnitude,* prestimuli also modify startle onset and peak latency. Reflex latencies are reduced ("latency facilitation") by prestimuli,

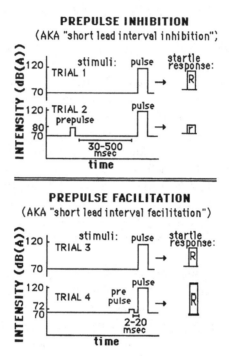

Figure 6.1. Acoustic startle reflex short lead stimulus modification: Discrete lead stimuli 5–15 dB above background presented 30–500 msec prior to the pulse (*top,* trial 2) typically cause reflex inhibition, while weaker prepulses at shorter lead intervals (*bottom,* trial 4) typically yield reflex facilitation.

particularly when lead intervals are relatively short (e.g., less than 100 msec). The relative independence of lead stimulus-induced changes in reflex magnitude and latency is suggested by the fact that normal latency facilitation occurs even in humans (with Huntington's disease) and rats (post-apomorphine) who exhibit little or no PPI, and by the fact that normal differences in PPI across groups (e.g., men vs. women) are not accompanied by group differences in latency facilitation. Relatively little is known about the neural substrates of latency facilitation, although it is thought to reflect lead stimulus effects relatively early within the startle circuitry (Davis, 1980). Because latency facilitation is intact within several neuropsychiatric populations (Braff, Grillon, & Geyer, 1992; Cadenhead, Geyer, & Braff, 1993; Swerdlow, Benbow, Zisook, Geyer, & Braff, 1993; Swerdlow, Paulsen, Braff, Butters, Geyer, & Swenson, 1995), and since it is not modified by several major classes of psychotropic agents (including psychotomimetics), this chapter will focus on lead stimulus effects on startle magnitude and, primarily, on PPI.

Much of what we know about the neurophysiology of short lead interval startle modification comes from studies in infrahumans, particularly rats. While specific anatomical substrates regulating startle modification likely differ across species, studies in humans with known brain "lesions" – including Huntington's disease, Parkinson's disease, and temporal lobe epilepsy – as well as studies involving drug administration in humans, suggest striking similarities in the regulatory substrates in humans and rats.

2. The Primary Startle Circuit and Discrete Lead Stimulus Effects

The primary mammalian acoustic startle circuit (Koch, Lingenhohl, & Pilz, 1992) includes serial connections linking the auditory nerve, the ventral cochlear nucleus, the nucleus reticularis pontis caudalis, and the spinal motor neuron (see Chapter 5). Since PPI in the rat is evident with lead intervals as short as 15 msec, the circuitry that mediates the actual inhibitory effect of the lead stimulus cannot deviate from the primary startle circuit by more than one or two neurons (e.g., 7.5 msec "out" and 7.5 msec "back" to the primary startle circuit). The most likely scenario is that the first acoustic stimulus (the "prepulse") activates the ventral cochlear nucleus and nucleus reticularis pontis caudalis; one of these regions then directly or indirectly activates cells in the pontine tegmentum, in the area of the pedunculopontine nucleus. Pedunculopontine nucleus cells directly innervate and apparently inhibit the nucleus reticularis pontis caudalis such that its response to a subsequent stimulus (the "startling stimulus") is reduced (Koch, Kungel, & Herbert, 1993). Thus, the actual circuitry that mediates PPI is likely very simple, and is integrally related to the "primary" startle circuit. For this reason, PPI persists despite transcollicular decerebration (Davis & Gendelman, 1977).

This simple "startle modification circuit" is regulated by higher brain circuitry that descends into the pontine tegmentum (Fig. 6.2). Activity within this forebrain circuitry, transmitted to the pontine tegmentum, appears to "set the gain" for PPI. The forebrain regulation of PPI involves, at least, limbic cortical inputs to the striatum, striatal connections with the pallidum, and pallidal inputs to the pontine tegmentum, as discussed below. Within this forebrain circuitry, several different neurotransmitter systems are capable of regulating the amount of sensorimotor inhibition. In addition to this descending segmental regulation of PPI, it is possible that more "direct" lines of regulation exist, per-

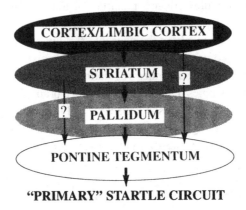

"PRIMARY" STARTLE CIRCUIT

Figure 6.2. General schematic representation of descending forebrain influences that may regulate prepulse inhibition of acoustic startle. Thick arrows signify serial connections between cortical and subcortical influences; thin arrows and "?" signify possible parallel direct influences converging within the pontine tegmentum.

haps even via uninterrupted monosynaptic cortico–pontine projections, by which forebrain circuitry can modify the "gain" of pontine startle circuitry.

Some studies suggest that forebrain circuitry regulates the *contralateral* facial effectors of PPI. Sequential projections from limbic cortex → striatum → pallidum → pontine tegmentum → nucleus reticularis pontis caudalis maintain an *ipsilateral* relationship, but the degree to which this nucleus reticularis pontis caudalis → facial motor nucleus (CN7) projection crosses the midline increases phylogenetically: In rats, nucleus reticularis pontis caudalis cells project bilaterally to innervate both sides of CN7, whereas this projection becomes predominantly contralateral in cats, and even to a greater degree in higher species (Takeuchi, Nakano, Uemura, Kojyuro, Matsushima, & Mizuno, 1979; Hinrichsen & Watson, 1983; Panneton & Martin, 1983; Holstege, Tan, Van Ham, & Bos, 1984). Studies of PPI in humans typically record the eyeblink component of the startle reflex, using *unilateral* electromyographic (EMG) recordings from orbicularis oculi. For example, PPI deficits in patients with schizophrenia, schizotypal personality disorder (see Chapter 11), Huntington's disease, and obsessive-compulsive disorder have all been reported in studies using measures of *right* eyeblink EMG (Braff et al., 1992; Cadenhead et al., 1993; Swerdlow et al., 1993; Swerdlow et al., 1995), and thus may reflect abnormalities in descending forebrain activity within the *left* hemisphere. Deficits in other groups, including enuretic children (Ornitz, Hanna, & de Traversay, 1992), were identified in measures using only *left* eyeblink startle, which is likely regulated by descending forebrain activity within the right hemisphere. Data from bilateral measures of PPI might be particularly important in understanding the neural bases for PPI deficits in specific disordered populations: Neuroimaging studies and neuropsychological measures indicate that dysfunction in several major neuropsychiatric disorders is either lateralized within cortico–striato–pallido–pontine substrates, or is characterized by a loss of normal structural asymmetry (Bracha, 1987; Early, Relman, Raichle, & Spitzmagel, 1987; Conrad, Abebe, Austin, Forsythe, & Scheibel, 1991; Shenton, Kirkinis, & Jolesz, 1992; Zigun & Weinberger 1992; Rauch, Jenike, Alpert, Baer, Breiter, & Fischman, 1994; Yasgan, Peterson, Wexler, & Leckman, 1995; Schwartz, Stoessel, Baxter, Martin, & Phelps, 1996).

Compared with PPI, the neural substrates of prepulse facilitation are considerably less well understood. Since prepulse facilitation is evident when very short lead intervals are used, it is possible that some prepulse facilitatory effects on startle are mediated very "early" in the reflex arc, perhaps even within the cochlea. However, potent prepulse facilitation has been reported with crossmodal prestimulus effects (e.g., vibrotactile lead stimulus and acoustic startle stimulus), and it would be difficult to explain such findings on the basis of cochlear involvement (Blumenthal & Gescheider, 1987). Other studies have reported that, within the pedunculopontine nucleus, there are two distinct sets of cell populations that differ in their response sensitivity to auditory clicks (Reese, Garcia-Rill, & Skinner, 1995). One cell group has a lower response threshold and shorter response latencies (less than 10 msec), whereas a second cell group has a higher response threshold and longer response latencies (greater than 10 msec). Thus, it is conceivable that the different cell groups within the pedunculopontine nucleus regulate both startle facilitation (maximal with weak prestimuli at very short lead intervals) and inhibition (maximal with more intense prestimuli at relatively "longer" short lead intervals).

3. Neurochemical Regulation of Short Lead Interval Startle Inhibition

Evidence from systemic drug studies supports a role of dopamine (DA), glutamate, serotonin, and acetylcholine in the neurochemical regulation of PPI (see Fig. 6.3). Other evidence appears to be emerging in support of a peptidergic influence on PPI, at least in part via modulatory interactions with major neurotransmitter substrates (Feifel, Dulawa, Taaid, & Swerdlow, 1995; Feifel & Minor, 1997). Evidence from studies of the neural circuit substrates

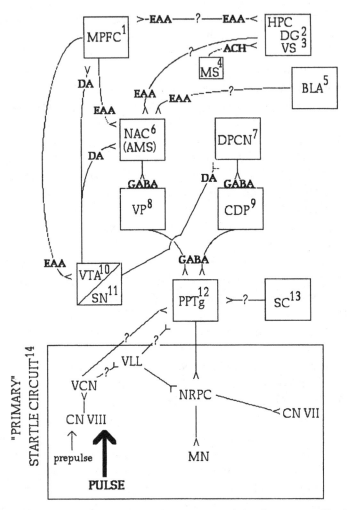

Figure 6.3. Detailed schematic representation of neural circuitry proposed by different investigative groups to regulate prepulse inhibition of acoustic startle. The basic elements of this neural circuitry have been identified in anatomical studies by numerous different investigators; they were first described in relation to the regulation of PPI by Swerdlow et al. (1992), based on a heuristically driven model proposed by Swerdlow and Koob (1987). This figure is meant for illustrative purposes only, and is certainly not thought to be complete; structures and neurotransmitters are indicated as supported by presently available experimental data (see text): (1) MPFC (medial prefrontal cortex: Bubser & Koch, 1994b; Koch & Bubser, 1994; Ellenbroek et al., 1995a; Swerdlow et al., 1995a); (2) DG (dentate gyrus: Caine et al., 1991, 1992; Koch, 1995); (3) VS (ventral subiculum: Lipska et al., 1995; Swerdlow et al., 1995a; Wan et al., 1997); (4) MS (medial septal nucleus: Koch, 1995); (5) BLA (basolateral amygdala: Decker et al., 1995; Wan & Swerdlow, 1997); (6) NAC (nucleus accumbens: Swerdlow et al., 1986,

of PPI implicate other neurotransmitters, such as gamma-aminobutyric acid (GABA), in the regulation of PPI, via actions within specific segments of the PPI regulatory circuitry (see below).

3.1. Dopamine

In rats, PPI is reduced by drugs that facilitate DA activity, including the direct DA agonist apomorphine (Swerdlow, Geyer, Braff, & Koob, 1986; Mansbach, Geyer, & Braff, 1988; Schwarzkopf, Mitra, & Bruno, 1992; Schwarzkopf, Bruno, & Mitra, 1993; Swerdlow & Geyer, 1993; Hoffman & Donovan, 1994; Swerdlow, Braff, Taaid, & Geyer, 1994) and the indirect DA agonists d-amphetamine (Mansbach et al., 1988; Swerdlow, Mansbach, Geyer, Pulvirenti, Koob, & Braff, 1990) and cocaine, and these effects are reversed by DA receptor antagonists (Mansbach et al., 1988; Swerdlow, Keith, Braff, & Geyer, 1991; Schwarzkopf et al., 1993; Swerdlow & Geyer, 1993; Swerdlow et al., 1994). The D2 receptor may mediate the apomorphine disruption of PPI, since this effect of apomorphine is blocked by the D2 antagonists raclopride and spiperone (Swerdlow et al., 1991). Evidence in our laboratory (Peng, Mansbach, Braff, & Geyer, 1990; Wan & Swerdlow, 1996) and others (Hoffman & Donovan, 1994) does suggest that D1 and D2 receptors may interact in the regulation of PPI, but that D1 receptors do not serve as an independent substrate for changes in PPI.

We reported that the ability of antipsychotics (including atypical antipsychotics) to normalize startle gating in apomorphine-treated rats correlates significantly with their clinical efficacy ($r = 0.99$) (Swerdlow et al., 1994). The putative D4 antagonist NGD 94-1 also restores PPI in apomorphine-treated rats, despite the fact that it is inactive in traditional preclinical measures of antipsychotic action (Cassella et al., 1994). Furthermore, PPI is reduced by the putative D3 agonist PD 128907 (Varty, Hayes, & Higgins, 1995). Thus,

Caption to **Figure 6.3** (*cont.*)
1990a, b, 1992a, 1994; Kodsi & Swerdlow, 1994, 1995; Wan & Swerdlow, 1994, 1996; Wan et al., 1994, 1995a; Reijmers et al., 1995); (7) DPCN (dorsal posterior caudate nucleus: Kodsi & Swerdlow, 1995); (8) VP (ventral pallidum: Swerdlow et al., 1990a; Kodsi & Swerdlow, 1994, 1995); (9) CDP (caudodorsal pallidum: Kodsi & Swerdlow, 1995); (10) VTA (ventral tegmentum: Zhang et al., 1995); (11) SN (substantia nigra: Swerdlow et al., 1986; Morton et al., 1995); (12) PPTg (pedunculopontine tegmental nucleus: Leitner et al., 1981; Koch et al., 1993; Swerdlow & Geyer, 1993; Kodsi & Swerdlow, 1997); (13) SC (superior colliculus: Fendt et al., 1994); (14) "primary" startle circuit: cf. Davis et al., 1982; Koch et al., 1992.
(ACH) acetylcholine; (DA) dopamine; (EAA) excitatory amino acid; (GABA) gamma-amino-butyric acid; (?) unknown or speculative connection or neurotransmitter

converging evidence supports the important involvement of dopaminergic systems, acting via D2-family (i.e., D2, 3, and 4) receptors, in the control of PPI. A dopaminergic regulation of PPI in humans is supported by the apomorphine-disruption of PPI in Parkinson's disease patients (Morton, Chaudhuri, Ellis, Gray, & Toone, 1995).

3.2. Glutamate

The major neurotransmitter used by cortico-striatal efferents is glutamate. Since evidence supports both limbic cortical and striatal regulation of PPI (see below), one would expect brain glutamate systems to be important in the regulation of PPI. PPI is reduced or eliminated in rats by systemic administration of noncompetitive *N*-methyl-D-aspartate (NMDA) antagonists, such as phencyclidine (PCP), dizocilpine (MK-801), and ketamine (Mansbach & Geyer, 1989). In humans, this class of drugs produces symptoms that mimic some forms of schizophrenia (Javitt & Zukin, 1991), and ketamine reduces PPI in normal subjects (Karper, Grillon, Charney, & Krystal, 1994). Studies in our laboratory suggest that the PPI-disruptive effects of PCP are reversed by the atypical antipsychotics clozapine (Bakshi, Swerdlow, & Geyer, 1994), olanzapine (Bakshi & Geyer, 1995), and Seroquel (Swerdlow, Bakshi, & Geyer, 1996), but not by haloperidol (Keith, Mansbach, & Geyer, 1991) or selective D1 or D2 antagonists (Bakshi et al., 1994).

3.3. Serotonin

Ascending serotonergic (5HT) fibers innervate much of the limbic cortex, and it is possible that this circuitry is one substrate for the serotonergic regulation of PPI. PPI is reduced in rats by 5HT releasers (Mansbach, Braff, & Geyer, 1989; Kehne et al., 1992) and by direct agonists for 5HT1A, 5HT1B, and 5HT2 receptors (Rigdon & Weatherspoon, 1992; Sipes & Geyer, 1994). The PPI-disruptive effects of 5HT releasers are reversed by pretreatment with the 5HT reuptake inhibitor fluoxetine, and the PPI-disruptive effects of direct 5HT receptor agonists are reversed by pretreatment with corresponding receptor subtype-specific 5HT antagonists (Sipes & Geyer, 1994).

3.4. Acetylcholine

PPI can be increased by stimulation of nicotinic cholinergic receptors via systemically administered nicotine or nicotine agonists (Acri, David, Popke, & Grunberg, 1994). The locus of action for these nicotinic effects is not known, but hippocampal nicotinic receptors have been implicated in the regulation of sensory gating in the dual-click P50 event-related potential gating paradigm (Adler, Pachtman, Franks, Pecevich, Waldo, & Freedman, 1993). This hippocampal substrate is of particular interest, because studies suggest that some schizophrenia patients – as well as unaffected family members – exhibit both sensory gating deficits and abnormalities in the alpha-7 subunit of the nicotinic receptor complex; this deficit is highly linked to a dinucleotide polymorphism at chromosome 15q14 (Freedman et al., 1997). A nicotinic regulation of PPI is also of particular interest to investigators studying PPI abnormalities in schizophrenia patients because there is both theoretical and empirical evidence that PPI measures can be altered by heavy levels of smoking in these patients (Kumari, Checkley, & Gray, 1996). The impact of smoking or smoking cessation (nicotine withdrawal) on PPI measures in psychiatric patients is thus an issue being intensively studied by several groups. Muscarinic cholinergic receptors in the hippocampus also regulate PPI, but activation of these receptors reduces PPI, in contrast to the effects of nicotine or nicotinic agonists (see below) (Caine, Geyer, & Swerdlow, 1991).

4. The Neurochemical Regulation of Short Lead Interval Facilitation of Startle

In the context of an investigation of the PPI-disruptive effects of the NMDA antagonist ketamine, Mansbach and Geyer (1991) observed that lead intervals of 30 msec tended to elicit lead stimulus facilitation from saline-treated rats – in particular, early in the test session – and that this lead stimulus facilitation effect was significantly potentiated by ketamine. These same doses of ketamine significantly disrupted PPI, and the authors suggested that the appearance of lead stimulus facilitation might reflect the removal of the inhibitory processes that normally "mask" the presence of lead stimulus facilitation. Thus, it is conceivable that the facilitatory effects themselves are not regulated by glutamate antagonism, but rather, the ketamine-induced disruption of PPI was "permissive" and allowed the emergence of lead stimulus facilitation. Others have reported that both PPI and prepulse facilitation are disrupted by low doses of MK-801 (Al-Amin & Schwarzkopf, 1996), although higher doses appeared to disrupt PPI, but not prepulse facilitation.

Some findings support the notion that short lead prestimuli generate a facilitatory effect on the startle response that under some conditions is obscured by more powerful inhibition, resulting in a "net" measurement of PPI. Some drugs in rats that potently disrupt PPI – such as the mixed D1/D2 agonist apomorphine or the D2-family agonist quinpirole – also "unmask" these facilitatory effects, manifesting prepulse facilitation (Wan & Swerdlow, 1994); interestingly, however, it has been reported in one study that apomorphine blocks not only PPI but also lead stimulus facilitation (elicited by very short interval lead stimuli) (Schwarzkopf et al., 1993). Other evidence for a balance of facilitatory and inhibitory lead stimulus effects exists in human studies. Under some conditions, lead stimuli that elicit only PPI in normal controls elicit only lead stimulus facilitation in Huntington's disease patients (Swerdlow et al., 1995) or in normal women in the midluteal phase of the menstrual cycle (Swerdlow, Hartman, & Auerbach, 1997).

5. Descending Forebrain Tonic Influences on Lead Stimulus Modification

The neuroanatomical substrates regulating PPI appear to be organized in serial segmental and perhaps parallel direct pathways linking limbic cortical regions with the pontine tegmentum, via connections in the striatum and pallidum.

5.1. Limbic Cortex

Significant changes in PPI follow experimental manipulations of the hippocampus, the medial prefrontal cortex (MPFC), and the basolateral amygdala.

5.1.1. The Hippocampus

Some evidence for the involvement of the hippocampus in regulating PPI has been found in humans: PPI is significantly reduced in patients with temporal lobe epilepsy and psychosis, compared with temporal lobe epilepsy patients without psychosis (Morton, Gray, Mellers, Toone, Lishman, & Gray, 1994). In rats, PPI of both acoustic and tactile startle is reduced or eliminated by intrahippocampal infusion of the cholinergic agonist carbachol, and this carbachol effect is reversed by co-infusion of the antimuscarinic atropine (Caine et al., 1991). This hippocampus cholinergic regulation of sensorimotor gating may be a normal function of the septo-hippocampal projection, since PPI is reduced by alpha-amino-3-hydroxy-5-methyl-4-isoxazole propionic acid (AMPA)-activation of the septal nucleus, and this effect is reversed by intrahippocampal infusion of atropine (Koch, 1996). Cholinergic activation of the hippocampus may impair PPI by stimulating glutamate release in the nucleus accumbens via hippocampal-accumbens glutamate fibers, as suggested by observations that PPI is disrupted by intra-accumbens infusion of glutamate (Swerdlow, Caine, Braff, & Geyer, 1992) or the glutamate agonists NMDA (Reijmers, Vanderheyden, & Peeters, 1995) or AMPA (Wan, Taaid, & Swerdlow, 1995), and by reports that intrahippocampal carbachol infusions cause behavioral activation that is blocked by intra-accumbens infusion of glutamate antagonists (Mogenson & Nielsen, 1984). PPI is also disrupted by NMDA infusion into the ventral subiculum, and this effect is reversed by co-infusion of the NMDA antagonist AP5 (Wan, Caine, & Swerdlow, 1996). A link between the hippocampal and ventral striatal regulation of PPI is suggested by findings that ibotenic acid lesions of the hippocampus in adult rats result in the development of "supersensitivity" to the PPI-disruptive effects of the DA agonist apomorphine (Swerdlow et al., 1995). Other studies suggest that the "supersensitive" apomorphine disruption of PPI is mediated via the ventral striatum (see below).

5.1.2. The Medial Prefrontal Cortex

In rats, PPI is reduced by interventions that decrease MPFC DA "tone," such as depletion of MPFC DA by infusion of 6-hydroxydopamine (6OHDA) (Bubser & Koch, 1994b; Koch & Bubser, 1994), or intra-MPFC infusion of D1 or D2 antagonists (Ellenbroek, Budde, & Cools, 1995). Reduced MPFC DA transmission might disrupt PPI via disinhibition of descending gluta-matergic fibers, resulting in subcortical increases in nucleus accumbens DA transmission. Such a model is consistent with the finding that the PPI-disruptive effects of MPFC 6OHDA lesions are blocked by systemic injection of haloperidol (Koch & Bubser, 1994). Also consistent with this model is the fact that cellular lesions of the MPFC result in the development of "super-sensitivity" to the PPI-disruptive effects of the DA agonist apomorphine, perhaps via the loss of a descending tonic facilitatory influence on subcortical DA activity (Swerdlow, Lipska, Weinberger, Braff, Jaskiw, & Weinberger, 1995).

5.1.3. The Basolateral Amygdala

The central nucleus of the amygdala has been implicated in the regulation of fear-potentiated startle, in elegant experiments by Hitchcock and Davis (1991). Decker, Curzon, and Brioni (1995) demonstrated that large radio-frequency lesions of the amygdala significantly reduced PPI. We have demonstrated that small cell-specific quinolinic acid lesions of the basolateral amygdala potently reduce PPI (Wan & Swerdlow, 1996). These lesions did not significantly reduce basal startle magnitude, but significantly disrupted fear-potentiated startle, raising the possibility that two structurally different forms of startle modulation – that produced by discrete, "phasic" 20-msec acoustic prestimuli (PPI), and that produced by a "tonic" state of fear elicited by a sustained 4-s visual cue (fear potentiation) – may share some overlapping neural substrates.

5.2. Striatum

Studies of the regulation of PPI by forebrain dopaminergic terminal regions have focused on the nucleus accumbens and the anteromedial striatum.

5.2.1. Nucleus Accumbens

Within the nucleus accumbens, there is a convergence of glutamatergic fibers from the hippocampus, MPFC, amygdala, and cingulate gyrus, and of dopaminergic fibers from cells in the ventral tegmentum. As such, the nucleus accumbens is a key subcortical integrative "hub," connecting forebrain and limbic structures that control cognition and behavior (Swerdlow & Koob, 1987).

The effects of DA agonists on PPI may be mediated by increased DA activity in the nucleus accumbens. First, low doses of apomorphine that do not decrease PPI in control rats potently disrupt PPI in control rats potently disrupt PPI in rate that are surgically altered to have "supersensitive" accumbens DA receptors (Swerdlow et al., 1986). Second, the loss of PPI induced by the indirect DA agonist amphetamine is reversed by depletion of accumbens DA (Swerdlow et al., 1990). Third, PPI is disrupted in rats by infusion of the D2 agonist quinpirole or DA into the nucleus accumbens or anteromedial striatum (but not the orbital cortex, amygdala, or posterior striatum) (Swerdlow et al., 1992; Wan, Geyer, & Swerdlow, 1994). The effects of intra-accumbens quinpirole or DA infusion on PPI are reversed by systemic treatment with D2 antagonists (Wan & Swerdlow, 1994). Thus, overactivity of nucleus accumbens DA may be a substrate for the loss of PPI in rats.

This is not to say that the nucleus accumbens is the *only* region supporting the dopaminergic regulation of PPI. In fact, dopaminergic activity in other areas – including the anteromedial striatum – appears to regulate PPI (see below). Furthermore, there is no clear evidence that the neuroleptic restoration of PPI in DA agonist-treated rats reflects the action of these neuroleptics within the nucleus accumbens. In fact, the effective dose of haloperidol needed to restore PPI in apomorphine-treated rats is similar, whether the haloperidol is administered subcutaneously or directly into the nucleus accumbens (or the MPFC, ventral hippocampus, caudate nucleus, or ventral tegmentum) (Hart, Zreik, Carper, & Swerdlow, 1996). Obviously, identifying the site of action of neuroleptics in restoring PPI in DA agonist-treated rats might be very important for the development of antipsychotic agents.

The nucleus accumbens is functionally heterogeneous, with lateral core and medial shell subregions characterized by distinct neurochemical, anatomical, and behavioral properties; this heterogeneity is also evident in the neurochemical regulation of PPI. The dopaminergic regulation of PPI is distributed across the nucleus accumbens: For example, PPI is reduced by quinpirole infusion into any one of several different nucleus accumbens locations, with only a small potency gradient favoring lateral core over medial shell regions (Wan et al., 1994). The same is true of the regulation of PPI by non-NMDA receptors in the nucleus accumbens: AMPA infusion into either the nucleus accumbens core or shell subregions reduces PPI (Wan et al., 1995; Wan & Swerdlow, 1996). However, interactions between DA and glutamate substrates regulate PPI only within the lateral accumbens core region, but not within the shell. Within the core, the PPI-disruptive effects of AMPA are DA-dependent: They are blocked by either 6OHDA lesions or systemic haloperidol injections (Wan et al., 1995). In contrast, the PPI-disruptive effects of intrashell AMPA infusion are not reversed by DA blockade (Wan & Swerdlow, 1996). These results suggest that, within the core, activation of non-NMDA receptors causes a reduction in PPI via a facilitatory effect on presynaptic DA release. Such a mechanism is consistent with our findings that blockade of non-NMDA receptors in the accumbens core with 6-cyano-7-nitroquinoxaline-2,3-dione (CNQX) prevents the PPI-disruptive effects of intracore infusion of the DA releaser amphetamine (Wan et al., 1995). This effect is also restricted to the nucleus accumbens core subregion: Intrashell infusion of amphetamine reduces PPI, but this effect is not opposed by co-infusion of CNQX (Wan & Swerdlow, 1996). Thus, in contrast to the core, within the nucleus accumbens shell, DA and non-NMDA glutamate transmission appear to regulate PPI independently.

5.2.2. Anteromedial Striatum

DA activity in striatal areas other than the nucleus accumbens also appears to regulate sensorimotor gating. First, PPI is disrupted by low doses of apomorphine in rats that have surgically induced "supersensitive" DA receptors in the striatum (Swerdlow et al., 1986). Supersensitivity to the PPI-disruptive effects of apomorphine is also reported in patients with Parkinson's disease (Morton et al., 1995). Second, DA infusion into the anteromedial striatum significantly disrupts PPI (Swerdlow, Braff, Masten, & Geyer, 1992). Third, Huntington's disease patients show profound deficits in PPI of both acoustic and tactile startle (Swerdlow et al., 1995), as do rats with quinolinic acid lesions of the dorsal posterior striatum (Kodsi & Swerdlow, 1995).

5.3. Pallidum

Decreased PPI after nucleus accumbens DA activation might reflect reduced activity in GABAergic fibers projecting from the accumbens to subpallidal regions. This striato–pallidal projection forms the next segment of a pervasive neural circuit regulating central inhibitory mechanisms in mammals (Mogenson & Nielsen, 1984). Some studies also suggest abnormalities in metabolism (Early et al., 1987) and cell number (Bogerts, Ashtari, Degreef, Alvir, Bilder, & Lieberman, 1985) in the ventral or internal pallidum in schizophrenia patients. The PPI-disruptive effects of nucleus accumbens DA infusion or accumbens cell lesions in rats are reversed by subpallidal infusion of the GABA agonist muscimol, and are reproduced by subpallidal infusion of the GABA antagonist picrotoxin (Swerdlow, Braff, & Geyer, 1990; Kodsi & Swerdlow, 1994). This accumbens–subpallidal GABAergic projection is a substrate for other behavioral effects of accumbens DA activation, and may translate the effects of activity in the hippocampus to lower motor circuitry.

5.4. Pontine Tegmentum

While it is not yet clear how decreased subpallidal GABA activity is translated to the primary startle circuit to modulate PPI, one possible route is via efferents to the pedunculopontine nucleus. Electrolytic or quinolinic acid lesions of the pedunculopontine nucleus eliminate PPI in rats (Swerdlow & Geyer, 1993; Kodsi, Taaid, Hartston, Zisook, Wan, & Swerdlow, 1995), as does muscimol infusion into this nucleus (Kodsi et al., 1995). There may be cytoarchitectural abnormalities in the pedunculopontine nucleus in some schizophrenia patients (Karson, Garcia-Rill, Biedermann, Mrak, Husain, & Skinner, 1991), and developmental dysfunction in this region is thought to occur in patients with nocturnal enuresis, who also exhibit reduced PPI (Ornitz, Hanna, & de Traversay, 1991). The pedunculopontine nucleus innervates the nucleus reticularis pontis caudalis, which is ultimately responsible for the elicitation of startle responses (Davis, 1984). It is also conceivable that the pedunculopontine nucleus might regulate PPI via ascending cholinergic projections to the thalamus.

5.5. Other Brain Regions

Because PPI is regulated by descending segmental projections linking the limbic forebrain with the pons, it is likely to be influenced by numerous other brain structures that "feed into" this circuitry. For example, the ventral tegmentum provides the dopaminergic innervation of the nucleus accumbens and receives descending glutamatergic inputs from the MPFC. Not surprisingly, PPI is reduced by chemical stimulation of the ventral tegmentum (Zhang, Engel, Hjorth, & Svensson, 1995). Similarly, the mediodorsal thalamus provides a dense glutamatergic input to the MPFC, and receives GABAergic projections from the ventral pallidum. Given its intimate relationship with the MPFC and ventral pallidum, it would not be surprising to find evidence for a mediodorsal thalamus regulation of PPI. PPI is significantly reduced after neurotoxin lesions of the superior colliculus, an effect thought to result from the loss of projections from the superior colliculus to the pedunculopontine nucleus (Fendt, Koch, & Schnitzler, 1994b). Thus, several brain structures other than those "neatly" arranged within descending segmental cortico–striato–pallido–pontine circuitry appear to regulate PPI.

6. The Forebrain Regulation of Lead Stimulus Effects: Relationship to Models of Psychopathology

The forebrain control of sensorimotor gating may have particular relevance to mechanisms regulating information processing and cognition, both in normal individuals and in specific neuropsychiatric disorders.

6.1. Human Studies

Interest in PPI as a measure of sensorimotor gating grew from the observation that human disorders with known dysfunctions in PPI "regulatory circuitry" are accompanied by impaired cognitive or sensorimotor inhibition. PPI deficits have been reported in patients with schizophrenia (see Chapter 11), obsessive-compulsive disorder (Swerdlow et al., 1993), Huntington's disease (Swerdlow et al., 1995), nocturnal enuresis and attention-deficit disorder (Ornitz et al., 1992), Tourette's syndrome (Castellanos et al., 1996), and temporal lobe epilepsy with psychosis (Morton et al., 1995). These disorders are all characterized by a loss of gating in sensory, motor, or cognitive domains, and by abnormalities in cortico–striato–pallido–pontine circuitry that modulates PPI. Importantly, PPI deficits are not unique to a single form of psychopathology but, instead, are the result of abnormalities within a specific, defined brain circuit.

It can be hypothesized that both clinical signs and reduced PPI in several disorders result from the same underlying neural deficit. While much more work is needed to address this issue, it has been shown that PPI deficits in schizophrenia patients correlate significantly with neuropsychological measures as distinct as perseverative responses on the Wisconsin Card Sorting Task (Butler, Jenkins, Geyer, & Braff, 1991; see Chapter 13) and pathologically elevated thought disorder (Perry & Braff, 1994; see Chapter 11). PPI deficits in schizophrenia patients correlate with certain indices of illness severity, including the number of hospitalizations, chlorpromazine equivalents, and global scores of negative symptoms (Braff, Perry, Cadenhead, Swerdlow, & Geyer, 1995). PPI is also significantly reduced in nonpatient controls who have a Minnesota Multiphasic Personality Inventory (MMPI) profile associated with specific neuropsychological deficits (Swerdlow, Filion, Geyer, & Braff, 1995). Thus, PPI is a measure of sensorimotor gating abilities that may correlate with, and perhaps contribute to, important determinants of information processing in both patients and nonpatient controls. It appears that PPI can be used to study neural circuitry that regulates normal cognitive processes and which is defective in several distinct neuropsychiatric disorders.

Importantly, the amount of PPI exhibited by any individual is not by itself predictive of pathology: Normal women exhibit significantly less PPI than do normal men (Swerdlow, Monroe, Hartston, Braff, Geyer, & Auerbach, 1993). These sex-linked differences in startle modulation are limited to PPI: No sex differences were found in startle magnitude, habituation, or latency. Others have reported greater startle response probability in women than in men when prepulses are used (Blumenthal & Gescheider, 1987), which may reflect greater PPI in men, and greater inhibition in men compared with women is seen in the P50 event-related potential measure (Hetrick, Sandman, Bunney, Gin, Potkin, & White, 1996), which is conceptually related to PPI.

6.2. Developmental and Genetic Studies

Sensorimotor gating deficits in schizophrenia patients – unlike PPI deficits in apomorphine-treated rats – are not an acute drug response, but are instead a reflection of longitudinal and complex interactions of genetic, developmental, social, and environmental forces. For this reason, it is important that startle gating in rats appears to be sensitive to these same forces. Studies also indicate that development and stress may significantly alter startle gating in rats. For example, Geyer, Wilkinson, Humby, and Robbins (1993) indicate that isolation-reared rats that exhibit elevated nucleus accumbens DA activity also demonstrate a neuroleptic-reversible deficiency in PPI.

Since PPI appears to develop in children between ages 5 and 8 (see Chapter 12), it is conceivable that abnormal developmental processes may contribute to PPI deficits in adult schizophrenia patients. In one finding of direct relevance to neurodevelopmental theories of schizophrenia (Weinberger, 1987), we have noted impaired PPI and enhanced sensitivity to the PPI-disruptive effects of apomorphine in postpubescent rats that had received neurotoxin lesions of the hippocampus as neonates (Lipska, Swerdlow, Geyer, Jaskiw, Braff, & Weinberger, 1995). It will be critically important to identify the peripubertal neural circuit changes that occur in neonatal hippocampal-lesioned rats that are responsible for the development of this supersensitive DA-mediated loss of PPI in adulthood. Thus, PPI studies can be used to examine the contribution of developmental processes to the pathophysiology of sensorimotor gating deficits in schizophrenia.

Genetic factors may also be critical determinants of sensorimotor gating in rats, since strain-related differences in the dopaminergic modulation of PPI have been reported (Rigdon, 1990). If susceptibility to the gating-disruptive effects of DA agonists is genetically controlled in rats, these studies might offer critical insight into genetic factors mediating the susceptibility to and development of schizophrenia in humans (Weinberger, 1987). Ellenbroek, Budde, and Cools (1995) utilized pharmacogenetic inbreeding to produce strains of rats that were either sensitive (APO-SUS) or insensitive (APO-UNSUS) to the behavioral effects of apomorphine. Rats descended from an inbred APO-SUS strain exhibited significantly less PPI, compared with rats descended from an inbred APO-UNSUS strain; this difference was also particularly evident with weak prepulses. Apparently, the physiological substrates that regulate the behavioral sensitivity to apomorphine (presumably some feature related to DA receptor sensitivity) are associated with substrates that regulate PPI, and these substrates are transmitted genetically. APO-SUS rats have elevated numbers of striatal D2 receptors and increased responsivity of both the hypothalamic-pituitary adrenal axis and dopaminergic systems. Certainly, the inheritance of reduced PPI might reflect the expressed inheritance of any one, or a combination of several, of these characteristics.

Another genetic strategy has recently been applied to understanding the normal physiological substrates regulating PPI (Dulawa, Hen, Scearce, & Geyer, 1995). PPI was compared between wild-type (WT) mice and mice that had been genetically engineered to lack serotonin-1B receptors – so-called 5HT1B "knock-outs" (5HT1BKOs). Basal PPI was slightly but significantly elevated in 5HT1BKOs compared with WTs, supporting a tonic regulation of PPI by 5HT1B receptors. Furthermore, PPI was significantly reduced in WT mice by the 5HT1A/1B agonist RU24969, but RU24969 did not reduce PPI in 5HT1BKOs. This work demonstrates a clear utility of applying genetic knock-out techniques toward understanding the physiological substrates of behaviors and processes such as sensorimotor gating. Similar strategies are currently being applied toward understanding the dopaminergic substrates of PPI, using D4 knock-out mice (Grandy et al., 1995).

7. Summary

Animal and human studies of PPI have been aimed at understanding the basic physiological and neurochemical substrates regulating sensorimotor gating. This effort has been motivated in part by the awareness that several neuropsychiatric disorders are characterized both by deficits in PPI and by clinical evidence of impaired inhibition of cognitive, sensory, or motor information. The convergence of information from preclinical and clinical studies supports the notion that brain regions frequently implicated in the pathophysiology of these disorders – the limbic cortex, ventral striatum, pallidum, and pontine tegmentum – also critically regulate PPI.

The structure of complex systems has been studied across scientific disciplines – from quantum physics to ecology – by measuring the changes in system "output" that follow the application of controlled, orderly forces. By systematically studying lead stimulus modification of the startle reflex, this same strategy can be applied toward understanding central nervous system organization. This paradigm has been effectively used to study the normal physiology of "gating circuitry," applying the sophistication of anatomical and pharmacological manipulations to parse apart complex neural circuit interaction, such as the dopamine–glutamate interactions within different subregions of the ventral striatum. In the process, it has also been possible to identify the particular perturbations of normal brain function at each level of this circuitry that might yield deficits in PPI – such as those observed in schizophrenia and other disorders – and, conversely, what interventions might act at each level of the circuitry to enhance or restore normal levels of sensorimotor gating. Presumably, this functional gating circuit "map" will become increasingly valuable, as neuroimaging and neuropathological findings draw us closer to identifying the specific brain disturbances associated with these disorders.

ACKNOWLEDGMENTS

This work was supported by MH 48381, MH 42228, MH 52885, MH 53484, and MH 01436 from the National Institute of Mental Health. The authors gratefully acknowledge the many contributions to our work by Dr. David Braff and our other colleagues in San Diego. Although some of the material and concepts raised in this chapter are addressed in works previously published by the authors (e.g., Swerdlow, 1996; Swerdlow & Geyer, 1996; Dawson et al., 1997), many new themes of the present work are not duplicated in other writings by the authors.

PART III

Psychological Mediation of Startle Modification

Implications of Blink Reflex Research for Theories of Attention and Consciousness

STEVEN A. HACKLEY

ABSTRACT

Neuroscientists such as Kandel (1978) and Thompson (1986) have exploited the behavioral and neuranatomical simplicity of reflexes in their development of reductionistically approachable model systems of learning and memory. It is argued in this chapter that the field of attention and performance would similarly benefit from the development of a simple model system based on startle and related reflexes. Representative studies are reviewed with respect to the three attentional subsystems distinguished by Posner and Petersen (1990) – the orienting, alerting, and executive networks. To integrate data from reflexology into the broader field of cognitive neuroscience, information processing models that incorporate a vertical architecture are recommended.

1. The Relevance of Reflexology

Contrasts can help us to grasp amorphous concepts. We may be unsure as to what exactly consciousness is, for example, but we are confident that the comatose patient lacks it, whereas an alert, healthy person has it. Approaching this poorly defined concept from the perspective of several distinct contrasts has helped bring it into clearer view: Experimental comparisons between wakefulness versus sleep, alertness versus anesthesia, masked versus supraliminal priming, ocular dominance versus suppression, blind sight versus visual awareness, and evoked potentials to attended versus ignored stimuli have provided a wealth of relevant data. It is the thesis of this review that direct comparisons of voluntary and reflexive reactions can also provide valuable insights into the neural bases of attention and consciousness.

Neurobehavioral research on reflexes has continued uninterrupted for a quarter of a millennium (e.g., Whytt, 1751, reviewed in Fearing, 1930). What

Michael E. Dawson, Anne M. Schell, and Andreas H. Böhmelt, Eds. *Startle modification: Implications for neuroscience, cognitive science, and clinical science.* Copyright © 1999 Cambridge University Press. Printed in the United States of America. All rights reserved.

can the venerable discipline of reflexology contribute in the present era of functional neuroimaging? One answer is *cost-effective reductionism.*

Memory researchers have successfully exploited this possibility. Neuroscientists such as Kandel (1978) and Thompson (1986) have adapted simple reflex paradigms to study learning and memory in small, inexpensive laboratory animals. Reflexes are used because the underlying circuitry is simple enough to be defined on a cell-by-cell basis. Inexpensive lab animals are used so that the massive research effort can be distributed among a large number of research groups, including many that pursue their work without federal grant support. By contrast, the current focus within the neurobiology of attention emphasizes complex tasks performed by monkeys (e.g., Moran & Desimone, 1985). These animals are expensive to acquire, maintain, and train. Consequently, such research is necessarily restricted to a few well-funded labs. More important, the neural pathways that underlie the tasks in question (e.g., visual search by macaques for feature conjunctions), are orders of magnitude more complex than conditioned eyeblink in rabbits or the gill-withdrawal reflex in *Aplysia.* In view of this complexity, the reduction of higher attentional processes to the circuit, synaptic, and molecular levels may be presumed to lie only in the distant future.

The possibility of developing reflex paradigms for the study of attention has been discussed sporadically in the literature since the time of Dodge (1931, pp. 43, 99). Systematic research on the topic began with the work of Frances Graham (1975; Bohlin & Graham, 1977), Howard Hoffman (Del-Pezzo & Hoffman, 1980), and their respective associates. A number of potentially useful paradigms have now been developed. As is the case with simple system models of learning and memory, the degree to which findings can be generalized to higher brain function varies considerably. Some reflex paradigms may reflect the same mechanisms that underlie attention effects on voluntary reactions (e.g., selective orienting effects on the acoustic startle-blink reflex). Others may index ancillary pathways that are only of indirect relevance to the attentional phenomena studied by cognitive psychologists (e.g., suppression of lid closure during the perceptual analysis of a new stimulus). Still other paradigms involve reflex processes that may either be directly ancestral to, or ancient analogs of, phylogenetically more recent mechanisms (e.g., response competition at spinal vs. neocortical levels). The degree of relevance to higher brain function will be more apparent as specific reflex data are reviewed.

This review of representative studies of startle and other reflexes will be organized around the tripartite attention theory of Posner and Petersen (1990; Posner, 1995). According to their theory, one of the three anatomically circumscribed systems involves parietal, pulvinar, and midbrain structures. This "posterior attention network" is responsible for both overt and covert orienting of attention to sensory stimuli. The second system functions to initiate and maintain an alert state; it is mediated by brain-stem monoamine and cholinergic pathways (i.e., the ascending reticular activation system) and by as yet undefined right hemisphere structures. Finally, the third system mediates executive functions, such as target detection, control of working memory, and the scheduling of competing responses. This "anterior attention network" has been linked to lateral and mesial prefrontal cortex.

2. Reflex Studies of the Orienting Network

2.1. Direct Effects on Startle

In the cognitive literature, the term "orienting" refers to the selective focusing of perceptual resources on an object or location. It can be triggered by the sudden appearance of a new perceptual object, a phenomenon termed *exogenous orienting*. Alternatively, a symbolic cue can instruct the subject to voluntarily direct attention to a specific object or location, a process referred to as *endogenous orienting* (Yantis & Hillstrom, 1994). These two modes of selective attention have distinguishable properties, but both result in improved perception of stimuli within the attended channel (Yantis & Jonides, 1990). Hemodynamic imaging (Corbetta, Miezin, Dobmeyer, Shulman, & Petersen, 1991) and event-related potentials (ERPs; Mangun, 1995) have revealed cortical level changes that are likely to underlie such effects. Research on brainstem reflexes may help to identify relevant subcortical processes.

A study of the acoustic startle-blink reflex illustrates the application of reflex psychophysiological methods to the investigation of endogenous orienting (Hackley & Graham, 1987; for more comprehensive reviews, see Anthony, 1985; Putnam, 1990; Hackley & Graham, 1991; and Chapters 4 and 15). On each trial in the Hackley and Graham study, subjects received a visual warning stimulus that was unpredictive of the location of the target, a 100-dB startle stimulus. The lead time between the warning stimulus and the startle stimulus varied randomly from 1 to 4 s. The startle stimulus was delivered over headphones at either the left, midline, or right location and its duration varied randomly between 50 and 75 msec. In balanced blocks of trials, subjects attended to one designated location and made an unspeeded verbal report regarding startle-stimulus duration, "short" or "long." The eyeblink component of acoustic startle reflex (onset, approximately 50 msec) was recorded electromyographically from the upper eyelid of both eyes.

Consistent with the assumption that orienting can produce a preset bias within selected auditory pathways, the onset latency of the blink reflexes evoked by either left- or right-ear stimuli was speeded when attention was directed to that position relative to when it was directed to the other ear. The effect was not significant for the midline tones, a finding that is consistent with ERP studies of auditory attention (e.g., Schwent, Snyder, & Hillyard, 1976): Larger attention effects on the amplitude of the N100 component have been observed for lateral (left- or right-ear) tones than for midline tones, presumably due to overlap of the attentional "spotlight" onto neighboring locations.

The key finding was that the onset latency of startle blinks to left-ear tone pips was facilitated when attention was focused on the left stimulus channel, whereas reactions to right-ear stimuli were speeded when attention was directed to the right channel. This location specificity suggests a modulatory effect within the afferent limb of the reflex arc, that is to say, a selective facilitation or inhibition at some point prior to the convergence of left- and right-ear sensory pathways onto the startle center (for reviews of related studies, see Anthony, 1985, and Putnam, 1990).

So little is known about the reflex arc for acoustic startle blink that one cannot even say whether the locus of modulation must be subcortical. Although animal studies have shown that the acoustic blink reflex persists after section of the brain at the intercollicular level (Hori, Yasuhara, Naito, Yasuhara, 1986), this does not rule out the possibility that a parallel pathway involving forebrain structures might supplement the brain-stem circuitry. In fact, a comparison of spinal-level startle responses to left- and right-ear stimuli in patients with lesions of auditory cortex on the left or right side indicates that such a long-loop pathway may exist (Liegois-Chauvel, Morin, Musolino, Bancaud, & Chauvel, 1989): Smaller startle effects were observed in these patients when the evoking stimulus was presented at the ear contralateral to the lesion. Because cortical-level attention effects can be manifested in auditory ERPs as early as 15–20 msec after stimulus onset (Woldorff, Hansen, & Hillyard, 1987; Hackley, Woldorff, & Hillyard, 1990), modulation of a long-loop pathway could occur quickly enough to influence startle blink.

To test this possibility, Hackley, Woldorff, and Hillyard (1987) examined the effects of highly focused attention on a reflex that occurs too quickly to be mediated by a transcortical loop – the postauricular component of startle (onset latency, 9–11 msec). The results indicated that attention has no direct effect on the sensory pathways that trigger this trisynaptic reflex.[1] Therefore,

---

[1] However, an indirect effect of attention that appeared to be mediated via short-lead interval inhibition – to be discussed later – was quite reliable. Also, an effect of attention on the

it is possible that attentional modulation of sensory processes at cortical rather than brain-stem levels could account for the Hackley and Graham (1987) findings.

Both the Hackley and Graham (1987) and the Hackley et al. (1987) studies evaluated the effects of within-modality manipulations of orienting on acoustic reflexes. Using between-modality manipulations of orienting (e.g., attend tone vs. attend air puff), reliable effects have been observed for the cutaneous as well as the acoustic blink reflex. Effects on air puff-evoked blinks reached significance for onset latency in one study (Hackley & Graham, 1983) and for amplitude in another (Haerich, 1994). (In general, these two measures are highly correlated, but they can be dissociated by manipulations that differentially influence the mechanisms responsible for triggering a reflex versus adjusting its size and duration in accordance with stimulus parameters; Blumenthal & Berg, 1986; Manning & Evinger, 1986.)

Whether attention effects on air puff-evoked blinks are due to modulation of subcortical or cortical sensory pathways is uncertain. The comparison of blink reflexes to left versus right trigeminal nerve stimulation in patients with lesions of somatosensory cortex on the left and right side (reviewed in Kimura, 1992) suggests that a long-loop pathway may contribute to the cutaneous blink reflex. Therefore, the possibility that attention effects on the cutaneous blink reflex involve modulation of cortical-level pathways cannot be ruled out.

In contrast to the acoustic and cutaneous startle response, the evidence to date indicates that the reflex arc for the photic blink reflex does not include a long-loop pathway. (For another type of visual blink reflex, the startle/defensive reaction to threat of imminent collision, cortical circuits probably do play a role; see discussion in Hackley & Boelhouwer, 1997.) The claim that there is no long-loop pathway for photic blink is based on an experiment analogous to those that did indicate the participation of cortex in acoustic and cutaneous reflexes. Comparisons in patients with lesions of visual cortex on the left or right side showed that the photic blink reflex to left versus right hemifield stimulation did not differ (Fig. 7.1; see Hackley & Johnson, 1996).

Consistent with the hypothesis that attentional orienting effects are limited to cortical or at least forebrain levels (Hackley, 1993), no incontrovertible effects of attention on the afferent limb of the subcortical reflex arc for photic blink have been documented. No study that has controlled gaze direction, accommodation, and/or emotional valence across conditions has obtained

motor limb of the reflex arc was documented. The postauricular muscle on the side to which the subject oriented exhibited larger reflexes, regardless of whether the evoking stimulus was presented to the attended or ignored ear.

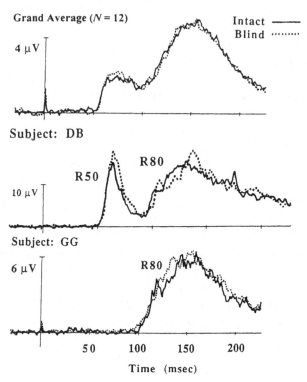

Figure 7.1. Signal-averaged electromyographic responses to intense visual stimuli within the blind or intact hemifield of patients with unilateral visual cortex damage. (*Top*) A grand average across 12 patients; (*middle, bottom*) data for two individual patients who denied any awareness of strobe flashes within their scotomata. Subject GG, shown in *bottom,* lacks an R50 component, but this is probably unrelated to his neurological status. About 15% of normal adults lack the early component of the photic blink reflex. (Copyright 1996, The Society for Psychophysiological Research. Adapted with permission of the publisher from Hackley and Johnson, 1996.)

evidence for selective modulation of the afferent limb of the photic blink reflex arc (Bradley, Cuthbert, & Lang, 1990; Hackley, Woldorff, & Hillyard, 1990; Hackley & Burke, 1992; Burke & Hackley, 1997; but cf. Anthony & Graham, 1983, 1985; Balaban, Anthony, & Graham, 1985, who did not control these factors). Taken together, the studies of acoustic, cutaneous, and photic startle reviewed in this section suggest that attention effects on reflexes may be limited to sensory pathways involving the forebrain. These experiments certainly cannot be regarded as definitive, but their findings converge with those obtained using a very different methodology, startle modification by a nonreflexogenic lead stimulus.

2.2. Indirect Effects via Startle Modification

The ability of a weak visual lead stimulus, or "prepulse," to inhibit the startle response to a subsequent strong stimulus apparently requires an intact visual cortex. A visual lead stimulus that is presented within the scotoma of patients with unilateral striate cortex damage does not produce inhibition of the amplitude of startle to a subsequent reflexogenic stimulus (Hilgard & Wendt, 1933; Burke & Hackley, 1997; see also Ison, Bowen, & O'Connor, 1991). However, these studies also indicate that the ability of a visual lead stimulus to facilitate the latency or magnitude of startle is preserved following loss of visual cortex. For startle modification by acoustic lead stimuli, the involvement of cortex appears to depend on the type of prepulse. Amplitude inhibition by a gap within an otherwise continuous background noise does require cortex, whereas inhibition by an onset or offset transient does not (Ison, O'Connor, Bowen, & Bocirnea, 1991; latency facilitation was not evaluated).

When a person orients to a short-interval lead stimulus because that stimulus is inherently interesting for biological reasons (e.g., photos of opposite-sex nudes or mutilated bodies; Bradley, Cuthbert, & Lang, 1993) or because it is relevant to the task at hand (DelPezzo & Hoffman, 1980; Hackley & Graham, 1987), the ability of that lead stimulus to produce prepulse inhibition is enhanced. If the only value of this finding were an incremental gain in our understanding of eyelid oculomotor control during attentional orienting, it would have attracted little interest among psychophysiologists. The phenomenon is of broader interest for three reasons. First, because almost any stimulus can serve as a prepulse and because short-interval inhibition is automatic, this paradigm can be used to unobtrusively probe the allocation of attentional resources. Second, because the effect is at least partly mediated within the brainstem, this phenomenon offers a window on orienting processes that are not easily accessible to neuroimaging or ERP methods. Finally, this attention effect is important because it is apparently absent in schizophrenics (Dawson, Hazlett, Filion, Nuechterlein, & Schell, 1993) and in normal subjects who manifest certain aberrations of perception or thought, indicating that they are at risk for developing schizophrenia (Schell, Dawson, Hazlett, & Filion, 1995).

A study by Sonnenberg, Low, and Hackley (1996) will illustrate the general methods and findings. This particular study was based on an orienting paradigm that is popular among cognitive psychologists (e.g., Posner, 1980). On each trial, a centrally located arrow either correctly or incorrectly precued the location of a subsequent target stimulus. These valid- and invalid-precue trials occurred randomly with a probability of 80% and 20%, respectively.

The target stimulus was the illumination of a red, light-emitting diode, located 25 degrees to the left or right of fixation. Subjects made an unspeeded oral report regarding target duration, "short" or "long" (300 or 500 msec), regardless of whether the target appeared on the cued or uncued side.

Not surprisingly, this perceptual discrimination was more accurate (as measured by d') when the subject's attention was correctly oriented to the location of the target than when attention was misdirected to the wrong side. Consistent with prior ERP studies (e.g., Mangun, Hansen, & Hillyard, 1987), cortical potentials evoked by the target stimuli were enhanced on valid compared with invalid trials. More important, the results showed that short lead interval inhibition also was modulated by visuospatial attention. This was determined from trials on which an intense but task-irrelevant noise burst was presented 150 msec after onset of the target stimulus. The inhibition of startle-blink magnitude to this noise burst was significantly enhanced when the location of the lead stimulus (i.e., the target) was validly precued as compared with trials in which attention was misdirected to the other side.

Similar effects have been demonstrated within the auditory modality. For example, directing attention to the same versus a different location than that of an acoustic lead stimulus reliably modulates the ability of that lead stimulus to inhibit the response to a subsequent reflexogenic stimulus (Hackley & Graham, 1987; Hackley, Woldorff, & Hillyard, 1987). Dawson and colleagues have obtained similar results for selective attention to the pitch of the lead stimulus (e.g., Filion, Dawson, & Schell, 1993). In the Dawson paradigm, subjects are presented with a series of long-duration tones that randomly vary between two different pitches. They are instructed to keep a running count of the number of longer than usual (7 s as opposed to 5 s) tones of one designated pitch while ignoring tones of the other pitch. Task-irrelevant noise bursts are unpredictably presented during attended and ignored tones, typically at asynchronies of 60, 120, 240, or 2000 msec relative to tone onset. The amount of inhibition or facilitation of startle blink is determined by comparison with noise-alone control trials. In normal young adults, inhibition of startle in the 120-msec condition and facilitation in the 2000-msec condition is greater for attended tones than for ignored tones (e.g., Filion et al., 1993, 1994).

The variation in startle modification as a function of orienting toward or away from the lead stimulus can be interpreted in the context of Graham's (e.g., 1975) theory of short lead interval inhibition. According to her theory, startle subserves a reset function, interrupting ongoing perceptual-motor processes so that the organism can better evaluate and respond to the abrupt/intense evoking stimulus (e.g., a predator). Vision is interrupted by the eyeblink component of startle, and audition (in most mammals) by the pinna-flexion component of startle, also known as the postauricular reflex. The purpose of short lead interval inhibition is to prevent such disruptions during the course of perceptual analysis of any new stimulus (i.e., the lead stimulus). Keeping the pinnae motionless and the eyes wide open following detection of a new stimulus has obvious adaptive value. Under the present interpretation, attentional orienting to the lead stimulus enhances the duration (Bradley et al., 1990) and magnitude (e.g., Hackley & Graham, 1987; Filion et al., 1993, 1994) of the inhibition it triggers. If a stimulus has inherent motivational value or is relevant to the organism's immediate goals, it is all the more important that perceptual processing be protected from interruption.

What happens after perceptual analysis of that stimulus is completed? According to one popular theory (Posner & Cohen, 1984), there is a tendency to avoid reorienting to a location that has recently been attended, a phenomenon known as *inhibition of return*. If a sudden stimulus in the visual periphery captures attention, the voluntary reaction to a target stimulus appearing at that location during the next 50–150 msec is speeded. However, at longer lead times (e.g., 400–2000 msec), the latency of voluntary reactions to targets at that location is inhibited as compared with targets presented at other locations.

In an experiment with normal subjects, Burke and Hackley (1997) obtained a pattern of results for photic blink that was similar to reaction time (RT) measures of inhibition of return. On each trial, a startle-blink reflex was evoked by the discharge of one of two strobe lamps, located 25 degrees to the left and right of fixation. Each lamp was encircled by four light-emitting diodes, the illumination of which served as the lead stimulus. Both the startle and lead stimuli were irrelevant to the subject's task, which was to monitor a central fixation light for occasional flickering. The diode-to-strobe lead times varied randomly among the values 1200, 600, 120, 70, 45, 20, and −50 msec (the negative onset asynchrony indicates that diode illumination followed the strobe flash). On half of the trials, the location of the lead and startle stimulus was concordant, and on the other half, the two stimulus were presented on opposite sides of fixation.

Consistent with RT data regarding inhibition of return (e.g., Posner & Cohen, 1984), blink onset was delayed when the lead stimulus and strobe locations were the same versus when they were different. The concordance effect was maximum at a lead time of 600 ms. These results might be explained in terms of the close physiological (Evinger, Shaw, Peck, Manning, & Baker, 1984) and neuroanatomical (Schmidtke & Büttner-Ennever, 1992) linkage between lid- and eye-movement control mechanisms. Because both eyeblinks and saccades momentarily disrupt vision, their scheduling is tightly synchronized. We usually saccade when we blink and we usually suppress spontaneous blinking when we attentively fixate a stationary object or when our *eyes smoothly pursue* a moving object (Webb & Obrist, 1970; Evinger et al., 1984). Inhibition of return is believed to involve an active suppression of evoked saccades toward a recently attended location (Posner & Cohen, 1984; Posner, Rafal, Choate, & Vaughan, 1985). If reflexive as well as spontaneous blinks are subject to oculomotor control factors, then the observed pattern of inhibition of return effects on photic blink would be expected.

Although the reflex data appeared similar to prior RT data with respect to inhibition of return, this was not true with regard to attentional orienting per se. In contrast to findings for voluntary RT (e.g., Posner & Cohen, 1984; Posner et al., 1985), reflex latencies were not facilitated when the strobe flashed at the same location as the lead stimulus in the 45-, 70-, or 120-msec conditions. The absence of an attention capture effect at short lead times (less than 200 msec) within an experiment demonstrating inhibition of return is surprising, but it does corroborate previous failures to obtain an effect of visuospatial orienting on the photic blink reflex (Hackley et al., 1990; Hackley & Burke, 1992). Perhaps the facilitatory, but not the subsequent inhibitory, effects of exogenous attention are limited to cortical pathways that mediate voluntary reactions to visual stimuli. Alternatively, the putative inhibition-of-return findings of Burke and Hackley may have been due to some local sensory–sensory interaction rather than attentional orienting.

The apparent dissociation between the putative inhibition of return and attentional orienting effects on eyeblink underscores an important point. Reflex measures are not redundant with RT data, or with other physiological measures. The study of startle blink and lead stimulation effects offers a unique perspective on brain function during orienting, as well as during other attentional processes.

3. Reflex Studies of the Alerting Network

The sudden appearance of a lead stimulus not only activates the orienting system, it can also trigger alerting. For example, a task-irrelevant tone pip delivered at around the same time as a visual reaction stimulus reliably speeds choice RT (e.g., Bernstein, Rose, & Ashe, 1970). It is generally agreed that this *accessory stimulus effect* is generated by a brief surge of arousal that nonspecifically facilitates some postsensory process (e.g., Posner, 1978, pp. 128–131; Sanders, 1980). It is also agreed that the alerting effects of an accessory stimulus are closely related to those produced by a neutral warning stimulus. This conclusion is based on similar patterns of interactions with other experimental variables (Sanders, 1980) and on the fact that the facilitation of RT by both warning and accessory stimuli is often accompanied by a compensatory increase in error rate (Posner, 1978, p. 137).

The main disagreement within the cognitive literature concerns which particular stage or stages within the chain of processing that extends from stimulus to response is influenced by alerting. Of the two most prominent theoretical accounts, Sanders (1980) has argued that alerting facilitates a late, low-level motor process, whereas Posner (1978, pp. 128–131) appears to assume that alerting influences a decision-level mechanism. Studies of alerting effects on reflexes could help resolve this controversy for two reasons. First, decision processes that are capable of arbitrarily assigning particular voluntary responses to particular stimuli play no role in the mediation of reflexive reactions.[2] Consequently, evidence that alerting effects on voluntary and reflexive reactions involve a single common mechanism would argue against Posner's theory. Second, there is some overlap among the pathways that mediate voluntary and reflexive reactions at the lowest levels of the motor system (at the very minimum, shared use of alpha motor neurons and muscle fibers). Animal neurophysiology research has shown that alerting effects on reflexes involve modulation of low-level motor processes (e.g., Young, Cegavsge, & Thompson, 1976; Stafford & Jacobs, 1990). Therefore, evidence that a common mechanism underlies alerting effects on voluntary and reflexive reactions would support Sanders's assumption of a locus for alerting effects at a relatively late motoric stage.

To test the degree of overlap between alerting effects on voluntary and reflexive reactions, Low, Larson, Burke, and Hackley (1997) directly compared choice RT and photic-blink reflexes to intense flashes of light. Alerting was manipulated using both accessory stimuli (a nonstartling tone pip delivered at a 40-msec lead time with respect to the strobe flash) and neutral warning stimuli (the illumination of a diode either 1.5 or 4.0 s prior to strobe onset). Both manipulations of alerting speeded reflexive as well as voluntary reactions. However, a number of dissociations were observed. For example, warning and accessory effects were additive for blink latency but strongly interactive for choice RT. Similarly, the magnitudes of these alerting effects on voluntary and reflexive reactions were not correlated across subjects. Discrepancies were also noted by Sollers and Hackley (1997) between the pat-

---

[2] It would be a violation of common usage to designate a response as *reflexive* if that response could be mapped to any arbitrarily designated experimental stimulus. However, it is argued in Section 4 that decision-making can play a role in reflexive behavior when two or more responses are concurrently elicited.

tern of warning interval effects on simple RT versus the postauricular and eye-blink components of acoustic startle. Together, these data imply a divergence in the mechanisms that underlie alerting effects on voluntary and reflexive reactions.

Brain ERPs have now more definitively localized the effects of alerting on voluntary reactions. Valle-Inclan and Hackley (1996) used the onset of the lateralized readiness potential (LRP) as a temporal landmark to split mean RT into two segments, the time interval from stimulus onset until onset of hand-specific motor cortex activation (stimulus-to-LRP), and the interval extending from LRP onset until movement onset (LRP-to-movement). As expected, choice RT to a visual stimulus (the letter S or T) was speeded when the reaction stimulus was accompanied by an acoustic accessory stimulus (30-msec lead time). Analyses of the ERPs showed this effect to be entirely localized to the stimulus-to-LRP time interval; the duration of motor processes subsequent to lateralized motor cortex activation was unaffected by alerting. A similar pattern of LRP results was obtained by Smulders, Kenemans, and Kok (1995) in a study of temporal uncertainty effects that were assumed to have been mediated by alerting.

When Posner originally theorized that alerting does not speed RT by facilitating low-level motor processes, one of his arguments was that a neutral warning stimulus has no effect on the time interval extending from onset of EMG activity until onset of the physical movement (Botwinick & Thompson, 1966, cited in Posner, 1978). The data of Smulders and colleagues and of Valle-Inclan and Hackley simply push this line of evidence further upstream: Alerting also does not affect the time interval extending from the onset of response-specific motor cortex activation cortex until onset of the physical movement.

Sanders's (1980, 1983) theory, on the other hand, appears to predict that alerting should influence the LRP-to-movement interval. Although his theory is articulated in cognitive rather than neuroanatomical terms, he does indicate that the effect of alerting is localized to the same stage at which variations in tonic, instructed muscle tension influence voluntary RT. We know from studies using magnetic stimulation of cortex in humans and from motor neuron studies in animals (discussed in Murray, 1992) that at least part of the tonic muscle effect occurs downstream from motor cortex, including the spinal cord. Therefore, the stage that Sanders postulates as the locus of alerting effects is probably downstream from the stage associated with LRP onset. In summary, converging evidence from reflex, LRP, and direct motor stimulation studies argues against Sanders's theory that alerting speeds RT by facilitating low-level motor pathways. The exact stage or process that alerting does facilitate (e.g., making a decision from among several task-relevant responses) remains to be determined.

4. Reflex Studies Relevant to the Executive Network

Much behavioral and ERP research on the executive network (anterior attention system) has focused on the resolution of conflict among simultaneously activated responses. Competing voluntary responses can be elicited by distinct stimuli, as in studies of the psychological refractory period or Eriksonian interference, or they can be triggered by separable attributes of a single stimulus, as in studies of the Stroop or Simon effects. Functional neuroimaging studies (Pardo, Pardo, Janer, & Raichle, 1992) implicate frontal lobe structures, especially the anterior cingulate cortex, in the resolution of response competition.

Any influence of the anterior cingulate is, of course, absent in the isolated spinal preparations that have traditionally been used to study competition among reflexive responses. Nonetheless, the patterns of interactions that have been observed among simultaneously evoked reflexes (e.g., Sherrington, 1906, chap. 4) are similar to those that have been observed during competition between voluntary responses (e.g., Coles, Gratton, Bashore, Eriksen, & Donchin, 1985). For example, Sherrington (1906, p. 114) notes, "Antagonistic reflexes interfere, one reflex deferring, interrupting, or cutting short another, or precluding the latter altogether from taking effect on the final common path." The nature of interactions among overlapping reflexes is strongly determined by their onset asynchrony, a fact emphasized in a series of studies by three Nobel prize-winning reflexologists (Eccles & Granit, 1929; Eccles & Sherrington, 1930). Similarly, stimulus onset asynchrony has proven critical in accounting for prioritization, scheduling, and interference among voluntary reactions (e.g., Pashler, 1984; de Jong, Coles, Logan, & Gratton, 1990).

The similarity between voluntary and reflexive reactions with regard to response competition suggests that comparable mechanisms may be involved. As noted in Section 1, the circuits that resolve conflicts among spinal reflexes may be either directly ancestral to, or else ancient analogs of, phylogenetically more recent structures that mediate response selection among voluntary behaviors. The advantage of studying response selection among reflexes is that the underlying circuitry is simpler. Much progress has been made, for example, in defining the neural pathways that mediate a spinal cord decision between scratching at two different locations, or between scratching an itch versus withdrawing from a painful shock (Stein, 1989).

As findings from reflexology are integrated with the cognitive neuroscience of response selection, it will be important to develop *vertical models* of executive functions. Such models will address the coordination of lower sensorimotor behavior with cortically mediated perception and voluntary behavior. The importance of the distinction between vertical versus horizontal models is illustrated by recent developments within the field of robotics.

Until about ten years ago, as noted by Brooks (1991), control systems for robots were organized into a horizontal array of functional modules. Similar to the models developed by cognitive psychologists (e.g., Sternberg, 1969), the flow of information from sensors to effectors typically involved a linear progression through such stages as perception, planning, task execution, and motor control. Unfortunately, the enormous computational demands of perceiving and modeling the environment with enough sophistication to meet the requirements of multiple behavioral tasks often left these robots "lost in thought" for hours. To develop robots that could think on their feet, Brooks (1986) developed real-time control systems with predominantly vertical architectures.

In these systems, control is decomposed into task-achieving behaviors rather than general purpose information-processing stages. Each horizontal layer receives sensory input and can directly generate some part of the robot's behavior. The lower layers are purely reflexive in character, such as the network designed to *Avoid bumping into things and avoid being bumped into.* Intermediate layers are more similar to instincts or fixed action patterns, such as *Wander, Actively explore,* and *Monitor for changes in the environment.* The highest layers have a primitive cognitive quality – primitive in sense that they are not based on symbols, as are traditional artificial intelligence systems. An example of a such a layer in one of Brooks's machines is *Reason about the behavior of identifiable objects.*

Both the engineering development of these layers and the resulting interlaminar relationships can be viewed as a metaphor for the evolution of the nervous system. New, more sophisticated task layers are added on top of existing layers, with conservation of established behavioral competencies. Because each horizontal layer has independent access to motoric structures, there must be a method for conflict resolution. Response competition is resolved by a fixed priority arbitration scheme. Lower layers are oblivious to the function of higher layers, but a higher layer can suppress the motor output of the next-lowest layer when it wishes to take control. There is no central executive system, no shared global memory, and no unified perceptual representation of the world. Nevertheless, a coherent, integrated behavior emerges. For example, the insect-like robot Attila, which was designed for unmanned planetary surface exploration (Brooks, 1989), appears to exhibit a degree of intelligence comparable to that of some real insects.

For 20th-century robotics – which differ sharply from 20th-century science fiction – that is an achievement worth noting. Whereas artificial intelligence has long served as an inspiration for model construction within cognitive psychology, and connectionism is currently enjoying a similar influence within some branches of neurobiology, reflexologists and other sensorimotor researchers may find robotics to be a fruitful source of testable hypotheses.

5. Definitions for Volition and Consciousness

Models with vertical architectures, whether for robotics or cognitive neuroscience, are naturally organized along the spectrum of automatic-controlled processing. Lower-level networks receive minimally analyzed sensory input and provide rapid, minimally variant responses. An illustration would be the prompt lid closure and slight eyeball retraction that is reliably elicited by corneal stimulation. Intermediate layers offer greater flexibility by sacrificing a degree of automaticity. For example, the eyeblink component of the sneeze reflex can be blocked while one is driving a car by suppressing the entire reflex with pressure to the gums, or else the eyeblink component can be selectively reduced in amplitude by tonically contracting the levator palpebrae muscle. The highest levels achieve maximum adaptability by abandoning the speed and reliability of automatic motor behavior for the flexibility of ad hoc stimulus-to-response mapping. An example would be the use of a brief, unilateral lid closure to signal a private understanding between two individuals.

Of course, it is the highest levels that are associated with the phenomena of volition and awareness. Farber and Churchland (1995) argue persuasively that, given our present level of understanding, it would be premature to subject these terms to precise definitions. However, provisional definitions are surely necessary both for guiding research on this topic and for interpreting the resulting data. With this in mind, the following tentative definitions are offered:

- A response may be considered as *voluntary* provided that (1) it can be arbitrarily mapped to a designated stimulus, and (2) the subject can withhold the response if signaled to do so.
- Similarly, *conscious awareness* of a stimulus may be assumed if it is the case that (1) the stimulus can be arbitrarily mapped to a designated response, and (2) the subject judges the stimulus to be present rather than absent.

Under these definitions, neither the ability to comply with verbal task instructions nor the ability to verbally report the presence of a stimulus is assumed; therefore, consciousness and volition in infants, adult aphasics, and animals are not ruled out a priori. In fact, the definition offered for awareness is based on experimental criteria developed by Cowey and Stoerig (1995) for the study of unconscious visual perception, or "blindsight," in cortically lesioned monkeys. In human studies of blindsight, patients with lesions of striate cortex can make discriminant, arbitrarily mapped responses to visual stimuli of which they claim to have no awareness (Weiskrantz, 1986). Cortically lesioned monkeys can also make such discriminant responses, but, of course, they cannot verbally report their degree of awareness of the stimuli. However, monkeys that have been trained to press one button when a stimulus is absent on a trial and another when it is present will press the "absent" button when that same stimulus is displayed within the blind portion of their visual field. Regarding voluntary versus involuntary reactions, note that the suggested definition of volition might be inadequate for classifying certain automatized responses. However, it should appropriately classify behaviors lying more toward the extremes of the involuntary–voluntary continuum (e.g., a discriminant conditioned response performed by an isolated spinal preparation would be categorized as involuntary, based on the response-withholding criterion; cf. Beggs, Steinmetz, & Patterson, 1985).

An example of an exteroceptive response that is both involuntary and unconscious is the R50–R80 photic blink complex. This reaction represents a nonarbitrary stimulus–response mapping because the EMG burst latencies and morphology are specific to the lid reaction evoked by sudden illumination (reviewed in Hackley & Boelhouwer, 1997). Furthermore, neither the R50 nor the R80 can be withheld, as, for example, when subjects are instructed to oppose the reflex by widening their eyes in response to the reflexogenic flash of light (Hackley, Sollers, & Stafford-Segert, 1991). Finally, when intense strobe lights were discharged either within or outside of the blind hemifield of 12 patients with unilateral visual cortex lesions, five patients denied any awareness of the blind-hemifield flashes, yet R50 and R80 were invariant across hemifield of stimulation (Fig. 7.1; see Hackley & Johnson, 1996). These results would seem to refute the hypothesis, which has been around since the Pflüger-Lotze debate of the 1850s (e.g., Fearing, 1930), that *all* neural functions are associated with some degree of conscious awareness.

6. Vertical Models of Attention and Consciousness

The photic blink reflex is specifically noted within one recent example of a neurobehavioral model that incorporates a predominantly vertical architecture (Stoerig, 1996). With respect to Posner and Petersen's (1990) tripartite theory of attention, Stoerig's model is of some relevance to the executive network, in the sense that it deals with simultaneous access to multiple response systems. Her model is also relevant to the orienting network if the assumption is true, as will be argued below, that the boundary between visual processes that do or do not have access to conscious awareness is the same as the boundary between visual processes that are or are not influenced by attentional orienting. There are other vertical models that deal more specifically with orienting, two of which will be briefly noted. So far as the present author is aware, no vertical model of the alerting network has yet been proposed.

The goal of Stoerig's model is to explain the variations in residual vision across patient groups with lesions at different sites within the central nervous system. She distinguishes seven levels or stages of visual competency, the lowest being neuroendocrine function (e.g., photic entrainment of sleep–wake rhythms in individuals with complete blindness). The second level mediates visually evoked brain-stem reflexes, such as photic blink, and these functions may be preserved even after neocortical death (Keane, 1979). The third level is implicit visuomotor performance, such as modulation of RT by a task-irrelevant accessory stimulus presented within the blind hemifield. The fourth level can mediate reliable forced-choice guessing regarding the location or basic features of an unseen stimulus within the visual field defect (e.g., Weiskrantz, 1986). Competency at levels 3 and 4 is preserved in some patients with lesions of striate cortex.

These first four levels are unconscious. The subsequent levels 5, 6, and 7 (which are distinguished by lesions in extrastriate pathways) entail, respectively, conscious awareness of a phenomenal image, segregation of the image into distinct objects, and recognition of the meaning of individual objects. Analogous to the sensorimotor control layers of Brooks's (1986) robotic insects, the functions of each level within Stoerig's primate vision model depend on the integrity of the pathways that make use of the information. "If the muscles that close the lid in the photic blink reflex are paralyzed," she points out, the corresponding "visual information is processed to no effect." It is important that the transition from unconscious to conscious visual processing is specifically localized between levels 4 and 5. Lesions of striate cortex or of lower levels prevent conscious access to visual information, whereas lesions at higher, extrastriate levels do not.

Stoerig reached this conclusion based on lesion studies of responses to visual stimuli. Electrophysiological studies of attention effects on voluntary and reflexive reactions may offer converging evidence. As noted by many psychologists and neuroscientists, there is a close (Crick, 1994, pp. 14–19) or even isomorphic (Cowan, 1995, chap. 7) relationship between attention and awareness: The degree to which we are conscious of a stimulus is directly determined by the amount of attention that we allocate to that stimulus. Within the visual modality, ERPs that are generated at or prior to primary visual cortex do not vary as a function of whether the evoking stimulus is attended or ignored, whereas potentials evoked at subsequent, presumably extrastriate levels, are modulated by attentional orienting (Hackley, Woldorff, & Hillyard, 1990; Clark & Hillyard, 1996). Identical conclusions were reached using transcranial optical recordings of evoked striate and extrastriate cortical activity (Gratton, 1997).

As reviewed in Section 2, reflexology provides supporting evidence regarding the differential sensitivity of cortical versus subcortical pathways to attentional orienting. The photic blink reflex is apparently mediated entirely at levels below that of striate cortex (Hackley & Johnson, 1996), and transmission within the sensory limb of the reflex arc does not vary as a function of whether the eliciting stimulus is attended or ignored (Hackley et al., 1990; Hackley & Burke, 1992). Conversely, the ability of a weak visual lead stimulus to inhibit the startle reflex does require an intact visual cortex (Ison, Bowen, & O'Connor, 1991; Burke & Hackley, 1997) and in this case orienting does have an effect. The amount of inhibition is greater when the subject selectively attends to the lead stimulus as compared with when attention is directed to a different location (Sonnenberg et al., 1996).

To account for the varying effects of attentional orienting on reflexes and ERPs that are mediated at different levels of the neuraxis, Hackley and colleagues (1987; Hackley, 1993) proposed a model with a predominantly vertical architecture. The lowest levels (e.g., within the hindbrain) are assumed to process information in a fully automatic mode. That is to say, reflexes and evoked potentials mediated at these levels are obligatory (they cannot be withheld) and they do not benefit from attentional resources. For example, the postauricular reflex and auditory Wave III are the same size and latency regardless of whether the evoking stimulus is attended or ignored. By contrast, processing at intermediate levels exhibits partial automaticity. To continue with illustrations from the auditory modality, the startle-blink reflex, the inhibition of startle by a lead stimulus, and the radially oriented subcomponent of the N100 potential are all examples of obligatory responses, but they can be modified by attention. At the highest levels – those levels that mediate voluntary behavior and certain endogenous (task-dependent) ERPs – information processing is controlled rather than automatic.

A similar vertical model incorporating top-down influences on acoustic startle and prepulse inhibition circuits has recently been proposed by Dawson, Schell, Swerdlow, and Filion (1997). This schema elegantly summarizes the current wealth of neuroanatomical data concerning startle modification, much of which has accumulated since the 1987 model described by Hackley, Woldorff, and Hillyard. The more recent model makes it clear that top-down processes (e.g., attention and emotion) originating in neocortex represent only the tip of the iceberg. The hindbrain circuitry that underlies startle is integrated with higher brain functions by means of descending control from limbic, striatal, pallidal, and mesencephalic structures, in addition to neocortical areas. For an even more complete picture, future neuroanatomical research on this topic should attempt to forge links with the sophisticated vertical models that have been developed to account for oculomotor control at forebrain, midbrain, and hindbrain levels (e.g., Gouras, 1985). After all, the eyelids are part of the eyes, and eyelid movements are known to be mediated by some of the same neural pathways that control ocular movements (Schmidtke & Büttner-Ennever, 1992).

The relevance of these reflex and ERP data to Stoerig's (1996) hypothesis regarding the unconscious-to-conscious transition depends on the assumption of a tight association between attention and awareness. However, if it could be shown that an unconsciously detected stimulus can capture attention, that assumption would be undermined.

Hawley,[3] Hackley, and Johnson (unpublished data) tested this possibility in a study of seven patients with unilateral visual cortex damage. In a choice-RT task, subjects responded with a speeded keypress to the letter H or S presented near fixation within the intact hemifield. On 20 percent of the trials, a task-irrelevant distractor was presented unpredictably in the blind or intact hemifield at a lead time of 88–132 msec. A prominent warning stimulus (a cross) was presented at fixation with a fixed lead time of 412 msec to enhance alertness. Consequently, the irrelevant stimulus could provide little benefit by serving as a warning or accessory stimulus. Rather, the irrelevant stimulus was intended to distract attention from the letter discrimination task and thereby impair performance. To this end, the distractor was designed to be perceptually salient. Specifically, it consisted of a small grid that either flickered off and on, darted toward the edge of the screen, or reversed in color. Not surprisingly, when this distractor was presented within the intact hemifield, reactions to the parafoveal target letter were slower and tended to be less accurate than on control trials. By contrast, distractors presented within the blind hemifield had no effect on performance. This failure to demonstrate a

---

[3] Prior to the completion of the study, Dr. Kevin Hawley passed away. The untimely death of this gifted and personable young psychologist is deeply mourned by his friends and colleagues in the field.

dissociation between attention and conscious awareness supports the assumption that ERP, neuroimaging, and reflex studies of orienting are relevant toward understanding the distinction between conscious and unconscious sensory processes.

7. Concluding Comments

When students first encounter Kandel's (e.g., Kandel & Schwartz, 1985) account of the molecular basis of learning and memory in *Aplysia,* they are unlikely to appreciate the amount of essential work that preceded it. These cellular and molecular studies were made possible by a sequence of hard-won discoveries that followed Pavlov's initial report that reflexes can be used for the objective study of associative learning. The essential previous discoveries include discriminative conditioning, sensitization, alpha conditioned responses, and the truly random control condition – to mention only contributions from within psychology.

The study of attention using reflexes is currently at a stage analogous to the early post-Pavlov era. Graham and Hoffman have already established that simple, short-latency reflexes can be used to investigate the effects of attentional orienting on motor behavior (Bohlin & Graham, 1977; DelPezzo & Hoffman, 1980). The problem now is to identify one or a few optimal paradigms, analogous to discriminative alpha conditioning in memory research or fear-potentiated startle in emotion research. These paradigms should exhibit important general features concerning the ability of attention to improve performance, such as the speeding of response latency, selectivity in sensory analyses, and the resolution of conflict among competing response tendencies. As soon as a few key paradigms have been identified that are as suitable for small lab animals as for humans, neurobiologists can commence their analyses at the cellular and molecular levels.

ACKNOWLEDGMENTS

Thanks are extended to my colleagues whose collaborative work is described in this review. Our research was supported by grants from the U.S. National Science Foundation, the U.S. National Institutes of Health, and the Spanish Ministry of Education.

CHAPTER EIGHT

Affect and the Startle Reflex

MARGARET M. BRADLEY, BRUCE N. CUTHBERT,
AND PETER J. LANG

ABSTRACT

Brief startle probes presented while people perceive emotionally evocative
events are systematically and differentially modulated according to the affective valence of the foreground stimulus content: Unpleasant stimuli evoke a
potentiated reflex to the startle probe that exceeds the normal reaction; pleasant stimuli occasion a relative inhibition of reflex magnitude. This chapter
reviews theory and data relevant to affective modulation of the startle reflex.
Properties of the startle probe (including sensory modality, intensity, aversiveness, task, timing, laterality, and response) and of the perceptual stimulus
(including duration, repetition, blocking, intensity, and semantic or emotional
category) are discussed as they impact on the pattern of affective startle modulation. Taken together, these studies elucidate further the nature of affective
startle modulation, and provide support for the idea that the startle reflex is a
useful measure of motivation and emotion.

1. Introduction: Affect and the Startle Reflex

The purpose of this chapter is to review data and theory relating to a relatively
new phenomenon in the study of human emotional experience. Brief startle
stimuli, presented as probes while people perceive emotionally evocative
events, are systematically and differentially modulated according to the affective valence of the foreground stimulus content. Unpleasant stimuli evoke an
augmented, potentiated reflex to the startle probe that exceeds the normal
reaction; pleasant or appetitive stimuli occasion a relative inhibition of reflex
magnitude.

Over several years of study, affective modulation of the startle reflex has
proven to be highly replicable – a relatively rare event in psychological science. This reliability has made it a useful tool in investigating many critical
issues in the study of emotion. For example, affective modulation of startle

Michael E. Dawson, Anne M. Schell, and Andreas H. Böhmelt, Eds. *Startle modification:
Implications for neuroscience, cognitive science, and clinical science.* Copyright © 1999
Cambridge University Press. Printed in the United States of America. All rights reserved.

varies with fear and phobia (Hamm, Cuthbert, Globisch, & Vaitl, 1997; Chapter 9) and may help to discriminate among anxiety disorders (Grillon, Ameli, Goddard, & Woods, 1994; Cuthbert, Strauss, Drobes, Patrick, Bradley, & Lang, 1997). It has been used to investigate hypotheses regarding affect deficits in psychopathy (Chapter 10), schizophrenia (Schlenker, Cohen, & Hopmann, 1995), and in the neurologically impaired (Morris, Bradley, Bowers, Lang, & Heilman, 1991), and to explore emotional development (Balaban, 1995; McManis, Bradley, Cuthbert, & Lang, 1997) and individual differences in emotionality (Cook, Hawk, Davis, & Stevenson, 1991; Grillon, Ameli, Foot, & Davis, 1993; Blumenthal, Chapman, & Muse, 1995; Collins, Hale, & Loomis, 1995; Corr, Wilson, Fotiadou, & Kumari, 1995). The use of affective startle modulation to address these clinical, temperamental, neuropsychological, and developmental questions regarding emotion relies on a firm understanding of the mechanism underlying these modulatory effects. In this chapter, we discuss important methodological and theoretical issues in the study of affective startle modulation.

Certain features of the affect–reflex relationship should be noted at the outset: First, startle reflex measurement is not a direct measure of emotion's psychophysiology. Rather, it is an example – perhaps in its most basic form – of motivational priming (Lang, Bradley, & Cuthbert, 1990, 1997). That is, the affective quality of a foreground content modulates the response to a wholly independent stimulus event – the startle probe. Second, affective modulation of startle is in no sense a conscious or "controlled processing" mechanism, and is not, furthermore, part of social-affective communication – as is, for example, facial expression. The blink reflex occurs 30–40 msec after probe presentation, at a latency that implies "preattentive processing," and which does not support modulation by intentional mechanisms. Third, startle modulation research in human subjects is solidly grounded in an animal neurophysiological model (see Chapter 5). The neural structure of the basic startle circuit is well understood, as is the path through which subcortical structures (notably the central nucleus of the amygdala) modulate its output. Taken together, these properties suggest the startle probe may be a useful tool in the study of human emotion.

Two independent lines of research – animal studies of fear (Brown, Kalish, & Farber, 1951; Davis & Astrachan, 1978) and human studies of attention (Anthony & Graham, 1985; Simons & Zelson, 1985) – initially prompted the discovery that the startle reflex is modulated as a function of the emotional valence of a foreground context. Beginning in the early 1950s, conditioning studies involving both animals (e.g., Brown et al., 1951) and humans had determined that startle reflexes are *potentiated* in the context of a cue that signals aversive reinforcement, usually shock (see Fig. 8.1, top left). More recently, cognitive studies of reflex modulation were finding that the startle reflex was *inhibited* in contexts involving attention and interest. For example, Figure 8.1 (top right) illustrates data from an experiment in which reflex inhibition was obtained when humans viewed interesting (erotic) pictures, compared with viewing an uninteresting wicker basket (Simons & Zelson, 1985). Taken together, these data suggest that the startle reflex may be sensitive to emotional valence, with reflexes relatively inhibited when processing pleasant, interesting stimuli and potentiated in the context of aversive stimuli. The use of different populations (animal vs. human subjects), methods (conditioning vs. cognitive paradigms), and theoretical constructs (fear vs. attention) obscured for awhile the possibility that a common, unifying dimension of emotional valence may satisfactorily account for the pattern of obtained effects.

The hypothesis that blink magnitude is modulated by affective valence was subsequently tested and confirmed (Vrana, Spence, & Lang, 1988), and has been repeatedly replicated in many different laboratories. The prototypical paradigm has involved the presentation of an acoustic startle probe – usually a 50-msec intense burst of white noise – in the context of affective picture perception, with the probe presented several seconds after picture onset (i.e., "long lead" interval). Consistent with the idea that this basic reflex is sensitive to emotion, responses elicited when viewing unpleasant pictures are potentiated, and those elicited when viewing pleasant pictures are inhibited, compared with when an affectively neutral picture constitutes the foreground stimulus.

The picture perception paradigm has been extensively used in subsequent investigations of affective modulation of startle, due, at least in part, to the existence of the International Affective Picture System (IAPS; NIMH Center for the Study of Emotion and Attention, 1995), a collection of color photographs that greatly facilitates the tasks of stimulus selection and control. Each picture in the IAPS has been rated in terms of pleasure, arousal, and dominance – dimensions that have proven to be fundamental in organizing emotional language (Osgood, Suci, & Tannenbaum, 1957; Russell & Mehrabian, 1977), experience (Ortony, Clore, & Collins, 1988), and behavior (Schlosberg, 1952). The IAPS[1] currently comprises almost 600 pictures for

---

[1] The International Affective Picture System (IAPS, 1997) is available on CD-ROM and in photographic slide format. The IAPS and related technical manuals can be obtained on request from the authors at the National Institute of Mental Health Center for the Study of Emotion and Attention, Box 100165 HSC, University of Florida, Gainesville, FL, 32610.

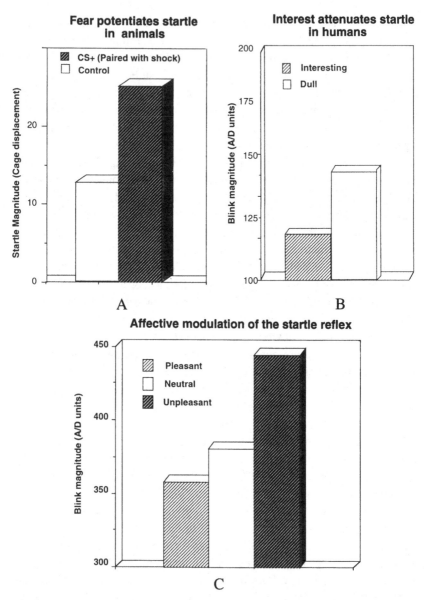

Figure 8.1. (*A*) Startle reflexes are potentiated in animals when a cue signals shock, compared with a no-shock control condition; (*B*) startle reflexes are inhibited when human subjects look at interesting compared with neutral pictures; (*C*) startle reflexes are potentiated when viewing unpleasant pictures as well as inhibited when viewing pleasant pictures, compared with neutral materials, producing affective modulation of the startle reflex. ((*A*) From Brown, Kalish, & Farber, 1951; (*B*) from Simons & Zelson, 1985; (*C*) from Vrana, Spence, & Lang, 1988.)

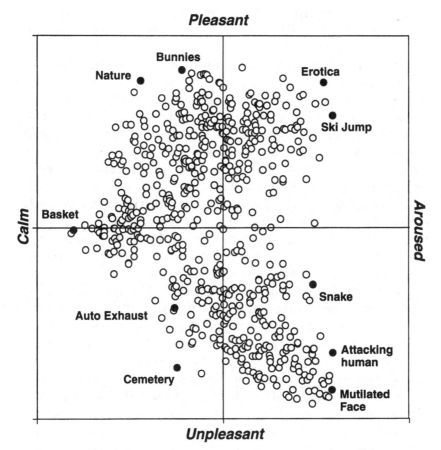

Figure 8.2. The IAPS (Center for the Study of Emotion and Attention, 1997) illustrates the placement of each of 600 pictures in two-dimensional space defined by subjects' mean pleasure and arousal ratings of each picture. Specific picture contents are labeled to illustrate the type of affective materials occurring in each corner of affective space.

which affective norms are distributed for both male and female subjects; subsets of these stimuli have been normed for use with children and the elderly as well (Lang, Bradley, & Cuthbert, 1995).

When pictures are plotted in the two-dimensional space defined by average pleasure and arousal ratings, the "affective space" depicted in Figure 8.2 results, which demonstrates that these materials span both the entire valence range (from pleasant to unpleasant), and vary widely in arousal. The basic shape of affective space is similar for sounds (Bradley, Zack, & Lang, 1994), words (Bradley, Cuthbert, & Lang, 1996), and brief films (Detenber, 1995), suggesting that this organization is fundamental in emotion, and not a specific feature of picture stimuli.

Pictures are evocative cues to emotional experience, as evidenced by studies indicating that a number of relevant physiological responses are elicited when people view these visual stimuli. Heart rate, blood pressure, skin conductance responses, event-related potentials, and facial electromyographic (EMG) responses in emotion-related muscles such as the corrugator (frown) and zygomatic (smile) muscle have all shown reliable covariation with the pleasure and arousal of affective pictures (Klorman, Wiesenfeld, & Austin, 1975; Winton, Putnam, & Krauss, 1984; Greenwald, Cook, & Lang, 1989; Lang, Greenwald, Bradley, & Hamm, 1993). In fact, it is rare that one would measure the startle reflex in the absence of other measures relevant to emotional response. These additional subjective and physiological indices allow one to confirm that affective engagement has been produced by the foreground stimuli, and constitute part of the three-systems data that are important when assessing emotional response (Lang, 1989). Thus, although the focus of this chapter is on the modulation of the startle reflex in the context of affective processing, data from other physiological systems will often facilitate the interpretation of the pattern of reflex modulation that is obtained.

In the picture/probe paradigm, there are two major components. First, foreground pictures that vary in affect are presented for a specific duration. Second, a startle stimulus is used to probe the attentional and emotional processing associated with the foreground event. Specific probe properties discussed below include modality, intensity, aversiveness, task, timing, laterality, and response; discussion of foreground properties include picture duration, repetition, blocking, intensity, and semantic or emotional category. Together, these studies elucidate further the nature of affective startle modulation, and provide convincing support for the idea that this simple reflex is a powerful new measure of emotion.

2. Probe Properties

2.1. Probe Modality: Motivational Priming and Selective Attention

Explorations of the effects of probe modality on affective startle modulation began almost immediately, as this variable was a key to discriminating among potential theoretical explanations of the basic effect. A hypothesis put forth by Lang and his colleagues (Lang, Bradley, & Cuthbert, 1990, 1997; Lang, 1995) suggests that affective startle modulation reflects motivational priming. In their view, startle is viewed as a defense reflex that is potentiated by an ongoing aversive/defensive state, and inhibited when elicited in an appetitive context. According to this account, emotions reflect the engagement of neural structures in biphasic appetitive or aversive motivation systems. When emotional circuitry is active, reflexes linked to the engaged motivational system are primed. Thus, the startle reflex – an independently evoked defensive reflex – is augmented when organisms are reacting to an aversive foreground stimulus (i.e., which evokes an unpleasant state); this same reflex will be reduced in amplitude when the organism is processing an appetitive foreground. In this view, the sensory modality in which the startle probe is presented – acoustic, visual, tactile, etc. – should not change the pattern of modulatory effects.

A second hypothesis focused on crossmodal attentional differences, and stemmed from data demonstrating that reflexes are inhibited when attention is directed away from the sensory modality in which a probe is presented, and facilitated when attention is directed toward the probe modality (Bohlin & Graham, 1977; Anthony & Putnam, 1985). If it is assumed that pleasant and unpleasant pictures differentially affect the direction of attention to the visual modality, crossmodal selective attention could explain the observed pattern. That is, if pleasant pictures direct attention toward the visual modality, reflexes elicited by a probe in a different (i.e., acoustic) channel should be inhibited. On the other hand, the augmented reflexes found for acoustic probes in the context of aversive visual stimulation could be explained only if attention were directed away from unpleasant pictures. The Sokolovian concept of a "defense response" (1958/1963) shutting down cortical "analysers," and Lacey and Lacey's (1970) idea of autonomically modulated stimulus rejection in the context of distressing input, provide a theoretical foundation for this explanation.

Critical tests of these hypotheses have involved manipulating the modality in which the startle probe is presented. To date, affective modulation in the picture perception paradigm has been investigated using acoustic (e.g., Vrana, et al., 1988), visual (Bradley, Cuthbert, & Lang, 1990; Erickson, Levenston, Curtin, Goff, & Patrick, 1995), and tactile (Hawk & Cook, 1997) startle probes. Regardless of probe modality, these studies have found a consistent pattern of reflex modulation during picture perception, in which augmented reflexes occur in the context of unpleasant picture viewing, and inhibited reflexes occur when viewing pleasant pictures. This pattern is not predicted by a selective attention hypothesis, but is consistent with a motivational priming account.

Other measures also suggest attention is not diverted away from the foreground stimulus when unpleasant stimuli are presented. Stimulus rejection is typically associated with heart rate acceleration, whereas "orienting" and attention are indexed by deceleration (Graham & Clifton, 1966). Significantly greater heart rate *deceleration* is reliably obtained during unpleasant pictures (Bradley et al., 1990; Lang et al., 1990) in the picture-viewing paradigm, with greater acceleration often obtained when viewing pleasant pictures (Greenwald et al., 1989), which would predict an opposite pattern of reflex modulation. In addition, unpleasant as well as pleasant pictures prompt larger event-related P300 components, are rated as more interesting, are voluntarily viewed for a longer duration of time, and are recalled better than neutral pictures, which does not support the interpretation that unpleasant pictures are implicitly rejected or subjected to less attentional scrutiny than pleasant stimuli (Bradley, Greenwald, & Hamm, 1993; Schupp, Cuthbert, Bradley, Birbaumer, & Lang, 1997).

Taken together, the data disconfirm a modality-driven attention interpretation of affective modulation. An unpleasant visual foreground is associated with augmented startle reflexes, and pleasant foregrounds prompt relative blink inhibition, regardless of the modality in which the startle probe is presented. Rather than due to modality-directed selective attention, blink modulation appears to be a synergistic augmentation, or inhibitory diminution that reflects motivational priming between the current affective state and the startle reflex.

2.2. Probe Intensity and Aversiveness

Preliminary data obtained using a visual startle probe (Bradley et al., 1990) suggested that probe aversiveness might contribute to affective modulation: Subjects who rated the visual probe as more aversive showed stronger modulation by the affective valence than those who rated it less aversive. To follow up this finding, the intensity of an acoustic startle probe was varied, under the assumption that a less intense probe would be rated as less aversive (Cuthbert, Bradley, & Lang, 1996). Acoustic probes consisted of 80- or 105-dB bursts of white noise; subjects reliably rated the 105-dB as highly aversive, whereas the 80-dB probe was generally rated as low in aversiveness. Despite differences in actual probe intensity and rated aversiveness of the probe, an identical pattern of reflex modulation was obtained for both probe intensities, suggesting that, at least for acoustic startle probes, physical intensity and rated aversiveness does not change the basic modulatory pattern.

2.3. Probe Task and Automatic Processing

According to a motivational priming account, the pattern of affective modulation of the startle reflex is obligatory, in the sense that associated reflexes are considered to be primed by the affective context well in advance of when the probe is actually presented. To the extent that priming occurs automatically in the picture perception context, affective modulation should not differ as a function of whether the startle probe is ignored or explicitly attended. A number of recent studies have supported this hypothesis. In these experiments, subjects were either attending to the startle probe and making an explicit detection response to it (Bradley, Drobes, & Lang, 1996), or attending to the startle probe without making an overt response (Cuthbert, Schupp, Bradley, McManis, & Lang, 1997). In both studies, the pattern of modulation as a function of affective picture content was identical to that obtained for unattended probes: Reflexes were augmented in the context of processing unpleasant pictures and inhibited for pleasant materials, regardless of the task-relevance or the overt response requirements of the startle probe.

It was expected that attending to the startle probe might augment the reflex in general, as a number of studies have demonstrated that startle responses are facilitated when attention is directed to the modality in which the probe is presented (Bohlin & Graham, 1977; Anthony & Putnam, 1985). However, in neither of the studies described above were startle responses significantly larger when the probes were attended, compared with when they were not. These data suggest that attention-related modulation of startle may be different for complex picture stimuli than for simple tones and lights, perhaps because simple modality effects are overridden in foreground contexts that are resource-demanding.

2.4. Probe Laterality and Hemispheric Specialization

The issue of whether affective processing is lateralized in the brain is a topic of current interest to researchers in a number of areas, including those in psychology, neurology, and psychiatry (e.g., Tucker, 1981; Kinsbourne & Bemporad, 1984; Gainotti, 1989; Heilman & Bowers, 1990; Davidson, 1992). Unilateral presentation of the startle probe is therefore an obvious avenue to explore in addressing these questions. To the extent that emotional processes engaged by the picture stimuli result in different patterns of reflex modulation for right and left monaural probes, a new methodology would exist for further examining hypotheses concerning laterality and emotion.

A number of studies have found a consistent pattern of differential modulation as a function of the ear to which an acoustic startle probe was presented: When startle probes are presented to the left ear (processed predominantly by the right neural structures), larger blink reflexes are obtained in the context of aversive, compared with pleasant, stimuli (Bradley et al., 1990, 1993). For probes presented to the right ear, significant effects of emotional context have not been reliably found. Across studies, effects of affective modulation appeared to be especially stable for left ear probes measured at the (contralateral) right eye.

Presentation of unilateral tactile, rather than acoustic, startle probes has been investigated as well, due to the fact that the neural circuitry for this modality is more completely lateralized (Hawk & Cook, 1997). For acoustic probes, the lateralization is incomplete, with approximately two-thirds of the afferent fibers in the acoustic system crossing the brain, whereas the remaining carry information ipsilaterally to higher centers. Using the picture perception paradigm, Hawk and Cook (1997) found that tactile probes (i.e., an air puff) presented to the left or right side of the face produced a similar pattern of affective modulation, with significant effects obtained for left side probes, and nonsignificant effects for probes presented to the right side of the face.

Using a paradigm in which subjects were under threat of shock, Grillon and Davis (1995) found a different effect, in which reflexes were somewhat larger for probes presented to the right, rather than the left, ear. If this pattern replicates, a reasonable hypothesis concerns the differences in the paradigms used, in which the subject is either anticipating an upcoming aversive stimulus (e.g., a shock) or perceiving one (e.g., an unpleasant picture). In fact, it appears that affective modulation of startle in the context of anticipation has a slightly different pattern of effects than that obtained during perception (Sabatinelli, Bradley, Cuthbert, & Lang, 1996).

2.5. Probe Timing: Attention and Emotion

The magnitude of the acoustic startle reflex in humans is modulated by factors other than the emotional context in which the startle-evoking sound occurs. For instance, when a nonstartle-eliciting stimulus (i.e., "prepulse") precedes the startle probe by a short duration, the probe blink reflex is attenuated, leading to a phenomenon known as "prepulse inhibition" (see Anthony, 1985; Graham & Hackley, 1991; Chapter 3). Graham (1980) attributes this phenomenon to processes that protect the initial "lead" stimulus from disruption by the startle probe during detailed cognitive analysis.

In paradigms involving simple lead stimuli (e.g., tones), maximum inhibition occurs with a short delay between the lead stimulus and the startle probe (e.g., 120 ms; Graham, 1975; see Chapter 3). On the other hand, affective modulation of startle was originally obtained when the emotional stimulus

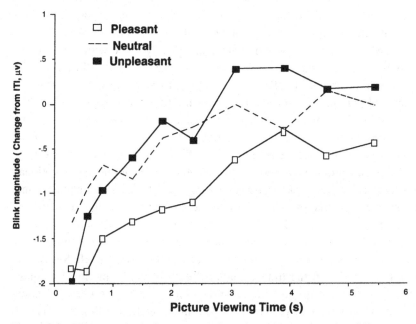

Figure 8.3. Blink magnitude for unattended startle probes presented at different temporal locations after picture onset show attentional and emotional modulation at different points in the viewing interval.

had been perceptually available for a relatively long duration (e.g., 3–6 s; Vrana et al., 1988; Bradley et al., 1990). A number of recent studies have bridged the gap between these two types of phenomena by presenting the startle probe at different temporal intervals before and after picture presentation, to assess the onset, development, and maintenance of emotional and attentional responses. These studies allow an assessment of whether startle reflexes show inhibition immediately after picture onset (i.e., "prepulse inhibition"), and when effects of affective valence on reflex modulation begin to appear.

Figure 8.3 summarizes these data (Bradley et al., 1993, 1996). Six findings are clear. First, strong inhibitory effects are obtained when blink reflexes are elicited immediately after picture onset. Second, reflex inhibition is maximal at 300 msec after picture onset, which is somewhat later than is typically found for simpler foreground stimuli. Third, at the point of maximum inhibition (300 msec), reflex inhibition is significantly larger for emotional pictures (pleasant or unpleasant), compared with neutral materials. Fourth, reflexes continued to be relatively inhibited, compared with responses elicited in the interpicture interval, for up to 3 s after picture presentation, at which time reflex magnitude appears to asymptote for all picture contents. Again, this is a somewhat longer inhibitory interval than typically found with more simple prepulse stimuli (Graham, 1975; Graham & Hackley, 1991). Fifth, by 500 msec after picture onset, reflexes are significantly augmented for unpleasant, compared with pleasant materials, suggesting that affective modulation has been initiated by this time. Affective modulation then continues throughout the picture-viewing interval. Sixth, although not depicted here, no significant effects of affective valence are found for reflexes elicited after picture offset.

These data provide a window onto the temporal development of emotional reactivity in the picture perception paradigm, and implicate both attention and emotion. Attentional processes are inferred on the basis of significant differences in the amount of prepulse inhibition. Whereas startle inhibition by a lead stimulus is typically considered an obligatory process (see Chapter 3), its magnitude is affected by "controlled" processes (Dawson, Schell, Swerdlow, & Filion, 1997). In the timing studies described here, emotional pictures resulted in more blink inhibition than neutral pictures for probes presented shortly after (300 msec) picture onset. Our interpretation of this effect is that the magnitude of blink inhibition in this region reflects the amount of processing resources allocated to encoding the picture contents. The greater the allocation to the foreground stimulus, the more inhibition to a startle probe. Interpreted within this scenario, greater attentional resources were allocated in the initial processing of arousing (pleasant or unpleasant), compared with neutral, materials, with correspondingly fewer available for processing the startle probe.

It is interesting that maximum blink inhibition occurs around 300 msec, as recent cortical studies of picture perception have determined that the first event-related component that reliably discriminates among picture contents is the P300 component, which not only occurs at the same temporal point, but is similarly larger for emotional (pleasant and unpleasant), compared with neutral, pictures (Cuthbert, Schupp, Bradley, Birbaumer, & Lang, 1997; Palomba, Angrilli, & Mini, 1997).

Affective modulation of startle also occurred very early in the viewing interval: By 500 msec after picture onset, reflexes were significantly larger for unpleasant, compared with pleasant, pictures and remained so for the duration of the viewing interval. In fact, obtaining affective modulation at this relatively short "lead interval" suggests that motivational relevance is a salient factor early in the encoding process, and is indexed by the magnitude of the blink reflex within a half-second after picture presentation. Particularly in terms of defensive reactions, quick activation of the aversive system is a functional tool that would have clear evolutionary significance.

2.6. Probe Response: Blinks, Reaction Time, and ERPs

Because the blink reflex shifts to a primary pattern of affective modulation within 500 msec of picture presentation, it cannot be used to index attentional resource allocation through much of the viewing interval. The use of a reaction time (RT) response as an index of resource allocation, on the other hand, has a long history in cognitive psychology. Secondary RT tasks usually consist of a simple detection procedure in which the appearance of an imperative stimulus (e.g., a tone or light) during a concurrent primary task signals a speeded reaction time response. Reaction time to the probe is taken as an index of the amount of attention allocated to the primary task: As more resources are utilized by a foreground task, reaction time to a secondary probe stimulus will increase. Clearly, the dual-task logic underlying the use of an RT probe is identical to that developed above for the reflex probe. A major difference concerns whether the response is voluntary – a button press – or involuntary – a reflexive blink.

A recent series of studies investigated both RT and blink responses to startle probes delivered at various temporal intervals after picture onset to further explore attentional and emotional processes in the picture paradigm (Bradley et al., 1996). In one study, the subject was instructed to press a button as fast as possible when the startle probe was presented. A second group of subjects received nonstartling tone probes, and were also instructed to make a speeded RT response on detection. Figure 8.4A illustrates the RT results from this experiment. The pattern of responses for both startle and tone probes was similar; although, as expected, RT was generally faster for the more intense startle probe. In both cases, RT was inhibited early in the picture interval, and more so for emotionally arousing (pleasant or unpleasant) pictures, compared with neutral. This pattern remained in effect throughout the picture-viewing interval, despite a general facilitation in RT as picture-encoding processes presumably finished. RT was asymptotic between 2 and 3 s after picture onset, which is comparable to when blink reflexes become asymptotic (Bradley et al., 1993), suggesting encoding processes may finish within this interval.

Effects of picture valence on RT responses for both the tone and startle probe were somewhat small later in the picture-viewing interval, possibly due to the simplicity of the probe task (e.g., floor effect) and the few attentional resources required after picture processing was complete. A similar pattern of

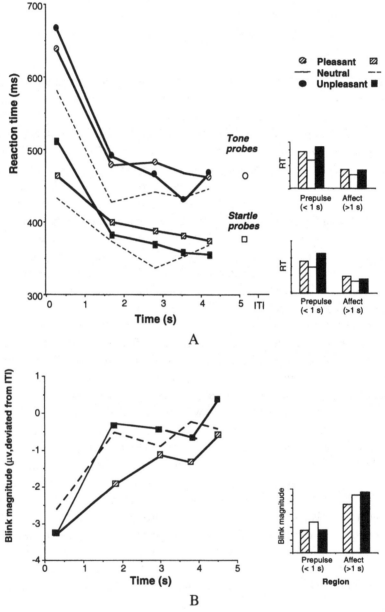

Figure 8.4. (*A*) Reaction time responses to tone or startle probes presented at different temporal locations after picture onset. For both probe types, responses are generally slower to affective (pleasant or unpleasant) pictures, compared with neutral, both early and late in the interval. (*B*) Blink responses to attended startle probes, requiring an RT response. The pattern of modulation is identical to that found for unattended startle probes.

RT modulation, but with larger differences between emotional and neutral pictures late in the interval, was obtained in a study in which reaction time to secondary probes was clearly off the floor (i.e., much slower), due to a more difficult probe decision (Bradley, Cuthbert, & Lang, 1996). In that study, the inhibitory effects of an emotional foreground context (pleasant or unpleasant), compared with neutral pictures, remained throughout the processing interval.

Figure 8.4B illustrates the pattern of blink modulation occurring for attended startle probes – those requiring a RT response – which turned out to be very similar to that found for ignored startle probes: Reflexes were inhibited at 300 msec after picture onset, and more so for arousing, compared with neutral, pictures, with affective modulation dominating the pattern throughout the rest of the viewing interval. Taken together, these data indicate that two concurrent responses to the same startle probe – RT and blink reflexes – appear to measure attentional and emotional processes in picture perception, respectively. A third response that can be measured to the startle probe – the P300 component of the ERP – also co-varies with the RT pattern and is similarly unaffected by whether the probe is attended or ignored (Cuthbert et al., 1997). That is, the P300 component elicited by presentation of a startle probe is smaller when emotional (pleasant or unpleasant), compared with neutral, pictures constitute the foreground stimuli. Smaller P300s and longer RTs to the startle probe when emotional pictures are the foreground stimuli are both consistent with the hypothesis that these motivationally relevant stimuli draw attentional resources, leaving less available for processing the secondary startle probe.

Greater inhibition of the blink reflex for arousing pictures, on the other hand, only occurred early in the processing interval. Similar modulation of prepulse inhibition by attentional factors has been obtained in studies that vary the task relevance of a lead stimulus (Filion, Dawson, & Schell, 1994). As attention to the lead stimulus increased, prepulse inhibition increased, as did reaction time, which is similar to the pattern we obtained for emotional pictures. Unlike the neutral stimuli used in many cognitive studies of attention, however, motivationally relevant pictures appear to *naturally* draw attentional resources, irrespective of task instructions or relevance (Lang et al., 1997). Processing resources appear to be automatically allocated to interesting, engaging stimuli that activate the appetitive or aversive motivational systems. Consistent with this interpretation, varying the task relevance of foreground pictures does not change the pattern of affective or attentional blink modulation (Vanman, Boehmelt, Dawson, & Schell, 1996).

Reaction time (as well as cortical P300) responses to a startle probe, therefore, appear to index attentional allocation, differing for emotional, compared with neutral, pictures, even late in the interval. On the other hand, by 500 msec after stimulus presentation, the startle response reflects activation of motivational systems associated with concurrent appetitive or aversive processes (Lang et al., 1990). Used as converging measures, different responses to the same startle probe provide an assessment of attentional and emotional processes in the context of affective perception.

3. Foreground Picture Properties

3.1. Foreground Duration

A 6-s picture presentation clearly allows assessment of both attentional and emotional processes involved in picture encoding. But, does affective modulation rely on a stimulus duration of this length? More important, the lack of affective startle modulation even very soon after picture offset (e.g., within 500 msec; Bradley et al., 1993) raises the issue of whether modulation relies on the presence of a perceptually available foreground. A number of recent studies have addressed these questions.

To investigate picture duration, Codispoti and colleagues (1996) used the same materials and probe times as in the startle timing studies described above, but each picture was presented only for 500 msec. The pattern of modulation was almost identical to that obtained when the foreground picture was actually present. In particular, strong effects of picture valence were found 1–4 s after picture presentation, despite the fact that no stimulus was perceptually available. Another study (Globisch, Hamm, Esteves, & Öhman, 1994) assessed a shorter picture presentation – 150 msec – and presented snake and spider pictures to participants reporting high fear of these materials. Reflexes were again potentiated for fear stimuli, compared with neutral, despite this very brief picture presentation. Both of these studies demonstrate that, in the absence of a perceptual masking stimulus, picture processing appears to proceed as if the stimulus was perceptually present, and the startle reflex is similarly modulated by affective valence.

The absence of affective modulation for reflexes elicited immediately after picture offset in the Bradley et al. (1993) study is presumably due to the fact processing was complete after a 6-s picture presentation, but not after the brief presentation periods described above. Picture processing could be extended, however, if the subject was instructed to continue to imagine that the picture was being displayed on the screen after actual offset. In two experiments investigating the effect of visual imagery instructions on the persistence of the picture stimulus (Cuthbert et al., 1997; Schupp et al., 1997), significant modulatory effects of picture valence were obtained when the subject was visually imagining the picture. For subjects who were not instructed to maintain a visual image of the picture, startle reflexes in the post-picture period were not affected by prior picture valence. These results are intriguing and suggest that reflex modulation by affective valence does not require the actual presence of a perceptual stimulus, but instead is an index of the mental processes associated with perception.

3.2. Foreground Repetition: Habituation and Modulation

Davis and his colleagues have proposed that two neural circuits affect the magnitude of a rat's startle response: a primary, obligatory circuit (from the cochlear nucleus through the nucleus reticularis pontis caudalis to the spinal cord), and a secondary, modulatory circuit based on projections to the reticular site from the central nucleus of the amygdala (see Chapter 5). Repeated presentation of a startle probe results in clear reflex decreases in both animals (e.g., Davis & File, 1984; Sanford, Ball, Morrison, & Ross, 1992) and human beings (e.g., Rimpel, Geyer, & Hopf, 1982), presumably due to habituation processes in the primary startle circuit. Whereas response decrement is clearly a salient factor in the output of the primary pathway, the nature and course of habituation processes in the modulatory circuit is less clear. Davis and File (1984) originally proposed that the modulatory circuit itself does not involve habituation (although they do suggest that *inputs* to this circuit might habituate), which suggests that affective modulation of startle should continue despite repeated presentation of the same pleasant and unpleasant pictures.

Habituation and affective startle modulation have been investigated in both within- and between-session designs. In one study, subjects were presented with the repetitive presentation of the same six pictures (including two unpleasant, two neutral, and two pleasant stimuli; Bradley, Lang, & Cuthbert, 1993). With repeated elicitation, the startle response showed a progressive, essentially monotonic reduction in amplitude, as expected. This pattern of steady change has frequently been found in both animals and humans, and encourages an explanation of startle habituation that emphasizes intrinsic factors, such as a progressive modification of supraspinal synaptic connections in the basic circuit (e.g., change in neurotransmitters) or effector fatigue (see Davis & File, 1984).

In contrast with this primary circuit reaction, affective modulation of the blink reflex displayed no habituation over trials. As found in previous studies, the blink response was potentiated when probes were presented during processing of unpleasant pictures (relative to neutral pictures) and reduced when viewing pleasant pictures, and this pattern was not affected by picture repetition. In fact, affective startle modulation was largest later in the experiment, suggesting that the effects of differing emotional foregrounds are easier to detect when some habituation in the primary pathway has occurred.

A second study investigated between-session habituation of affective modulation by presenting two sets of pictures in two different sessions conducted one week apart (Bradley, Gianaros, & Lang, 1995). For one group of subjects, the identical picture set was used; for another group, pictures were different on the two occasions. Results were the same for both groups: Whereas reflexes diminished from the first to second session, significant affective modulation of the startle reflex was found during both sessions, and did not change as a function of whether pictures were the same or different as those viewed in the first session. Taken together, these studies strongly support the hypothesis of dual startle circuits – basic and modulatory – put forward by Davis and File (1984) and, furthermore, demonstrate that in human beings there is clear independence in the habituation processes for these two reflex phenomena.

3.3. Foreground Blocking: Mood and Startle

Finding modulation by emotional content for the punctate presentation of a single 6-s picture in a completely intermixed series suggests that the strength of this modulatory effect is quite high. A stronger manipulation involves presenting a contiguous block of unpleasant pictures to create a more tonic, sustained mood state. To investigate reflex modulation during tonic exposure, a recent study presented blocks of 24 pleasant, neutral, or unpleasant pictures, and presented startle probes only during a 6-s interval between picture presentations (Bradley, Cuthbert, & Lang, 1996). Because affective modulation is not typically obtained after picture offset (in the absence of an explicit imagery instruction), effects in the interpicture interval could be attributed to carryover created by the presentation of a blocked series.

Results suggested that sustained exposure had clear effects: Startle responses were significantly modulated by affective state, with potentiated reflexes obtained for unpleasant, compared with pleasant, pictures, even though probes were presented only in the interpicture intervals. Startle reflexes did not, however, show an absolute increase in size from early to late in the unpleasant block, as one might expect if a cascade of unpleasant pictures produces an increasingly aversive state across the picture series. Rather, habituation in the primary circuit remains a factor influencing startle magnitude across repeated presentations, as usual. The effect of the mood-blocking manipulation was to sustain the affective response between perceptual picture presentations, consistent with the notion that a tonic mood state is created by sustained exposure to pleasant or unpleasant pictures.

3.4. Foreground Arousal

Most studies of affective startle modulation originally used stimuli that were highly arousing – both pleasant (e.g., erotica or sports) and unpleasant (e.g., violence or death) – and assessed reflex reactivity compared with affectively neutral stimuli that rated relatively low in arousal (e.g., household objects). The level of stimulus arousal is clearly not the moderating variable in these studies, as reflex magnitude is always most different for the most arousing – that is, pleasant and unpleasant – pictures. But if one assumes, as we do, that emotional activation can vary within separate appetitive and aversive systems (e.g., Lang et al., 1990, 1997), one pressing issue concerns how changes in arousal level might affect the pattern of affective reflex modulation. Based on the fact that highly emotional stimuli tend to be highly arousing, one hypothesis is that reflex modulation – potentiation in aversive foregrounds and diminution of responding in appetitive foregrounds – may be enhanced as the level of affective drive or activation increases.

This issue was addressed by using sets of pleasant, neutral, and unpleasant pictures that varied in terms of low, moderate, or high arousal, based on IAPS ratings (Cuthbert, Bradley, & Lang, 1996). Because of the fundamental nature of affective space (see Fig. 8.2), the range of arousal levels is not identical across different affective contents. In particular, neutral pictures tend to be lower in arousal than pleasant or unpleasant pictures. Furthermore, because few extremely unpleasant pictures with low arousal ratings exist, the range of arousal values is restricted for unpleasant, compared with pleasant, pictures. Thus, whereas direct comparisons can be made between categories at certain points (e.g., highly arousing pleasant and unpleasant pictures), the emphasis is on assessing the effects of increasing activation within each affective valence category on startle magnitude.

Figure 8.5 illustrates the data from this experiment. It is clear that reflex modulation – potentiation for unpleasant stimuli and inhibition for pleasant stimuli – is greatest for highly arousing stimuli. For stimuli that activate these motivational systems only weakly – those low in rated arousal – reflex modulation is absent. Figure 8.5 also illustrates that a reduction in blink magnitude was obtained for unpleasant pictures of moderate arousal, similar to that found for pleasant pictures in this arousal region. One hypothesis for this

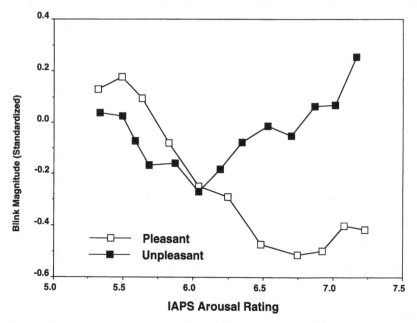

Figure 8.5. Startle potentiation for unpleasant pictures increases with increases in rated arousal, and blink inhibition for pleasant pictures increases with rated arousal, demonstrating that affective startle modulation is strongest for intense emotional pictures.

effect is that unpleasant pictures of moderate arousal engender an orienting disposition that overrides aversive activation – that is, the stimulus is as interesting as a pleasant picture. This hypothesis gains plausibility given the fact that the movie industry thrives on presenting violent and aversive images to a willing – even paying – audience. With increasing activation, however, aversive motivation outweighs attention and startle potentiation is obtained. Taken together, these data suggest that a threshold for aversive activation exists at which foreground stimuli begin to reliably activate the brain's primary motivational circuitry. The startle reflex can be used to index the mobilization of these appetitive and aversive systems, and to mark the threshold at which orienting to an unpleasant stimulus shifts to defense.

3.4.1. Manipulating Arousal in the Appetitive System

Effects of activation or drive on startle modulation in the appetitive system was recently investigated in a series of studies examining effects of food deprivation on startle magnitude when viewing pictures of appetizing food (Drobes, Hillman, Bradley, Cuthbert, & Lang, 1995). In the absence of deprivation, appetitive food cues are typically associated with the same pattern of inhibited startle reflexes as other pleasant materials. Two alternative hypotheses were assessed: From a motivational perspective, food deprivation might enhance the appetitive value of food cues, thereby causing a cue-specific reduction (i.e., even more inhibition than normal) in startle responding. Alternatively, exposure to food cues in an experimental context in which food consumption is not possible may elicit an affective response characterized by frustration among hungry subjects, with an associated augmentation of startle.

College subjects were randomly assigned to one of three levels of food deprivation (0, 6, or 24 hours). Food-deprived subjects showed an enhanced startle response during viewing of appetizing pictures of food, compared with subjects who were not food-deprived and compared with other pleasant materials. Food-deprived subjects also produced augmented skin conductance responses when viewing food cues, compared with other subjects, and their ratings of arousal were higher for these materials. Thus, the deprivation manipulation appeared to have been successful in increasing the subject's drive state (as measured by sympathetic reactivity and reports of arousal). The fact that startle reflexes were relatively potentiated in this high drive state for food stimuli, compared with nondeprived subjects, suggests that viewing appetitive cues in a deprived state may represent a situation of frustrative nonreward, which is characterized by an aversive, rather than appetitive, motivational state.

3.4.2. Manipulating Arousal in the Aversive System

The activating level of an unpleasant stimulus can be manipulated in a number of ways. When phobic subjects view pictures of their feared objects, potentiation of the startle reflex has been reliably obtained, compared with either nonphobic subjects viewing these pictures or phobics viewing pictures of other fearful scenes (Sabatinelli, Bradley, Cuthbert, & Lang, 1996; Hamm, Globisch, Cuthbert, & Vaitl, 1997). A second method involves increasing the aversiveness of an unpleasant picture by consistently following it with electric shock (Hamm, Greenwald, Bradley, & Lang, 1993; Hamm & Vaitl, 1996; Moulder, Bradley, Cuthbert, & Lang, 1996), which leads, as predicted, to further potentiation of the startle reflex over the level obtained prior to shock association.

3.5. Foreground Category

Thus far, the startle reflex has proved sensitive to a broad affective valence dichotomy, with larger reflexes elicited during unpleasant, compared with pleasant states. As noted above, arousal affects this relationship, with affective modulation occurring primarily for stimuli that are high in affective intensity. An important issue obviously concerns the extent to which the startle reflex might vary with specific categories of human experience or with specific emotional states.

In an early study investigating this question, reflexes were found to be potentiated for fearful, but not disgusting, pictures, compared with neutral stimuli (Balaban & Taussig, 1994). Subsequent studies have broadened the range of affective categories (Lang, Bradley, Drobes, & Cuthbert, 1995; Schupp, Cuthbert, Hillman, Raymann, Bradley, & Lang, 1996). In one study, for example, unpleasant categories included mutilated bodies, attacking animals, attacking humans, disasters, disgusting objects, sickness, grief, and pollution. Pleasant categories included male erotica, female erotica, erotic couples, romance, sports, adventure, nature scenes, food, and families. Neutral categories included household objects and mushrooms. Figure 8.6 illustrates these data, and shows that, as expected, there was significant startle modulation by affect. And replicating the effects found earlier when varying arousal, the largest difference in startle magnitude was found for the most highly arousing pleasant and unpleasant categories.

Differences among specific categories within each valence were clearly obtained. For unpleasant pictures, the greatest startle potentiation occurred for scenes involving danger and threat: Pictures depicting attacking people and attacking animals facilitated startle relative to other unpleasant categories, and did not differ from each other. This pattern of modulation is consistent with the hypothesis that startle potentiation reflects the activation of a defensive motivational system, which predicts that scenes involving direct threat produce the most potentiation. In the fear-potentiated animal literature, for example, the feared stimulus (e.g., shock) typically involves physical danger and sometimes pain. Startle reflexes were also relatively augmented during scenes of injuries and mutilations, compared with neutral scenes, and potentiation for both were significantly larger than blinks elicited during unpleasant pictures low in arousal, such as scenes of pollution. For pleasant categories, startle responses elicited when viewing any type of erotic stimulus were significantly smaller than those elicited when viewing pictures depicting other pleasant events. Again, this is consistent with the notion that stimuli that most strongly activate an appetitive motivational system produce the strongest startle inhibition in the picture-viewing context.

Although it appears that women tended to be more reactive to scenes involving attacking humans and disgust, compared with men, these differences were not significant. In general, although relative differences in startle size between men and women are sometimes seen, these differences are often

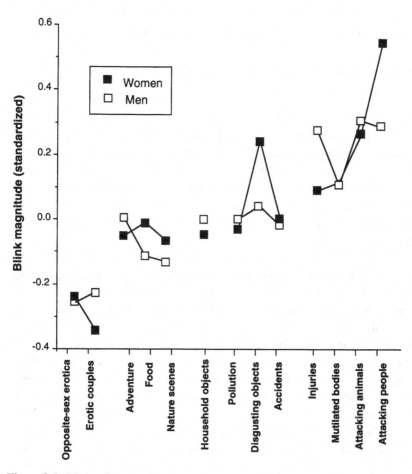

Figure 8.6. Blink reflex magnitude as a function of specific categories of human emotional experience. Scenes of threat produce the largest reflex potentiation and erotic scenes produce the largest reflex inhibition, consistent with the notion that affective modulation varies with arousal, and that reflex magnitude reflects activation of defensive or appetitive motivational systems.

not statistically reliable. Rather, a more typical finding across studies is a relative uniformity in affective modulation of the startle response for men and women, especially when compared with other physiological systems that are sensitive to emotion and often differ as a function of gender (Lang et al., 1993). On the other hand, a recent investigation assessing affective modulation in 7- to 9-year-old boys and girls found large, significant differences in the pattern of reflex modulation, with little girls showing the same pattern as adults, whereas little boys failed to show affective modulation (McManis, Bradley, Cuthbert, & Lang, 1997). Thus, the issue of gender differences in affective startle modulation remains an interesting avenue to investigate.

4. Beyond Pictures: Affective Modulation and Other Perceptual Stimuli

Use of the picture paradigm to study the mechanisms of affective modulation of the startle reflex has proven useful in defining attentional, temporal, cognitive, and emotional variables that affect the expression and size of this phenomenon. In addition, comparison across data sets is generally facilitated when the basic paradigm remains the same. On the other hand, use of a single perceptual stimulus – visual pictures – is insufficient for drawing the conclusion that affective startle modulation is a general phenomenon related to motivational priming.

Significant modulation of the startle reflex by affect has now been obtained using stimuli in a number of different perceptual activities, including viewing affective films (Jansen & Frijda, 1994), smelling odors (Miltner, Matjak, Braun, Diekmann, & Brody 1994; Erlichman, Brown, Zhu, & Warrenburg, 1995), listening to sounds (Bradley et al., 1994), and reading emotional texts (Spence & Lang, 1990). In each case, reflexes have been augmented when the affective valence of the perceptual stimuli is aversive, compared with when materials are pleasant. The roles of arousal, timing, and repetition have not yet been systematically studied in each modality, although preliminary evidence that arousal may again play an important role is suggested by data indicating that pleasant odors do not always result in significant startle inhibition (Erlichman et al., 1995), particularly when intensity is low (Miltner et al., 1994).

5. Imagery and Anticipation

The bulk of this chapter has focused on perceptual processing, in which the startle reflex is clearly modulated when one is perceiving an emotional stimulus. Other techniques for inducing emotional experience do not rely solely on perception of a foreground stimulus, such as narrative imagery or anticipatory anxiety paradigms. Is the startle reflex similarly modulated in these processing modes?

Early data investigating reflex modulation during emotional imagery found that the startle reflex was augmented during imagination of fearful, compared with neutral, narrative events (Vrana & Lang, 1990), as expected. Subsequent studies confirmed that the pattern of startle modulation during aversive imagery parallels that found during emotional perception, with arousing unpleasant images involving various emotions such as fear, anger, or disgust prompting significantly more potentiation than aversive images low in arousal (Bradley, Cuthbert, & Lang, 1995; Witvliet & Vrana, 1995). Also consistent with the picture data, imagery scenes involving physical danger prompted more potentiation than scenes that do not involve clear threat (Cuthbert, Strauss, Drobes, Patrick, Bradley, & Lang, 1997).

Using stimuli that included pleasant, as well as unpleasant, materials, the same monotonic pattern relating blink magnitude to affective valence that is found with pictures was first reported in the imagery paradigm (Cook, Hawk, Davis, & Stevenson, 1991). However, this pattern was not subsequently replicated in a number of different studies (Cuthbert, Bradley, York, & Lang, 1990; Miller, Levenston, Geddings, & Patrick, 1994; Witvliet & Vrana, 1995). Rather, results consistently indicated that, compared with neutral, nonarousing images, blink reflexes were augmented during imagery of both pleasant and unpleasant narrative events. Whereas some studies continue to find relative potentiation during unpleasant, compared with pleasant, imagery (e.g., Vrana, 1995; Witvliet & Vrana, 1995), other data indicate that the difference between unpleasant and pleasant images is attenuated or eliminated when highly arousing pleasant scenes are used (e.g., winning the lottery; Bradley et al., 1995) or when personally relevant pleasant scenes are constructed for each participant (Miller et al., 1994).

Studies involving anticipatory processing have consistently found that startle reflexes are potentiated in periods in which the subject is anticipating an electric shock, compared with a period when no shock is threatened (Grillon, Ameli, Woods, Merikangas, & Davis, 1991). Using pleasant as well as unpleasant pictures, some studies have found that startle responses during anticipation of picture stimuli show the predicted monotonic pattern of modulation by affective valence, with larger reflexes during anticipation of unpleasant, compared with pleasant, pictures (Erickson et al., 1995; Allen, Wong, Kim, & Trinder, 1996). On the other hand, at least one study suggests that, like narrative imagery, anticipation of both pleasant and unpleasant pictures potentiates startle responses, compared with anticipation of neutral material (Sabatinelli et al., 1996). Thus, the pattern of reflex modulation during anticipation, particularly for pleasant stimuli, is not yet clear.

6. A Motivational Priming Account of Affective Startle Modulation

Taken together, the data suggest that affective modulation of startle may be primarily a phenomenon of *motivated* attention. More specifically, reflex modulation by affective valence appears to occur in the context of perception of motivationally relevant cues. In a passive intake posture of this type, perceptual cues are processed for motivational significance, but the threshold necessary to produce overt action is not reached, and behavior not yet initiated. This mode is considered similar to that occurring in an animal as it stops and scans the environment for signs of prey or threat. Other physiological measures encourage this attentional view of affective modulation. For instance, in the picture-viewing context, one observes sustained cortical positivity, rather than the negative cortical potentials associated with the contingent negative variation (CNV) and anticipated responding. Picture viewing also prompts heart rate deceleration – largest for the most unpleasant images – which is a widely observed covariate of an attentive set (Graham & Clifton, 1966).

In keeping with a number of earlier theorists (Schneirla, 1959; Konorski, 1967; Dickinson & Dearing, 1979; Masterson & Crawford, 1982), motivated behavior is seen here as having an underlying biphasic organization, primitively based on functionally opposed approach and withdrawal reactions. The common assumption in this view is that emotion fundamentally stems from motivations involving (1) the appetitive system (consumatory, sexual, nurturant), prototypically expressed by behavioral approach, or (2) the aversive system (protective, withdrawing, defensive), prototypically expressed by behavioral escape and avoidance. When the motivational system is active, a modulatory effect is presumed to affect the brain's cognitive processing operations, with the most fundamental priming at the level of unconditioned reflexes. The startle response is a convenient defensive reflex that operates in this manner, potentiated during aversive states and inhibited during appetitive states.

This reflex priming appears to operate, however, in contexts in which overt action has not yet been initiated. Masterson and Crawford (1982), for example, describe a two-stage reaction to aversive stimulation in animals – a preparatory defense reaction in which the organism is vigilant for threat but passive, and a subsequent "alarm reaction" in which fight or flight are triggered. Fanselow (1994) describes a similar model, bolstered by neurophysiological evidence, with three progressive stages going from passive attention to action, based on predator imminence. Viewed in this way, startle potentiation during aversive perception represents a premature triggering of a defense response. The subject is primed by the foreground cue (as is an animal watching a distant predator), and this priming is enhanced progressively as the implied threat becomes more proximal or imminent. The startle probe, in effect, releases a defense reflex before the foreground cue is, itself, intense enough to cause overt fight or flight.

This view has several implications for understanding affective modulation of startle in human subjects. It explains, for example, why differences might be found between threatening events and those that are nonthreatening (e.g., injury to others), even when they are described as equally unpleasant. Furthermore, to the extent that different modes of processing – perception, imagination, anticipation, action – involve different degrees of preparation for responding, patterns of reflex modulation by affect will vary. In particular, this view predicts that startle modulation by emotion should be diminished or even absent in the context of overt behavior: When actively engaged in fleeing from the beast, priming of the startle reflex will no longer be functionally related to the defensive action. Consistent with this, preliminary data suggest that startle reflexes are not potentiated during anxiety-provoking social encounters (Blumenthal et al., 1995).

The hypothesis of differential affective modulation of startle during perception and action is also consistent with the reliable finding in the animal literature that "freezing" in the context of an aversive cue is correlated with potentiated startle (Leaton & Borszcz, 1985). That is, an exaggerated reflex response occurs in the immobile rodent, but is not generally observed in active animals (i.e., during fight/flight). Furthermore, there is evidence that the neural pathways leading to "freezing" and active defense behaviors differ, traversing either ventral or dorsolateral paths, respectively, through the periacqueductal central gray (Fanselow, 1994). Thus, startle potentiation appears to be an early stage in a defense cascade of autonomic and somatic responses (Lang et al., 1997), which indicates that threat has been detected and the defensive system activated, but appropriate action has not yet been instigated. The picture/probe paradigm, because it induces a posture of motivated attention, is excellent for assessing activation of the appetitive and aversive motivational system in humans by measuring affective modulation of the startle reflex.

ACKNOWLEDGMENTS

This work was supported in part by National Institute of Mental Health (NIMH) grants MH37757 and MH43975, and P50-MH52384, an NIMH Behavioral Science grant to the Center for the Study of Emotion and Attention, University of Florida, Gainesville. We thank the many students, postdoctoral associates, and collaborators whose contributions to the research described in this chapter are greatly appreciated.

PART IV

Individual Differences and Startle Modification

Affective Individual Differences, Psychopathology, and Startle Reflex Modification

EDWIN W. COOK III

ABSTRACT

Although affective modification of the startle reflex is a robust phenomenon, it does not occur universally. Research is reviewed suggesting that affective startle modification varies systematically in relation to affective trait dispositions and clinical diagnosis of anxiety, mood, and schizophrenia spectrum disorders. Evidence supports a reliable association between high trait fearfulness and enhanced startle modification by affective valence. Findings for other affective individual differences are thus far only suggestive. Despite the fact that much interest in startle stems from reports of exaggerated startle in posttraumatic stress disorder (PTSD), the precise pattern of startle reactivity and modification in this disorder remains uncertain. Nevertheless, recent studies of affective startle modification in PTSD, as well as in schizophrenia and depression, have yielded provocative results that may ultimately inform our understanding of these disorders. The review emphasizes the need to use a range of affect manipulations and modification paradigms, more powerful research designs, and more appropriate statistical comparisons in future research in this area.

1. Introduction

A decade has now passed since the original report of affective startle modification in humans (Spence, Vrana, & Lang, 1987), and startle potentiation during aversive compared with pleasant and/or neutral conditions has been repeatedly demonstrated. In one popular paradigm (e.g., Bradley, Cuthbert, & Lang, 1990, 1991, 1996), pictures evoke different affects, startle is elicited

Michael E. Dawson, Anne M. Schell, and Andreas H. Böhmelt, Eds. *Startle modification: Implications for neuroscience, cognitive science, and clinical science.* Copyright © 1999 Cambridge University Press. Printed in the United States of America. All rights reserved.

with brief noises, and the magnitude of the eyeblink startle response is measured. However, films (Jansen & Frijda, 1994), imagery (e.g., Vrana & Lang, 1990; Cook, Hawk, Davis, & Stevenson, 1991; Hawk, Stevenson, & Cook, 1992; Stevenson & Cook, 1997), shock threat (e.g., Grillon, Ameli, Foot, & Davis, 1993), and even odors (Miltner, 1994) similarly modulate acoustic startle magnitude; visual and tactile probes elicit startle blinks that also vary with affective state (Erickson, Levenston, Curtin, Goff, & Patrick, 1995; Hawk & Cook, 1997), and blink latency and cardiac acceleration show similar modulatory effects to those observed for blink magnitude (e.g., Cook, Davis, Hawk, Spence, & Gautier, 1992). Affective startle modification is clearly a robust phenomenon (see Chapter 8).

Accumulating evidence, however, also indicates that there are reliable individual and diagnostic group differences in affective startle modification, and these differences are the primary focus of this chapter. Findings are reviewed suggesting that affective startle modification varies systematically in relation to trait dispositions toward fear and anxiety, negative affectivity, schizotypy, and related characteristics. Studies of both nonclinical and clinical populations are considered, as clinical disorders are conceptualized here as extreme forms of normal individual variations.

1.1. Historical Background and Rationale

The studies described here have their roots in anecdotal clinical observations of exaggerated startle in survivors of combat and captivity, dating back at least to descriptions of "combat neurosis" in World War II (Bartemeier, Kubie, Menninger, Romano, & Whitehorn, 1946) and continuing in more recent descriptions of posttraumatic stress disorder (PTSD) resulting from a range of traumatic experiences (combat, captivity, technological disasters, and violent crime; see, e.g., Kalman, 1977; Langley, 1982; Kinzie, Fredrickson, Ben, Flec, & Karls, 1984; Russell, 1984; McCaughey, 1986; Hierholzer, Munsoon, Peabody, & Rosenberg, 1992). However, until recently, reports of associations between startle and anxiety disorders were based entirely on self-report and informal observation. In 1988 when we began researching individual differences in startle modification, there were no published studies of startle and PTSD in which the reflex had actually been measured.

Startle is an exceptional tool for the study of emotion and psychopathology. It is readily elicited by a variety of sensory stimuli and can be measured from several response systems. These characteristics convey practical advantages and also suggest that central information processing mechanisms are involved. Startle continues to be a topic of basic neurophysiological research, including studies of brain structures and neurotransmitter systems hypothesized to be involved in anxiety and affective disorders as well as schizophrenia (see Chapters 5 and 6). Behavioral observations and diagnostic practice link exaggerated startle to these same disorders. Startle is similarly modified by attentional and emotional variables in animals and humans, facilitating mechanistic research on these variables. In historically "soft" areas of psychology, such as psychopathology and emotion research, startle provides a reliable dependent variable measured on an interval scale. It is difficult to identify a psychophysiological response that is better grounded in basic behavioral and neurophysiological research, shows such a consistent pattern across human and animal studies, and is also behaviorally implicated in psychiatric disorders.

1.2. Brainstem and Modulatory Startle Circuits: Baseline Startle Magnitude and Affective Startle Modification

Because the theme of this book is startle modification, there is little need to elaborate the principle that the brain-stem startle circuit and the various modification circuits are dissociable (see Chapters 5 and 6). However, startle measured under any particular experimental conditions reflects activity in both the brain-stem circuit and descending modulatory pathways. Individual differences in baseline startle magnitude are typically quite large, relative to modulatory effects. As a result, startle magnitude measured under particular experimental conditions is heavily influenced by baseline magnitude, arguing in favor of within-subject designs for the study of modification effects. (Berg & Balaban, in Chapter 2, consider further the impact of baseline on startle modification scoring.)

Different modification "circuits" may also be discernible for different affective influences on startle. We follow Lang, Bradley, and Cuthbert (1990; see also Chapter 8) in focusing on two orthogonal affective dimensions: valence (pleasantness) and arousal. These dimensions have a long history in the conceptualization of emotion (e.g., Osgood, Suci, & Tannenbaum, 1957) but they are only one of several ways to conceptualize affective states. The negative affect and positive affect (Watson & Tellegen, 1985) dimensions represent an alternative dimensional system that startle researchers have pursued (e.g., Cook & Gautier, 1992; Witvliet & Vrana, 1995). Another alternative focuses on discrete categories rather than dimensions, and an unresolved question is whether particular affective states (e.g., fear) potentiate startle more than others that occupy the same region of "affective space" (e.g., anger and disgust; cf. Cook et al., 1991; Hawk et al., 1992; Balaban & Taussig,

1994; Stevenson & Cook, 1997). Thus, alternative conceptualizations of emotion can serve as useful starting points for understanding emotion effects on startle. Nevertheless, in attempting to understand how affective startle modification varies with personality and diagnosis, the valence X arousal model has most frequently been applied and appears to be more useful than alternatives for unifying results across paradigms, as discussed below.

Two recent studies from our laboratory illustrate typical paradigms used to assess startle modification by affective valence and arousal. Hawk, Cook, and Goates (1995) used the Lang group's three-content picture paradigm with an unselected group of 68 subjects, whereas Stevenson and Cook (1997) administered the Cook et al. (1991) imagery paradigm to 97 individuals selected to vary widely in fearfulness and positive schizotypy – two personality characteristics related to psychopathology. As in the typical picture paradigm, Hawk et al. (1995) compared startle responses elicited in the context of pleasant/interesting, unpleasant/interesting, and neutral/dull pictures. Stevenson and Cook used brief scripts as prompts for imagery of situations that elicited fear, anger, joy, pleasant relaxation, and sadness. Figure 9.1 maps the materials used to manipulate affect in these studies onto the valence and arousal dimensions, using the research participants' own ratings. Differences in the magnitudes of startles elicited under pleasant versus unpleasant conditions (represented by the vertical axes) indicate the effect of emotional valence. Likewise, differences in the magnitudes of startles elicited under high versus low arousal conditions (represented by the horizontal axis) indicate the effect of emotional arousal (or, in the case of pictures, a related dimension, such as interest or attention; see Hawk & Cook, 1997, for discussion of this issue).

In both studies, valence and arousal modification of startle appear to be independent (see Fig. 9.2), suggesting that these two types of startle modification reflect independent neuropsychological mechanisms. In further support for this view is the differential sensitivity of valence and arousal modification to certain experimental manipulations. For example, arousal-(or attention-) related startle modification decreases over trials, consistent with reduced impact of or attention to emotional stimuli over time; valence modification does not show this decremental effect (Hawk et al., 1992; Bradley, Lang, and Cuthbert, 1993; Hawk & Cook, 1997; Stevenson & Cook, 1997).

In the following review, four groups of studies are considered. The relationship between individual differences in fearfulness and startle reflex modification is first considered. A range of other individual difference dimensions that have been correlated with startle modification is then reviewed. The third set of studies relate startle responding to specific anxiety disorders. Finally,

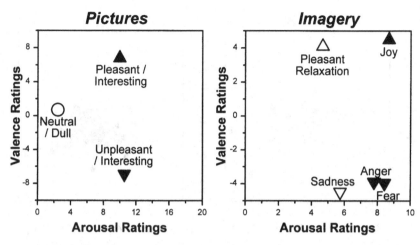

Figure 9.1. Manipulation of affective valence and arousal in the picture and imagery paradigm (data from Hawk et al., 1995, and Stevenson & Cook, 1997). Each panel presents mean ratings of the sets of materials used to manipulate emotion, and illustrates the a priori contrasts used to assess the two startle modification dimensions. For assessment of valence modification, startles elicited during pleasant picture viewing or imagery (upward-pointing triangles) are contrasted with startles elicited during unpleasant picture viewing or imagery (downward-pointing triangles). For assessment of arousal modification, startles elicited under high arousal conditions (solid symbols) are contrasted with startles elicited under low arousal conditions (open symbols). Note that the rating scales used in the two studies are not directly comparable: Hawk et al. (1995) used the Self-Assessment Manikin (Hodes, Cook, & Lang, 1985; Lang, 1980); whereas Stevenson & Cook (1987) used numeric ratings (in each case, the range illustrated corresponds to the full range of the rating scale).

preliminary evidence for relationships between affective startle modification and the schizophrenia spectrum disorders is summarized.

2. Fearfulness and Affective Modification of Startle

In a series of studies we have examined relationships between affective startle modification and the trait tendency toward situational fear. We initially chose this dimension because situational fear is a core characteristic of PTSD and might therefore account for exaggerated startle responses that are historically associated with that disorder. In our research, fearfulness is operationally defined as total score on the Fear Survey Schedule (FSS; Wolpe & Lang, 1964; Arrindell, Emmelkamp, & van der Ende, 1984). For most stud-

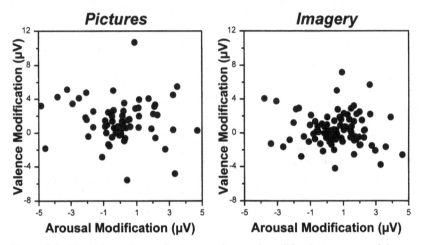

Figure 9.2. The independence of valence and arousal modification across participants in the same Hawk et al. (1995) and Stevenson and Cook (1997) studies for which ratings are presented in Fig. 9.1. Each point represents an individual subject. Valence modification is computed as the mean magnitude of startles elicited during unpleasant imagery or picture viewing minus the mean magnitude of startles elicited during pleasant imagery or picture viewing. Thus, subjects with positive valence modification scores had larger startles during unpleasant compared with pleasant conditions. Arousal modification is computed as the mean magnitude of startles elicited during high-arousal imagery or picture viewing (averaged across pleasant and unpleasant valence) minus the mean magnitude of startles elicited during low-arousal imagery or picture conditions (averaged across pleasant and unpleasant valence for imagery, or simply the neutral condition for pictures). Thus, positive and negative arousal modification scores correspond to startle potentiation and inhibition, respectively, during high arousal compared with low-arousal imagery or picture viewing.

ies the high- and low-fear samples are not extreme – they include subjects varying widely within the upper and lower 30 to 40 percent of each gender's distribution. Regression analysis is generally used to assess relationships of startle modification to fearfulness because it preserves information about differences within as well as between the high-and low-fear groups. Bursts of white noise (typically 100–110 dB, 50 msec duration, less than 3 msec rise/fall) are delivered by headphones under varying affective conditions to elicit startle and assess its affective modification.

2.1. Valence Modification and High Fear

In the first study in this series, Cook et al. (1991) probed startle responses in high- and low-fear subjects while they imagined situations designed to elicit five different emotions: fear, anger, sadness, joy, and pleasant relaxation. (A neutral imagery condition was also included in this initial study but did not contribute to the modification measures.) Valence and arousal modification was assessed as previously described. As shown in Figure 9.3 (Experiment I), valence modification varied with individual differences in fearfulness. High-fear subjects showed reliable startle potentiation during aversive compared with pleasant imagery, whereas startle responses of low-fear subjects during pleasant and aversive imagery were statistically identical.

Cook et al. (1992) investigated the relationship between fearfulness and startle modification using a different affect manipulation and additional startle measurement. Subjects viewed pictures that had been previously rated as either aversive or neutral. In addition to blink magnitude, blink latency as well as "cardiac startles" (short-latency heart-rate accelerations; Graham, 1979; Cook & Turpin, 1997) were also measured. Again in this study high-fear subjects showed reliable affective startle modification, and this effect appeared in all three measures: Fearful subjects had larger startle blinks (Fig. 9.3, Experiment II) and reduced blink latencies while viewing aversive compared with neutral pictures; cardiac startles occurred only during the aversive pictures in this group. In contrast, low-fear subjects showed no reliable effects of emotion on any startle measure. While these findings were generally consistent with those of Cook et al. (1991), clear separation of valence and arousal modification effects was not possible because only aversive and neutral materials were used in this study (see Fig. 9.1).

Stevenson and Cook (1997) selected subjects for high, moderate, or low fear and tested them sequentially in both imagery and picture paradigms. Valence modification during imagery increased monotonically with fearfulness score (see Fig. 9.3, Experiment III): Low-fear subjects showed no effect ($F < 1$) and moderate-fear subjects showed a trend ($p = .12$); only high-fear subjects showed reliably larger startles during aversive compared with pleasant imagery. Despite substantial habituation, women but not men continued to show a positive relationship between fearfulness and startle valence modification during the subsequent picture procedure.

More robust fearfulness differences in the three-content picture paradigm are suggested by two additional studies. Cook, Goates, Hawk, and Palmatier (1996) selected high- and low-fear subjects using the same criteria as Stevenson and Cook (1997). Hawk and Cook (1993) split their sample of unselected subjects on FSS total score. In both of these studies (Fig. 9.3, Experiments IV and V) high-fear compared with low-fear subjects showed greater valence modification of startle. In addition to further replicating the fearfulness-startle relationship, Hawk and Cook extended the finding to a tactile (air-puff) probe.

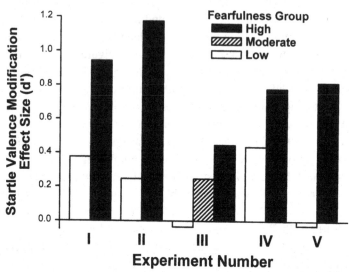

Figure 9.3. Startle valence modification in subjects with low, moderate, and high fear from five affective modification studies. Experiment I: Cook et al., 1991; Experiment II: Cook et al., 1992; Experiment III: Stevenson and Cook, 1997; Experiment IV: Cook et al., 1996; Experiment V: Hawk & Cook, 1993. In all experiments illustrated here the valence modification effect is significantly greater among high fear subjects compared with low-fear subjects. Startle valence modification was computed for each subject as in Fig. 9.2 and then converted to an effect size (d'; Cohen, 1988) using the mean and standard deviation for each group.

Studies based on median splits (e.g., Hawk & Cook, 1993) are in general less powerful than studies in which subjects are selected for more extreme scores on the FSS (e.g., Cook et al., 1991, 1996; Stevenson and Cook, 1997). However, several investigators using the median-split approach have obtained results that are generally consistent with our own. Greenwald, Bradley, Cuthbert, and Lang (1990) reported greater valence modulation among high- compared with low-fear subjects in the three-category picture paradigm, and Hamm, Greenwald, Bradley, and Lang (1993) reported reliable startle potentiation among high- but not low-fear subjects during pictures previously paired with electric shock (though in this case the overall Conditioning X Fear Group interaction was nonsignificant).

Thus, there are six studies demonstrating a statistically robust relationship between affective startle modification and high levels of trait fearfulness, and in one of these studies (Stevenson & Cook, 1997) the relationship was observed for both genders during imagery and for females (but not males) during subsequent picture-viewing, conducted after startle responding had substantially habituated. The relationship has been obtained with two affect manipulations (imagery and pictures), two types of probes (acoustic and tactile), and three startle measures (blink magnitude, blink latency, and heart rate). Hamm et al.'s (1993) data provide additional support, involving a third affect manipulation (aversive conditioning). Thus, the relationship between high trait fearfulness and enhanced affective startle modification, especially along the valence dimension, has been demonstrated with a variety of methods and measures.

Affective ratings are typically obtained from participants in these studies as a check on the affect manipulation, but ratings are also useful in interpreting the individual difference findings. Thus, in the Stevenson and Cook (1997) study, high- compared with low-fear individuals rated the unpleasant imagery and pictures as more aversive and the pleasant imagery and pictures stimuli as more pleasant. These data suggest that greater startle valence modification among high-fear subjects reflects a more general reactivity of these subjects to the emotional valence of stimuli.

2.2. Arousal (or Attentional) Modification and Low Fear

How can the relationships between fearfulness and valence modification of startle be explained? The absence of reliable valence modification in low-fear subjects raises the possibility that these subjects simply fail to follow task instructions or engage in affective processing. A related possibility is suggested by data of Cuthbert, Bradley, and Lang (1996), who found reliable valence modification of startle only with a subset of pictures within the pleasant and unpleasant categories that had been previously rated as most arousing (or, relatedly, to which subjects showed the greatest skin conductance responses). Thus, a lack of valence modification in low-fear subjects might reflect a failure to arouse an affective reaction in these subjects.

Data from the fearfulness studies, however, generally argue against this explanation. Consistently the high- and low-fear subjects show robust (and statistically equivalent) heart rate responses to the affective stimuli (i.e., greater deceleration to aversive than to neutral and pleasant pictures, and greater acceleration during aversive compared with pleasant imagery; Cook et al., 1991, 1992; Stevenson & Cook, 1997). Arousal ratings, on which the Cuthbert et al. (1996) findings were based, provide no evidence that low-fear subjects are less aroused by the affective materials than are high-fear subjects (Stevenson & Cook, 1997). Indeed, some data suggest that low- compared with high-fear individuals actually respond more to arousing affective materials. Cook et al. (1996) found greater arousal-related startle modification among low- compared with high-fear subjects in the three-content picture paradigm. Only the low-fear subjects showed significantly smaller startles on average while viewing pleasant and unpleasant pictures than during neutral pictures. (The combination of enhanced arousal modification and diminished valence modification in low- compared with high-fear subjects is illustrated in Fig. 9.4.) Although data analytic differences complicate comparisons, recent and preliminary data suggest similar findings (enhanced arousal modification, with or without valence modification) in the picture paradigm in other groups that were not selected specifically for low FSS scores, but might reasonably be characterized as low-fear: sensation seekers (Bradley & Lang, 1992; Muse, Weike, & Hamm, 1996), low harm-avoidant individuals (Corr et al., 1995), and psychopaths (Patrick, Bradley, & Lang, 1993; Patrick, 1994; Chapter 10).

The greater attenuation of startle during arousing pleasant and unpleasant materials (which are also more novel and interesting) may reflect greater attention to these stimuli among low-fear individuals. Startle inhibition in this context would presumably reflect a modality mismatch: With more attentional capacity devoted to the pictures, less is available for probes in the unattended acoustic modality (Chapter 4). A more direct test of this hypothesis, involving visual startle probes, has yet to be undertaken. An alternative interpretation of the pattern of findings is that low-fear subjects fail to potentiate startle during the aversive relative to the neutral pictures, resulting in an average for pleasant and unpleasant that falls below neutral. However, because neutral and aversive pictures differ on a range of dimensions (cf. Fig. 9.1), interpretation of separate comparisons of either pleasant or unpleasant to neutral is problematic.

The conventional picture paradigm was not designed to discriminate these competing hypotheses. However, two of our imagery studies (Cook et al., 1991; Stevenson & Cook, 1997) also support the hypothesis that low- compared with high-fear subjects process emotional materials with respect to their arousing properties rather than their valence. In both studies, significant arousal modification in the absence of valence modification was observed among low-fear subjects. Stevenson and Cook (1997) also observed greater arousal modification of skin conductance in the low- compared with the high-fear group.

Thus both picture and imagery studies suggest greater arousal modification of startle in ostensibly low- compared with high-fear subjects. Interestingly, the direction of the effect reverses between the imagery and picture par-

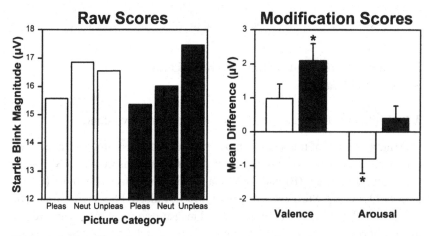

Figure 9.4. The effect of variations in both valence modification and arousal (or attentional) modification of startle between low-fear subjects (open bars) and high-fear subjects (solid bars). Data are from Cook et al. (1996). Valence and arousal modification scores were computed as in Fig. 9.2. Thus, only high-fear subjects showed significant (*: $p < .05$) potentiation during unpleasant compared with pleasant pictures (valence modification) and only low-fear subjects showed significant inhibition during high arousal (mean across pleasant and unpleasant) compared with low arousal (neutral) pictures (arousal modification).

adigms. In imagery the arousal effect involves startle potentiation, while during picture-viewing, highly arousing pictures occasion startle inhibition. This paradigm difference may explain a recent failure to observe a relationship between fearfulness and affective startle modification in our laboratory. Gautier and Cook (1997) administered an imagery paradigm that included only high-arousal aversive and low-arousal pleasant conditions. While affective startle modification along this "negative affect" dimension (Watson & Tellegen, 1985) is robust (Cook et al., 1991; Lang, Bradley, & Cuthbert, 1992), in the imagery paradigm it may be especially insensitive to fearfulness. That is, if high-fear subjects show greater valence modification (aversive greater than pleasant) and low-fear subjects show increased arousal modification (high greater than low), then both low- and high-fear subjects should show affective startle modification (aversive high arousal greater than pleasant low arousal), but for different reasons. This is indeed what Gautier and Cook (1997) observed: robust affective modification ($d' = .37$, cf. Fig. 9.3) in both fear groups. In contrast, in the picture paradigm startle modification by negative affect may be especially sensitive to fearfulness differences (cf. Fig. 9.3, Experiment II), because high fear should augment and low fear inhibit startle during aversive high-arousal compared with neutral low-arousal pictures. Such sensitivity is purchased, however, at the price of interpretive ambiguity.

3. Other Affective Individual Differences and Startle Modification

3.1. Trait Anxiety, Negative Affectivity, and Harm Avoidance

One interpretation of the relationship between fearfulness and startle modification casts the most commonly used fearfulness measure (the FSS) as a proxy for trait anxiety (Bradley & Vrana, 1993) or negative affectivity (Cook et al., 1991; Cook, Stevenson, & Hawk, 1993). Indeed, FSS scores are positively related to scores on commonly used measures of these constructs (e.g., the trait form of the State-Trait Anxiety Inventory and the PANAS-Gen Negative Affectivity scale).

Attempts to discover correlations between these measures and affective startle modification have met with partial success. Cook et al. (1991) split their mixed fearfulness sample on trait anxiety: High-anxiety subjects showed reliable startle valence modification during imagery, whereas low-anxiety subjects did not. A similar pattern of results was obtained by Cook and Gautier (1992), who selected subjects to vary widely in negative and positive affectivity on the PANAS-Gen scale (Watson, Clark, & Tellegen, 1988). Individuals high in negative affectivity showed significant valence modification, while low-scoring subjects did not. However, in neither of the two studies did the critical interaction effect (Valence X Trait Anxiety/Negative Affectivity) attain statistical significance ($p = .06$ and $.12$, respectively). Recently, however, Stevenson and Cook (1997) reported significant increases in startle valence modification with trait negative affectivity in their affective imagery procedure. Grillon et al. (1993), however, found no relationship between trait anxiety and fear-potentiated startle in a shock threat paradigm.

A preliminary conclusion from these studies is that startle valence modification is less strongly related to negative affectivity or trait anxiety than to fearfulness. These dimensions differ from fearfulness in focusing on subjects' modal emotional state (e.g., "tense," "distressed") rather than their reaction to potentially threatening stimuli. If startle is conceptualized as a protective or defensive response to a stimulus (Konorski, 1967; Lang et al., 1990), then fearfulness may come closer to matching the critical individual difference dimension that controls startle valence modification.

Fearfulness is also related to harm avoidance, a personality construct of particular interest because deficits in harm avoidance have been hypothesized to underlie psychopathy (Lykken, 1995), a diagnostic condition associated with reduced startle valence modulation (Patrick et al., 1993; Patrick, 1994; Chapter 10). Recently, Corr et al. (1995) investigated startle modulation in individuals who varied on a questionnaire measure of harm avoidance. Subjects scoring above the median showed potentiated startle during aversive compared with neutral pictures, while low harm-avoidance subjects showed inhibited startle during pleasant compared with neutral pictures. As noted previously, such comparisons confound contributions of valence, arousal, and selective attention, and thus are somewhat difficult to interpret. Valence modulation, though not tested, appeared to have been only slightly greater in high compared with low harm-avoidance subjects. Nevertheless, the theoretical importance of harm avoidance and these interesting preliminary results suggest further research with this dimension.

3.2. Depression and Positive Affectivity

In their mixed fearfulness sample, Cook et al. (1991) found that MMPI Depression scale scores were positively related to startle valence modification. Despite this encouraging initial finding, subsequent studies from our laboratory, employing larger samples, have not found any reliable relationships between affective startle modification and depression measured with either the Beck Depression Inventory (Beck, Ward, Mendelsohn, Mock, & Erbaugh, 1961) or the MMPI (Dahlstrom, Welsh, & Dahlstrom, 1972) Depression scale (Stevenson, Cook, & Hawk, 1991; Stevenson & Cook, 1997). Subjects selected by Cook and Gautier (1992) for low positive affectivity – a dimensional characteristic that distinguishes depression from anxiety (Tellegen, 1985; Watson, Clark, & Carey, 1988) – did show enhanced valence modification of startle during imagery, but this effect was restricted to high-arousal imagery conditions.

Recently, Allen, Trinder, and Brennan (1997) observed the opposite effect – diminished startle valence modification – in a clinically depressed sample. The three-content picture paradigm was administered to 14 individuals currently experiencing a major depressive episode and to an age- and gender-matched comparison group. Depressed subjects lacked potentiation of startle during the unpleasant relative to the pleasant pictures, and correlational analysis suggested that this effect was primarily due to increases in startle magnitude during pleasant picture-viewing among individuals with the highest depression scores (Beck scale). This finding suggests that clinical depression is associated with not just a lack of appetitive response, but even frank aversion to conventionally pleasant events. Longitudinal assessment of depression-prone individuals will help to clarify whether the aberrant startle observed in this study reflects the depressed state or a depression-prone trait.

3.3. Summary

Compared with research on startle modification and fearfulness, research on relationships between startle and other affective individual differences and disorders has produced inconsistent outcomes. Nevertheless, intriguing results (e.g., Corr et al., 1995; Allen et al., 1997) encourage further research. The studies reviewed previously in this chapter suggest that different emotion paradigms (e.g., imagery vs. pictures) can yield different outcomes. Preselection of subjects for specific characteristics would enhance future research in this area as well. In general, adequate evaluation of relationships between startle and additional affective characteristics depends on use of a range of emotion paradigms and more powerful research designs and statistical analyses than those typically employed thus far.

4. Anxiety Disorders and Affective Startle Modification

As noted previously, preliminary reports of exaggerated startle in anxiety disordered groups were a major impetus for research on affective individual differences and startle modification in nonclinical samples. The majority of these reports focused on PTSD, and we begin our review of startle responding in anxiety-disordered populations by considering the PTSD work.

4.1. Exaggerated Startle in PTSD

Exposure to traumatic events has long been associated with exaggerated psychophysiological reactivity (Bartemeier et al., 1946; Shalev & Rogel-Fuchs, 1993; Prins, Kaloupek, & Keane, 1995), and contemporary diagnostic criteria for PTSD (American Psychiatric Association, 1994, p. 428) suggest both chronic increases in arousal (including exaggerated startle) and phasic responses while "reliving" the traumatic event. Likewise, extant research on startle and PTSD can be divided into studies of baseline response and studies of startle modification by affective context.

Most investigations have focused on baseline responding, and results have been mixed. Grillon, Morgan, Southwick, Davis, and Charney (1996) observed no differences in startle response at baseline, and Ornitz and Pynoos (1989) actually reported smaller startles in six children with PTSD compared with six controls. However, the most common finding is that expected on the basis of self-report and clinical observation: larger startles in PTSD compared with healthy civilian or combat-exposed comparison groups (Butler, Braff, Rausch, Jenkins, Sprock, & Geyer, 1990; Morgan, Grillon, Southwick, Davis, & Charney, 1995, 1996; Morgan, Grillon, Southwick, Nagy, et al., 1995; Orr, Lasko, Shalev & Pitman, 1995).

Several authors have suggested that exaggerated baseline startle in PTSD is actually due to affective modification. Prins et al. (1995) attribute exaggerated startle in the absence of explicit threat cues to an increased frequency of aversive emotional states in PTSD and/or the elicitation of trauma-related fear by aspects of startle testing (e.g., memories of gunfire elicited by acoustic startle probes). Morgan, Grillon, Southwick, Davis, and Charney (1995) attempt to explain the discrepant findings for "baseline" startle on the basis of differences in laboratory contexts. To assess this hypothesis, Grillon, Morgan, Davis, and Southwick (in press) contrasted Vietnam veterans with PTSD with military and civilian controls in a two-session experiment. Session 1 involved only baseline startle assessment. Session 2 involved the same baseline procedure followed by a shock threat procedure in which two colored lights signaled shock-threat and safe conditions. Prior to each session, subjects were informed of the procedures, and thus two types of fear cues were present at various points in session 2 and totally absent in session 1: contextual cues (information that shock would be presented at some point during the session, attachment of the shock electrode), and the explicit cue (presence of the light signaling possible shock). There were no differences among groups in baseline startle magnitude in session 1, or in startle potentiation by the explicit fear cue in session 2. However, the PTSD group showed greater sensitivity to the contextual fear cues: increased startle from the session 1 baseline to the session 2 baseline (other groups decreased) and more of a further increase in startle magnitude with attachment of the shock electrodes. The authors suggest that increased sensitivity to contextual fear cues may be a distinctive characteristic of PTSD. This hypothesis is interesting in light of animal research suggesting different neural substrates of contextual and explicit fear cue conditioning (e.g., Phillips & LeDoux, 1992; Chapter 5), and holds promise for informing future research on affective startle modification as well as on the psychopathology and treatment of PTSD.

4.2. Startle Modification in Specific and Social Phobia

While specific phobia has not historically been associated with exaggerated startle, there are ample reasons to investigate startle in this group. Studies

reviewed earlier in this chapter document an association between trait tendencies toward phobic fear and enhanced affective startle modification.
Moreover, the intense fear and dread experienced by phobics exposed to their
phobic object provide a model system for investigating fear-potentiated startle in humans under extreme affective conditions.

Research with a variety of samples and research paradigms suggests that
phobia is associated with potentiated startle during various types of exposure
to the phobic object. Vrana, Constantine, and Westman (1992) found reliable
startle potentiation during phobia-relevant compared with neutral imagery in
one bird phobic and one dog phobic. Not surprisingly, clinically diagnosed
spider phobics show potentiated startle when confronted with live spiders relative to control stimuli (neutral objects and attractive food; see de Jong, Merckelbach, & Arntz, 1991, and de Jong, Visser, & Merckelbach, 1996; but cf.
de Jong, Arntz, & Merckelbach, 1993, for a failure to replicate this effect).

Hamm, Cuthbert, Globisch, and Vaitl (1997) compared animal-(snake/
spider) and mutilation-fearful women selected with specific fear questionnaires (Klorman, Weerts, Hastings, Melamed, & Lang, 1974) to a low-fear
comparison group in the three-content picture paradigm supplemented by a
fear-relevant condition (i.e., each subject viewed either snake, spider, or mutilation pictures, depending on his or her particular fear). Both high-fear groups
had larger startles while viewing their fear-relevant pictures, relative to neutral pictures; low-scoring subjects did not show this effect. In contrast, startle
potentiation during personally tailored fear imagery did not differ reliably
among specific phobics, social phobics, and nonphobic controls (Cuthbert,
Strauss, Drobes, Patrick, Bradley, & Lang, 1997). In neither the Hamm et al.
nor the Cuthbert et al. study did startle modification for standard picture and
imagery material differ significantly between groups.

If phobic fear potentiates startle in the presence of the phobic object, then
effective treatment of phobia should reduce or eliminate startle potentiation.
There is preliminary evidence that this occurs. Vrana et al. (1992) found that
treatment eliminated potentiation of startle during phobia-relevant imagery
relevant to neutral imagery. Similarly, de Jong et al. (1991) found that a single exposure-based treatment session reduced the magnitude of spider-
phobics' startles elicited in the presence of a spider, while startles elicited in
the presence of food were unchanged. The intriguing possibility that pretreatment startle responses predict treatment outcome was raised by de Jong
et al. (1996), who found that spider phobics whose startles were most potentiated at pretreatment by exposure to a live spider showed the least reduction
in self-reported spider fear at post-treatment and follow-up assessments.

4.3. Summary

Despite the long history of clinical observations relating disordered startle to anxiety, contemporary studies in which startle has been measured have thus far yielded few firm conclusions. Much effort has gone into testing differences in baseline or "unmodulated" startle, particularly in PTSD. Questions regarding chronic alterations of startle in particular diagnostic groups may remain elusive, however, particularly given the large individual differences in baseline startle magnitude that occur in even healthy populations. Moreover, there is little theoretical or empirical basis for interpreting such differences. In contrast, new data from Grillon et al. (1997; see also Grillon & Morgan, 1997) shed light on previous discrepant results by demonstrating that the experimental context can potentiate startle during a nominal baseline, even before explicit fear cues are presented.

Regarding specific phobia, it seems clear that startle is potentiated when phobia-related information (presented "live," as pictures, or in imagery) is processed. Such a finding for any particular diagnostic group is most interesting when placed in a more general theoretical context. A parsimonious view would be that, when other factors are held constant, startle is a reasonably good measure of a fearful or anxious state. This view implies that startle should be potentiated in all anxiety disorders, with the situation-specificity of startle potentiation matching the situation-specificity of the anxiety (e.g., low in generalized anxiety disorder and panic, high in specific phobia, and moderate in PTSD). To test this and related hypotheses, more studies are needed in which multiple patient groups are compared (e.g., Cuthbert et al., 1997) and additional anxiety disorder diagnoses (e.g., panic; cf. Grillon, Ameli, Goddard, Woods, & Davis, 1994) are considered.

The possibility that startle might serve as a supplemental measure or predictor of treatment outcome has been raised by several studies. As a basis for further explorations of this possibility, additional research on between- and within-session stability in affective startle modification needs to be undertaken (see Bradley, Gianaros, & Lang, 1995, and Hawk et al., 1995, for preliminary attempts to address these issues).

5. Schizotypy, Schizophrenia, and Affective Startle Modification

The possibility that affective startle modification is disordered in schizophrenia is of interest for several reasons. While thought disorder is generally considered the hallmark symptom of this disorder, affective dysfunction – including negative symptoms of schizophrenia such as ambivalence and affective flattening – are also widely recognized, and may be of greater prognostic significance (Knight & Roff, 1985). On the other hand, positive symptoms (delusions, hallucinations, catatonia, and formal thought disorder) are conceptualized as independent of affective impairment, and hence variations in these symptoms might be independent of affective startle modification, even while they are correlated with other forms of startle modification, such as prepulse inhibition (see Chapter 11). Finally, both positive and negative schizophrenia symptoms are also observed in PTSD, and preliminary evidence relates startle reactivity to schizotypal symptoms within the PTSD group, as discussed below.

5.1. Affective Startle Modification in Schizophrenia

Schlenker, Cohen, and Hopmann (1994) tested male schizophrenics and healthy controls in the three-content picture paradigm. A primary goal of this research was to investigate the relationship between affective flattening and affective startle modification. It was predicted that schizophrenics with more severe affective flattening would show less affective startle modification. Exactly the opposite effect was found: Greater affective modification of startle, particularly along the valence dimension, was observed in the high affective flattening compared with the low affective flattening subgroup. (Compared with healthy controls, the low affective flattening group showed the more distinctive pattern of startle modification.)

The relatively normal pattern of affective startle modification in the high affective flattening group is consistent with the hypothesis that affective flattening in schizophrenia is a phenomenon of affective expression rather than affective state (Kring & Neale, 1996). Interestingly, schizophrenics without significant affective flattening showed the startle modification pattern previously associated with temperamentally low-fear normals and emotionally detached psychopathy: inhibition during interesting and arousing pictures, relative to neutral pictures, regardless of their affective valence. The possibility that a common affective dimension might underlie the similar results from these disparate clinical and nonclinical samples remains to be determined.

5.2. Affective Startle Modulation and Schizotypal Symptoms

As noted previously in this chapter, initial research suggested that a number of negative emotional traits (fear, anxiety, anger-proneness, and depression) are associated with enhanced startle valence modification (Cook et al., 1991).

While suggesting a general relationship between affective startle modification and negative affective traits, the specificity of this relationship remained in question. Perhaps valence modification is a nonspecific covariate of deviance, unhappiness, or a global tendency toward psychopathology.

To begin to address this possibility, Stevenson et al. (1991) assessed startle modification by affective imagery in individuals selected for high scores on the Perceptual Aberration and Magical Ideation (Per-Mag) scales (Chapman, Chapman, & Raulin, 1978; Eckblad & Chapman, 1983) as well as low scores on the FSS. The Per-Mag scales are marker variables for "positive schizotypy" (Vollema & van den Bosch, 1995), and measure unusual perceptual experiences and beliefs. Hence, they seek to measure subclinical disorders of perception and cognition that are more profound in schizophrenia. A high FSS/low Per-Mag group was also tested, along with a group scoring low on both the FSS and Per-Mag scales. Stevenson et al. reasoned that if enhanced affective startle modification were primarily associated with excessive tendencies toward negative affect, then high-fear but not high Per-Mag subjects should show an enhanced modification effect. Alternatively, if affective startle modification was associated with general deviance or psychopathology, then both high Per-Mag and high-fear subjects should show enhancement of the effect.

Results supported neither alternative hypothesis. High Per-Mag subjects (selected in addition for low fear) showed robust affective modification of startle, whereas no reliable modification was observed in the high FSS/low Per-Mag or the low FSS/low Per-Mag groups. The failure to obtain enhanced affective modification in the high-fear group appeared to conflict with the results of Cook et al. (1991); however, the fact that high-fear subjects were also selected for low Per-Mag scores complicated the comparison of findings from the two studies. Contemporaneously, Butler et al. (1990) reported greater startle probabilities among men with PTSD who also showed positive and negative symptoms of schizophrenia. While procedures and methods were quite different in the Butler et al. and Stevenson et al. studies, both suggested a link between schizophrenia-related symptoms and increased startle reactivity.

Stevenson and Cook (1997) addressed this question in a larger sample, using both imagery and pictures to manipulate affect. Subjects were selected for low, moderate, or high fearfulness and low, moderate, or high schizotypy in a 3 × 3 between-subjects design; hence the confounding of fearfulness and schizotypy in Stevenson et al. (1991) was eliminated. High fearfulness was associated with enhanced valence modulation, as described previously (Fig. 9.3, Experiment III). In addition to high fear, high positive schizotypy was also associated with greater startle valence modification during imagery: The high Per-Mag group showed robust valence modulation, whereas subjects scoring in the low-to-moderate range on these scales did not. Per-Mag scores were unrelated to valence modification during the subsequent picture phase in this study and in a subsequent picture-viewing study (Cook et al., 1996).

Thus in two imagery studies from our laboratory, subjects reporting numerous schizotypal symptoms showed greater affective startle modification than subjects reporting few such symptoms. Two studies involving affective picture-viewing have not shown this effect. It is noteworthy in this regard that other investigators (Roedema & Simons, 1994) have also reported greater sensitivity of the imagery paradigm vis-à-vis the picture paradigm to psychopathologically relevant individual differences.

6. Summary, Conclusions, and Future Directions

We can now summarize the replicated results from the series of studies of individual and diagnostic group differences in affective startle modification.

1. Fearful subjects show greater modification of startle magnitude by affective valence than low-fear subjects. This phenomenon has been demonstrated with multiple affect manipulations, startle probe modalities, and startle reflex measures.
2. Low-fear subjects show a reliable paradigm-dependent arousal- or attention-related startle pattern. Thus, low-fear subjects show increased startle magnitude during high-arousal imagery, and decreased startle magnitude while viewing high-arousal pictures, regardless of affective valence.
3. Small-animal (snake and spider) phobics show potentiated startle responses while viewing phobia-relevant pictures compared with stimuli rated as equally aversive by nonphobic controls.
4. Subjects selected for positive schizotypy show enhanced valence modification of startle during affective imagery but not during affective picture-viewing.

Noteworthy by its absence from the list is a firm conclusion regarding startle and PTSD, despite considerable research activity in this area. The focus on chronic as compared with phasic startle potentiation in this group, coupled with substantial interindividual variability in baseline startle, may have acted to slow progress in this area.

Several of these conclusions are based on preliminary reports (conference presentations, unpublished manuscripts), and if one set a higher standard – two published supportive papers and no published reversals – only the relationship between fearfulness and valence modification would stand. In addition, we are aware of other failures to observe several of these effects, although some such null findings are inconclusive on the basis of low power to detect relationships due to unselected samples and/or insensitive statistical tests. Despite these cautions, it is not premature to conclude that where programmatic research has been undertaken, consistent differences among groups have emerged for affective startle modification.

To the extent that fear and anxiety are associated with potentiation of startle magnitude, we can reasonably question whether such effects represent a sensory or motor modulatory mechanism. For more than a decade, cognitively oriented research has sought to understand anxiety disorders on the basis of stimulus-processing characteristics. Thus, persons with anxiety disorders have been found to show greater attention to threat-related stimuli, whether external as in specific phobias (Mineka, 1992; Öhman, 1997) or internal as in panic (Clark, 1988). Such a theoretical perspective suggests the possibility that persons who are anxious (due to trait or state factors) respond more to startle probes because of some attentional, input-enhancing mechanism. Basic research on startle modification clearly demonstrates that attention to the probes enhances responding relative to attention directed away from the probes (e.g., toward an interesting stimulus in another sensory modality; see Chapter 4). If startle probes are themselves potentially threatening stimuli (due to their intensity and suddenness), then perhaps enhanced attention to threatening stimuli could be the mechanism that underlies greater fear-potentiated startle in anxious subjects, particularly when exposed to anxiety-enhancing or otherwise aversive experimental conditions.

Such a perspective on the data reviewed in this chapter warrants further research, although for two reasons we are not optimistic about this interpretation. First, an aversive probe is not necessary for startle elicitation, modification, or sensitivity to individual differences. It is true that the acoustic startle probe used in most investigations is aversive for most subjects (see, e.g., Bradley et al., 1990). However, air puffs to the face are judged as somewhat pleasant, but elicit robust startle responses (Hawk & Cook, 1997), the modification of which also varies with individual differences in fearfulness (Hawk & Cook, 1993). Second, recent research from our laboratory on spontaneous eyeblink suggests that the stimulus may be irrelevant. Palmatier, Goates, and Cook (1995) found that fearful subjects (selected as in the studies described above) showed increased rates of spontaneous blinking following aversive compared with pleasant pictures. Low-fear subjects do not show this effect, and thus fearfulness-related differences in spontaneous blink parallel those observed for elicited blink.

We would argue at this point that the startle potentiation phenomena described here are understood better on the basis of output facilitation than input enhancement. By this view, defensive or protective reflexes such as startle are primed by processing of aversive stimuli and contexts (Lang et al., 1990). Individuals who (due to a range of possible genetic and/or experiential factors) are disposed toward greater fear may more readily show this defensive response priming effect. Such a view is consistent with the finding of greater startle enhancement among fearful subjects regardless of the modality or affective quality of the startle-eliciting stimulus, and with our spontaneous blink data, obtained in the absence of a stimulus. Thus we tentatively conclude that affective startle modification is a motor modulatory phenomenon, and that individual and diagnostic group differences in this phenomenon are also likely to reflect motor modulatory mechanisms. Nevertheless, additional tests in additional samples are crucial before we can be confident in these interpretations.

ACKNOWLEDGMENTS

Research from my laboratory was supported by National Institute of Mental Health grant MH46701 and by Faculty Research Grants from the University of Alabama at Birmingham. Graduate students Clara Gautier, Larry Hawk, and Victor Stevenson collaborated on these projects and deserve much of the credit for the work described.

CHAPTER TEN

Psychopathic Traits and Intoxicated States: Affective Concomitants and Conceptual Links

CHRISTOPHER J. PATRICK AND ALAN R. LANG

ABSTRACT

Striking parallels are evident in the phenomena of psychopathic personality and acute alcohol intoxication. Both are characterized by disinhibited behavior (including heightened aggression, deviant sexual expression, thrill-seeking, and irresponsibility) and a disregard for the potentially harmful consequences of such actions. Both are hypothesized to involve disruptions of normal affective and cognitive processes. There is also substantial evidence for a relationship between antisocial personality traits and alcoholism.

This chapter reviews startle-probe investigations of emotional processing in criminal psychopaths and in alcohol-intoxicated normals. Its essential themes are that (1) core affective deficits are associated not with the disinhibitory behavioral features of psychopathy, but with the classic personality symptoms, and (2) alcohol appears to suppress emotional responsiveness not at a primary level, but indirectly, through its effects on higher cognitive processes. We argue for the probable existence of a significant subgroup of antisocial offenders who are analogous to intoxicated normal individuals in their proneness to disinhibited behavior, but are distinct from "primary" psychopaths in that they do not exhibit emotional detachment. Alcohol intoxication (as well as other pharmacological state manipulations) may provide a valuable heuristic for analyzing cognitive–emotional processes underlying persistent antisociality not attributable to a primary deficit in affective response capacity.

1. Overview: Disinhibitory Traits and States

Popular theories of behavioral deviance in antisocial personality rest heavily on the thesis that those exhibiting such behavior are deficient in their capac-

Michael E. Dawson, Anne M. Schell, and Andreas H. Böhmelt, Eds. *Startle modification: Implications for neuroscience, cognitive science, and clinical science.* Copyright © 1999 Cambridge University Press. Printed in the United States of America.

ity to react fearfully when circumstances warrant it. However, recent theoretical and empirical work suggests that the disinhibitory[1] behavioral features of psychopathy are dissociable from the emotional detachment that is regarded as the essence of the classic syndrome (Cleckley, 1976).

Lykken (1995) theorized that "primary psychopathy" is rooted in temperamental fearlessness, but that chronic antisociality is neither invariably nor exclusively the product of this disposition. Frick (in press) has presented evidence that "callous unemotional" traits in children – which are analogous to (and may be precursors to) psychopathic personality symptoms in adulthood, and which are associated with diminished fearfulness – typify only a portion of conduct disorder cases. Similarly, the present review of recent research employing the startle reflex as an index of negative emotional reactivity suggests that antisociality and fearlessness do not necessarily go hand in hand.

It is also becoming increasingly clear that fear and anxiety are not *directly* soluble in alcohol. Despite decades of research and theory predicated on this simple assumption, accumulating evidence – including the findings to be reviewed here – indicates that the drug has a rather diffuse effect on emotional reactivity, and that its role in disinhibiting behavior may depend upon a complex interplay of psychological and situational factors. We hypothesize (1) that the relative ineffectiveness of punishment in controlling the deviant actions of inebriates is secondary to an underlying alcohol-induced disturbance of higher order processes (e.g., contextual learning, declarative memory, attention allocation) required for appropriate regulation of behavior in complex situations, and (2) that analogous impairments in cognitive–emotional processing may underlie the disinhibited behavior of a significant portion of chronically antisocial individuals who are not classically psychopathic.

2. Emotional Processing: Theoretical Framework

2.1. Affective Dimensions and Levels

Our work is predicated on a multidimensional, multilevel conceptualization of emotion (see Chapter 8), in which affective states are viewed as action dispositions organized along broad dimensions of valence and arousal (Larsen & Diener, 1992; Russell, 1980) reflecting the operation of two primary brain

---

[1] We employ the term "disinhibition" in a purely behavioral sense, to refer to the exhibition of certain responses normally suppressed by controlling mechanisms.

motivational systems: an aversive system governing defensive reactions, and an appetitive system governing consummatory and approach behaviors (Konorski, 1967; Lang, 1995).[2] These motivational systems are presumed to be subcortically based, but through reciprocal connections to higher cortical regions they can influence and be influenced by more complex cognitive processes such as declarative memory, attention, and imagery (Lang, 1994; LeDoux, 1995).

While acknowledging the potential role of appetitive processing in the phenomena under consideration, the work reported here focuses primarily on fear-related emotion. Fear is widely presumed to play a key role in the inhibition of behavior, and it has been the most intensively studied affect in the literatures on antisociality and alcohol intoxication. In addition, fear has been the subject of considerable neuroscientific research in recent years, and a well-developed neural model of fear processing now exists.

Substantial evidence indicates that the subcortical amygdaloid complex is the heart of the defensive (fear) system (Fanselow, 1994; LeDoux, 1995; see Chapter 5). The amygdala's motor output system is the central nucleus, which projects to other structures directly mediating fear expression and behavior (e.g., central gray, lateral hypothalamus). The lateral nucleus of the amygdala, on the other hand, receives multimodal inputs from the sensory thalamus and from perceptual processing areas of the neocortex and is thus considered to be the amygdala's input substation.

Besides inputs from thalamic and cortical structures involved in stimulus recognition and discrimination, the lateral nucleus of the amygdala receives projections from higher associational systems, most notably the hippocampus. The hippocampal formation is a cornerstone of complex cognitive functions, including declarative memory (Squire, 1992) and related spatial, contextual, and associative functions (e.g., Nadel & Willner, 1980; Rudy & Sutherland, 1992). Connections between the hippocampus and the amygdala thus provide a mechanism by which higher-order cognitive activities can instigate or influence affective reactions, in a "top-down" fashion (LeDoux, 1995).

Relevant to this, recent studies have demonstrated striking dissociations between different fear learning capabilities in animals following surgical lesions of the hippocampus. Specifically, hippocampal lesions produce selective impairment of contextual fear conditioning without affecting explicit fear conditioning (Phillips & LeDoux, 1992; Kim, Rison, & Fanselow, 1993).

---

[2] The terms "emotion" and "affect" are used interchangeably here. The term "motivational" (connoting movement, or drive) is used in reference to those brain systems that instigate emotional action dispositions.

Control rats, after being placed in a distinctive new environment and receiving shock in the presence of a tone conditioned stimulus (CS), display a fear reaction not only to the explicit CS but also to the learning context, as evidenced by freezing behavior upon being returned to the training environment in which shock was administered. In contrast, rats with hippocampal lesions exhibit freezing to the tone CS, but not to the context itself. These data are consistent with the neuroanatomical model described above in that projections from the thalamus and auditory cortex to the amygdala can be viewed as sufficient to mediate fear conditioning to a simple tone cue, whereas associations between more complex environmental information and fear reactivity appear to depend on the integrity of hippocampal–amygdaloid connections (LeDoux, 1995).[3]

2.2. Fear-Potentiated Startle

So far, this neural model of fear has been based primarily on animal studies of fear conditioning, but some links have been forged with the human literature. One important point of contact is the phenomenon of fear-potentiated startle. In both animals (Chapter 5) and humans (Chapter 8), the acoustic startle reflex is enhanced during processing of aversive stimuli. Lang, Bradley, and Cuthbert (1990) theorized that this effect is due to a synergistic match between the ongoing (defensive) emotional state and the (defensive) reaction to the sudden nose probe. In parallel fashion, Lang et al. attributed the *reduction* in startle that reliably occurs during pleasant foreground stimulation (Vrana, Spence, & Lang, 1988) to a reciprocal inhibition of defensive reflex reactions during opposing appetitive states.

This response match/mismatch interpretation is easily reconciled with the neural circuitry underlying fear-potentiated startle, which has been precisely mapped in animals (see Chapter 5). The essential mechanism consists of a pathway from the central nucleus of the amygdala to the primary brain-stem startle circuit. Because the central nucleus projects to output systems including the pontine reticular node of the brain-stem startle circuit, fear-relevant

---

[3] It should be noted, however, that other emotion centers besides the amygdala could be involved in mediating contextual fear. Davis, Walker, and Lee (in press) have presented evidence that the bed nucleus of the stria terminalis – a structure that, like the amygdala, projects to output systems involved in negative affective expression and receives input from the hippocampus – plays a role in anxiety reactions not linked to simple, explicit cues. Although this research has focused on separate phenomena (i.e., light-enhanced startle; corticotropin-releasing hormone-enhanced startle), it is conceivable that this "anxiety" system is importantly involved in contextual aversive conditioning.

stimuli that activate the amygdala also prime the startle response. Further-more, the finding that benzodiazepine anxiolytics block fear-potentiated star-tle in both rodents (Davis, 1979) and humans (Patrick, Berthot, & Moore, 1996) is consistent with the notion that a common defensive state underlies this phenomenon in both species (Lang et al., 1990) and that potentiated star-tle can serve as an index of fear in humans.[4]

3. Affect and Startle Modification in Psychopathy

3.1. Two-Factor Model of Psychopathy: Emotional Detachment and Antisocial Behavior

Cleckley (1976) provided the classic clinical description of the psychopathic personality – what others (e.g., Lykken, 1957, 1995) have called the "pri-mary" psychopath. Cleckley theorized that the symptoms of psychopathy derived from a deep-rooted emotional deficit, and his 16 diagnostic criteria for the disorder centered around affective and interpersonal deviations. In Cleckley's view, the behavioral characteristics of psychopathy (e.g., irre-sponsibility, antisocial acting-out, failure to plan) were symptomatic of this underlying deficit. The Psychopathy Checklist (PCL) was developed by Hare (1980) to identify incarcerated criminal offenders who fit Cleckley's profile. The current, revised version (PCL-R; Hare, 1991) consists of 20 items. Fac-tor analytic investigations of the PCL (Harpur, Hakstian, & Hare, 1988; Harpur, Hare, & Hakstian, 1989) have identified two correlated dimensions underlying the scale – emotional detachment and antisocial behavior (Patrick, Bradley, & Lang, 1993) – that show markedly divergent relationships with other measures of personality and behavior.

Ratings on the emotional detachment factor, which is marked by items reflecting the central affective and interpersonal features emphasized by Cleckley, are correlated negatively with self-reported anxiety and positively with measures of social dominance, narcissism, and Machiavellianism (Harpur et al., 1989; Hare, 1991). Ratings on the antisocial behavior factor, which is defined by items describing a chronically deviant lifestyle, are posi-

---

[4] In contrast to fear-potentiated startle, the mechanisms underlying startle reflex inhibition during pleasant foreground stimulation are not well understood. Furthermore, this phe-nomenon may be less general than fear-potentiated startle. Specifically, it appears that pleasant activation may result in diminished startle reactivity primarily when the affect-evoking stimulus occurs in a perceptual context (e.g., picture viewing). This could indicate that attention plays a mediating role in this phenomenon (Lang, Bradley, & Cuthbert, 1997).

tively correlated with impulsivity, sensation seeking, and number of criminal charges (Harpur et al., 1989; Hare, 1991). Drug and alcohol abuse are also significantly associated with the antisocial behavior factor, but not the emotional detachment factor (Smith & Newman, 1990).

3.2. Psychopathy and Emotional Reactivity

Cleckley (1976) believed that the true ("primary") psychopath is incapable of deeply felt emotions, either positive or negative. Other theorists (e.g., Lykken, 1957, 1995) have argued that psychopathy reflects primarily a deficit in fear reactivity, with no impairment in capacity for pleasure. Most of the empirical studies on emotional reactivity in psychopaths have evaluated this low-fear hypothesis, and it has received substantial support. The best established results are that psychopathic individuals show diminished skin conductance activation in response to an anticipatory warning cue or a conditioned stimulus signaling noxious stimulation (e.g., shock or loud noise), and impaired passive avoidance learning (Lykken, 1957, 1995; Hare, 1978, 1986; Siddle & Trasler, 1981).

The evidence for diminished electrodermal reactivity to threat cues in psychopaths, however, is open to varying interpretation. Skin conductance is a nonspecific index of sympathetic arousal (Venables & Christie, 1973) that is subject to cortical influences (Tranel & Damasio, 1994) and that reflects negative affect only indirectly. Therefore, an alternative to the low-fear interpretation of this diminished electrodermal activity is the notion that it reflects a deficit in the vigilance and higher associative processing normally evident during anticipation of an emotionally potent event (Miller, Curtin, & Patrick, in press).

The finding of poor passive avoidance learning in psychopaths is also surrounded by interpretive ambiguities. The passive avoidance learning task is inherently a conflict paradigm, in that the participant must learn to inhibit a previously rewarded response in the presence of cues for punishment. Thus, a deficit in passive avoidance learning could reflect either an enhanced sensitivity to reward cues or a reduced sensitivity to punishment cues (Newman, Widom, & Nathan, 1985; Newman & Kosson, 1986; Patterson & Newman, 1993).

There are also indications that these effects may not be confined to individuals possessing the classic personality features of psychopathy. Raine (1993) reviewed the literature on aversive electrodermal conditioning in various criminal offender groups (including noninstitutionalized delinquents and unselected adult criminals as well incarcerated psychopaths) and concluded that "poor conditioning is related to the general development of antisocial behavior" (p. 220). Similarly, passive avoidance learning deficits have been observed in delinquents scoring high on questionnaire measures of antisociality (e.g., Minnesota Multiphasic Personality Inventory (MMPI) Psychopathic deviate (Pd) scale; Newman et al., 1985) and in adult offenders classified as "secondary sociopaths" (Lykken, 1957). These findings suggest some complexities in the relationships of these experimental paradigms to fear reactivity and to psychopathy.

3.3. Startle Modification during Affective Picture Processing

Recent research employing the startle probe reflex as an index of emotional reactivity has helped to clarify the relationship between psychopathy and fear. In an initial study by Patrick et al. (1993), eyeblink startle reactions to unwarned noise probes were recorded while criminal offenders, grouped using Hare's (1991) PCL-R, viewed pleasant, neutral, and unpleasant slides. The sample consisted of equal numbers of psychopathic (PCL-R $\geq$ 30), nonpsychopathic (PCL-R $\leq$ 20), and "mixed" (i.e., moderately psychopathic) adult male sex offenders ($n = 54$).

The slides were 27 color pictures (nine of each valence) selected from the International Affective Picture System (IAPS; Lang, Öhman, & Vaitl, 1988; see Chapter 8). Slides were presented for 6 s each, with variable (10–20 s) intertrial intervals. Acoustic probes were 50-msec, 95-dB(A) bursts of white noise, delivered binaurally through headphones at lead intervals of either 3.5, 4.5, or 5.5 s following slide onset. Blink responses to the startle probes were measured as electromyographic activity from the orbicularis muscle beneath the left eye (see Chapter 2).

The groups did not differ in overall startle response magnitude. To correct for disproportionately large responders, analyses of startle modulation effects were performed on scores standardized across trials within subjects. Statistical tests revealed that nonpsychopathic and mixed offenders both displayed a normal, *linear* pattern of startle modification, with blink responses larger during unpleasant slides and smaller during pleasant slides, relative to neutral. In contrast, psychopaths showed an abnormal *quadratic* startle pattern, with blink responses diminished during both pleasant and unpleasant slides relative to neutral.

In light of the animal and human evidence indicating that startle reflex potentiation during aversive cuing reflects defensive response priming (Lang et al., 1990) mediated subcortically (Davis, 1989), these data provided strong support for the hypothesis that psychopaths are deficient in fear reactivity.

Furthermore, Patrick et al. (1993) found that this deficit was related specifically to the emotional detachment component of the PCL-R: When individuals with high antisocial behavior ratings (i.e., at least two-thirds of the possible maximum) were subdivided into those low and high in emotional detachment, only the latter ("detached antisocial") group showed an abnormal pattern of startle modification. Individuals with elevated scores on the behavioral factor of psychopathy only ("simple antisocials" – most of whom, like the detached antisocials, met diagnostic criteria for antisocial personality disorder; Patrick, Cuthbert, & Lang, 1994) showed normal startle potentiation during aversive slide viewing (see Fig. 10.1).

Regarding positive (appetitive) emotional reactivity, psychopaths in this study did not differ from nonpsychopaths or mixed participants in their responses to pleasant slides: All groups exhibited normal startle reflex inhibition during pleasant as compared with neutral slide viewing. Overall, the findings of this experiment are consistent with the hypothesis that "primary" psychopathy is characterized by weak defensive responsivity, but at least normal reactivity to appetitive stimuli (cf. Fowles, 1980; Lykken, 1995).

3.4. Potentiated Startle during Noxious Stimulus Anticipation

A follow-up investigation (see Patrick, 1994) replicated and extended these findings by using a new experimental paradigm and diagnostic groups selected a priori on the basis of PCL-R factor ratings. Participants were 58 male inmates residents of a federal correctional institution selected from a larger sample evaluated for DSM-III-R antisocial personality symptoms and assessed for psychopathy using the PCL-R. Four groups were formed: (1) *nonpsychopaths,* rated low on both psychopathy factors ($n = 18$); (2) *detached* offenders, with high ratings on emotional detachment but low antisocial behavior ratings ($n = 14$); (3) *antisocial* offenders, with high antisocial behavior ratings only ($n = 8$); and (4) *psychopaths,* with high ratings on both factors ($n = 18$). The startle responses of these four study groups were assessed in an aversive anticipation procedure.

The experiment comprised two phases. In the first (baseline), participants viewed a monitor on which a simple cue (i.e., a string of asterisks) was presented intermittently for 6 s at a time. At varying times, a white-noise probe (50 ms, 95 dB) was introduced to elicit a startle-blink reaction, measured from the left orbicularis. The startle probe occurred during three of the six cue presentations (at lead intervals of either 3, 4, or 5 s), and during three of the intertrial intervals. In the second (anticipation) phase, the procedure was identical, except that a loud noxious noise blast (110 dB(A)) was delivered fol-

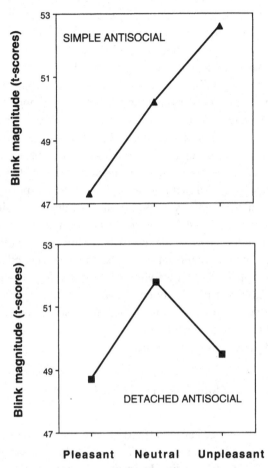

Figure 10.1. Mean startle reflex magnitude during pleasant, neutral, and unpleasant slide viewing in criminal offenders with high ratings on the PCL-R antisocial behavior factor only ("simple antisocial"; $n = 18$), and in offenders with high ratings on both the emotional detachment and antisocial behavior factors of the PCL-R ("detached antisocial"; $n = 17$). Startle magnitude is expressed in t-score units, computed by standardizing raw blink magnitude scores within participants.

lowing the offset of the visual cue; startle probes were presented during nine of 14 warning cue intervals (at 3, 4, or 5 s lead intervals), and during six of the intertrial intervals.

No group differences in overall startle reactivity were found, and in the baseline phase, startle blink magnitude during cue intervals did not differ from startle magnitude during intertrial intervals in any of the groups. As in non-prisoner controls (Patrick & Berthot, 1995), startle reactions to cue probes generally exceeded reactions to intertrial probes during the anticipation phase, when the cue signaled a forthcoming noxious event. However, the psychopathic and the detached groups both showed reduced startle potentiation during noise anticipation relative to the nonpsychopathic and antisocial groups. Furthermore, this group difference was evident within the initial trials of anticipation (see Fig. 10.2), indicating that the effect was not simply due to differential habituation to the threat of noise. (As the figure indicates, startle potentiation was greater for antisocial individuals than for nonpsychopaths, but with the small n in the former group this difference was not significant.)

These results further indicate that psychopathy is associated with a deficiency in fear reactivity and that this fear deficit is linked specifically to the classic affective/interpersonal symptoms of the disorder. Interestingly, and in contrast with Patrick et al. (1993), psychopaths in the noise anticipation study did not show an inhibition of startle reactivity during aversive (warning cue) periods relative to neutral (intertrial) intervals. It may be that reflex inhibition occurred in psychopaths during viewing of aversive slides because the foreground in this case was inherently engaging (i.e., unpleasant slides, along with pleasant slides, were rated as much more interesting than neutral slides) and attentional inhibition of startle (see Chapter 4) superceded the normal, defense-related potentiation of the reflex.

3.5. Psychopathy and Simple Antisociality: Features and Mechanisms

Relevant to the foregoing, Patrick (1995) reported correlations between the two PCL-R factors and temperament-related personality traits assessed by the Emotionality–Activity–Sociability–Impulsivity inventory (Buss & Plomin, 1975, 1984) and the Multidimensional Personality Questionnaire (Tellegen, 1982). The two psychopathy factors showed contrasting relationships with self-reported traits: Emotional detachment was positively linked to social dominance and negatively related to anxiety-related scales (Distress, Fear, Stress Reaction), whereas antisocial behavior scores were correlated positively with the latter. Antisociality scores were also correlated positively with scales measuring anger and aggressiveness, and negatively with indices of impulsivity and constraint. Overall PCL-R scores were positively related to social dominance and aggressiveness, and negatively related to inhibition and affiliativeness. Results consistent with these have been reported recently in clinic-referred children rated using a juvenile version of the PCL (Frick, in press).

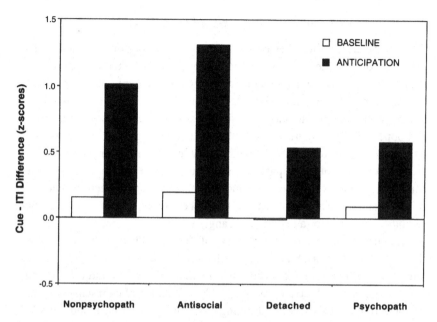

Figure 10.2. Mean blink magnitude difference scores (visual cue minus intertrial interval) during baseline and during block 1 of noise anticipation for four prisoner groups, defined according to scores on the two factors of Hare's (1991) Psychopathy Checklist – Revised. Startle magnitude is expressed in z-score units, computed by standardizing raw blink magnitude scores within participants. (From C. J. Patrick (1994), Emotion and psychopathy: Startling new insights, *Psychophysiology, 31,* 328; copyright 1994 by the Society for Psychophysiological Research. Reprinted with the permission of Cambridge University Press.)

These findings suggest that the emotional detachment and behavioral disinhibition components of psychopathy should be viewed as potentially coexisting, but empirically and conceptually separable entities. The data further suggest that while a primary fear deficit may underlie the former, it does not account for the latter. Our hypothesis is that some forms of chronic, impulsive antisociality reflect a deficit in higher information-processing systems that interact with primary motive systems, but which are anatomically and functionally distinct (LeDoux, 1995). In the next section, we review evidence indicating that the effects of acute alcohol intoxication on fear reactivity are also indirect, most probably operating via a disruption of higher processing systems, and we suggest that the alcohol challenge paradigm may provide a useful model for further investigation of mechanisms underlying chronic antisociality.

4. Alcohol and Emotion: A Startle-Probe Analysis

As with the disinhibitory behavioral features of psychopathy, alcohol-related disinhibition has often been attributed to suppression of affective reactivity at the level of primary brain motivational centers. For example, Pihl and his colleagues (Pihl & Peterson, 1993; Pihl, Peterson, & Lau, 1993) have argued that a major contributor to alcohol-related aggression (for a review, see Bushman & Cooper, 1990) is "fearlessness." More specifically, the anxiolytic effect of alcohol is thought to diminish the inhibitory influence of fear on the expression of behavior linked to past receipt of punishment or exposure to threat. Similar hypotheses have been advanced to account for connections between drinking and other behaviors, such as sexual expression, thought to be under inhibitory control (for a review, see Lang, 1985).

Of course, a direct suppressant effect of alcohol on fear is only one potential explanation of drinking-related behavioral disinhibition. Other theories have focused on alcohol-induced impairment of attentional and other cognitive processes (e.g., Steele & Josephs, 1990), alteration of pain sensitivity and motor activity occasioned by drinking (e.g. Pihl et al., 1993), and complex social learning variables that might influence drunken comportment (e.g., Lang, 1993; McAndrew & Edgerton, 1969). Furthermore, different mediators or combinations of mediators could be important for different types of behavior. This complexity is compounded by consideration of dose-related factors, individual response differences, and other contextual variables.

Nonetheless, "tension reduction" and "stress-response dampening" have been dominant themes in the alcohol literature for decades (see Conger, 1956, for the seminal theoretical statement). In view of this, one would expect the theoretical and empirical underpinnings of this perspective to be well developed. However, of the many analytic reviews of the relevant literature that have been undertaken (e.g., Cappell & Greeley, 1987; Sher, 1987), none has concluded that there is much support for the assertion that alcohol consistently reduces tension, anxiety, or fear, except perhaps in conflict situations.

Considering the lack of compelling evidence of a simple, direct tension- or stress-reducing effect of alcohol, an understanding of relationships between alcohol and emotion might benefit from an application of new conceptual and methodological approaches. We offer a summary of one such alternative here (see Stritzke, Lang, & Patrick, 1996, for a detailed presentation). Specifically, we describe the results of three recent studies that examined drug effects on human emotion using the startle modification paradigm. These data, combined with the broad literature on cognitive impairment and other effects associated with intoxication, may offer clues as to how affect mediates between drinking and disinhibited behavior in humans.

4.1. Intoxication and Emotion: Three Experiments

Most prior research on alcohol and emotion has focused exclusively on *negative* affect, typically operationalized in terms of autonomic arousal and/or self-report (for reviews, see Cappell & Greeley, 1987; Sher, 1987; Wilson, 1988; Pohorecky, 1991). In the first and, so far, only experiment (Stritzke, Patrick, & Lang, 1995) to manipulate positive as well as negative affect in a design based explicitly on a dimensional (valence/arousal) model of emotion (see Chapter 8), participants received either a moderate dose of alcohol (mean peak blood alcohol level = 0.071) or no alcohol prior to viewing pleasant, neutral, and unpleasant IAPS slides, with emotionally laden slides matched for arousal. Eyeblink reactions to acoustic startle probes (50-msec, 100-dB bursts of white noise), presented at lead intervals of 3, 4, or 5 s after slide onset, were used to index the valence of the evoked response disposition (cf. Vrana et al., 1988). Changes in emotional valence were also assessed via facial electromyographic (EMG) recording of corrugator ("frown") activity, while skin conductance responses to the slides were included as an index of physiological arousal. Heart rate responses during slide viewing were also recorded.

Results indicated that alcohol diminished the *overall* magnitude of startle probe reactions, and also phasic skin conductance responses, regardless of the valence of the foreground slides. However, the normal *emotional modification* of startle remained intact in the alcohol condition: Although mean startle magnitude during slide viewing was lower in the alcohol group, intoxicated participants (like controls) showed comparatively greater reactions for aversive slides and smaller reactions for pleasant slides, both relative to neutral. A similar linear valence effect for corrugator EMG reactions was also found in both groups. These results were contrary to the prediction, derived from tension reduction or stress-response dampening perspectives, that alcohol would selectively block reactions to aversive slides. Instead, the results suggested that "response dampening" by alcohol may be a more general phenomenon.

For the heart rate measure, initial deceleration following slide onset (i.e., orienting response; cf. Graham & Clifton, 1966) was somewhat greater in intoxicated individuals, although the fact that it was marked in all participants suggests that both beverage groups were attentive to the stimuli. However, analysis of the complete waveforms revealed a dramatic failure of intoxicated participants to show the normal secondary acceleration of heart rate later in the slide presentation. This could reflect alcohol's well-documented interference with higher cognitive processing, particularly elaborative encoding of visual and verbal information (Lister, Eckardt, & Weingartner, 1987).

In a follow-up experiment, Curtin, Lang, Patrick, and Stritzke (1997) presented sober or moderately intoxicated (*M* peak blood-alcohol level = 0.075)

individuals with a series of two-minute light cues denoting either the possibility that an electric shock could be delivered at any moment (red light =
"threat"), or that no shock would be administered (green light = "safe"; cf.
Grillon, Ameli, Woods, Merikangas, & Davis, 1991). During half of the cue
intervals of each type, pleasant photographic slides were presented periodically as distracters. Acoustic startle probes comparable to those used by
Stritzke et al. (1995) were delivered at varying unpredictable points during
the threat and safe intervals, some of them during slide distracters (at 3-, 4-,
or 5-s lead intervals). Autonomic activity (skin conductance, heart rate), corrugator EMG, and probe-elicited blink reactions were monitored throughout
the experiment.

Results showed that threat provoked expected increases in arousal, self-
reported distress, facial frowning, and startle magnitude. Yet despite evidence
of a general suppressant effect of alcohol on overall blink magnitude,[5] there
was no Threat/Safe X Beverage Condition interaction to suggest a selective
attenuating effect of alcohol on fear-potentiated startle. However, startle
reflex potentiation was blocked by alcohol in the condition involving inter-
position of a pleasant distracter with the threat cue (see Fig. 10.3). This, of
course, is the condition that placed the greatest cognitive demands on participants, particularly in terms of simultaneous allocation of attention or processing of competing stimuli. Such results, obtained using a more direct and
potent manipulation of threat, are consistent with those of Stritzke et al.
(1995) in suggesting that alcohol's anxiolytic effects may be limited to complex stimulus processing contexts.

A third study in this series (Patrick et al., 1996) serves to allay concern that
typical human startle paradigms might not be sensitive to fear-reducing
effects of common psychoactive substances. It also offers an opportunity for
comparison of the effects and possible mechanisms of a drug specifically pre-
scribed as an anxiolytic with those of alcohol. The methodology of this experiment paralleled that used by Stritzke et al. (1995), with two main exceptions:
(1) participants received a placebo or one of two doses (10 or 15 mg) of
diazepam, rather than alcohol, and (2) physiological responses, including
startle, were evaluated during presentation of slides that were either aversive
or neutral. No pleasant (appetitive) slide condition was included, and there-

---

[5] The general suppressant effect of alcohol on startle reactivity is a stable finding that has been
reported in animal studies as well (e.g., Pohorecky, Cagan, Brick, & Jaffe, 1976). The mechanisms of this effect at this point in time are unclear. One possibility is that this phenomenon is a by-product of alcohol's suppressant influence on sensory sensitivity or motoric activation. However, this effect could also reflect, at least in part, an arousal-dampening impact
of alcohol on central systems including the pontine reticular formation.

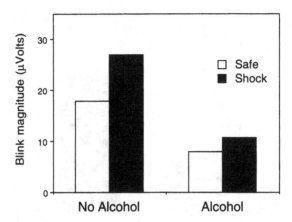

Figure 10.3. Mean startle response magnitude for intoxicated and nonintoxicated college students during "safe" and shock threat intervals under conditions of distraction (i.e., concurrent viewing of pleasant arousing slides). Shock intervals were designated by a red light indicating that an electric shock could be delivered at any moment; safe periods were designated by a green light indicating that no shock would be administered.

fore comparisons to Stritzke et al. (1995) are limited to effects on fear-potentiated startle.

Nonetheless, the results were quite striking. The main effect of drug condition was not significant, indicating that diazepam did not dampen *general* startle reactivity. However, the predicted dose-related reduction of *fear-potentiated* startle was observed. In other words, diazepam selectively reduced potentiated startle in the context of aversive slides, without dampening overall startle reactivity. This contrasts markedly with effects observed for alcohol in the Stritzke et al. (1995) study, wherein overall startle reactivity was diminished while robust fear potentiation was maintained (see Fig. 10.4). This suggests that a distinctly different mechanism probably underlies whatever anxiety-reducing or stress response-dampening effects alcohol may have. In particular, there is reason to believe that, unlike diazepam, alcohol does not act directly and selectively on the fear system.

4.2. Possible Mechanisms of Alcohol's Effects on Emotion and Their Relation to Disinhibition

If alcohol does not, at least at the doses tested, directly dampen fear, but does reduce overall arousal and reactivity, the question of how intoxication is related to emotion and disinhibition becomes more complex. Alternatives to

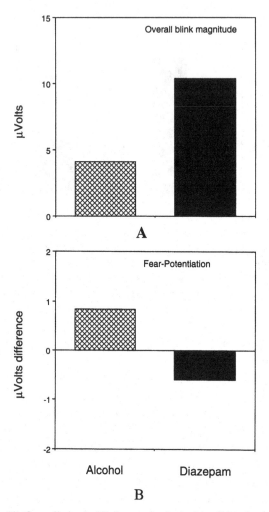

Figure 10.4. (*A*) Overall startle blink magnitude during slide viewing for .75 ml/kg alcohol-intoxicated college students and 15 mg diazepam-influenced participants (*n* = 18 per group). Each bar represents the average magnitude of scores across all slide viewing trials. (*B*) Startle blink potentiation for these same alcohol and drug groups. Each bar represents the mean startle magnitude for unpleasant slides minus the mean magnitude for neutral slides. Results are for 100-dB noise probe trials.

simple tension reduction theories have existed for some time (e.g., Pernanen, 1976; Hull, 1981), and in recent years more refined theories have emerged in the form of attention-allocation (Steele & Josephs, 1988, 1990) and appraisal-disruption models (Sayette, 1993; see Stritzke, Lang, & Patrick, 1996, for a detailed discussion of these perspectives). A common element in these proposals – and in the model of alcohol and aggression proposed by Pihl et al., 1993) – is the idea that alcohol's impact on affective responding is often "cognitively" mediated.

Certain aspects of information processing can be compromised even by relatively low doses of alcohol, whereas others are relatively unaffected. Peterson, Rothfleisch, Zelazo, and Pihl (1990) found that alcohol was detrimental to a number of higher-order functions involved in planning and transforming short-term information into long-term memory, whereas simple perception, recognition, and even reaction time were left largely intact. Others (e.g., Lamb & Robertson, 1987) have found that alcohol does not seem to affect overall attentional capacity, but it interferes with the ability to allocate attention to optimize performance.

These selected results correspond well to conclusions drawn from an extensive review of the recent literature on alcohol and human performance. Holloway (1994) concluded that impairment is greatest for "controlled" tasks involving selective or divided attention and/or a high level of complexity, whereas performance on "automatic" tasks is relatively less affected. It is interesting to juxtapose this conclusion with the observation by Cappell and Greeley (1987) that to the extent that alcohol reduces tension, it is primarily in conflict situations where the organism is faced with competing (appetitive and aversive) response contingencies.

This perspective implies that what alcohol does, perhaps related to its nonspecific arousal-reducing effects, is to differentially impair higher-order cognitive functions. In particular, the ability to allocate attention may be compromised, along with associative memory processes involved in processing complex situations, anticipating consequences, and selecting appropriate responses. Intoxication may impair the ability to make normal associations between cognitive and motivational elements of a stimulus situation, leaving the inebriate more inclined to attend to salient aspects of the immediate stimulus environment and to react accordingly. This conceptualization maps onto LeDoux's (1995) "top down" model of cognitive-emotional processing and suggests that the affective consequences of drinking may represent the byproduct of alcohol's impact on higher associational processes.

Two experiments by Zeichner and Pihl (1979, 1980) illustrate these points within the domain of disinhibition of aggression by alcohol. In the first of these, sober individuals were responsive to subtle feedback establishing a contingency between the intensity of shocks delivered and those received from a bogus competitor. However, intoxicated participants seemed oblivious to the contingencies, choosing instead to continue giving high-intensity shocks despite the adverse consequences for themselves. Parallel results were obtained in the second study: Unlike sober individuals, those given alcohol did not vary their shock selections when told that their opponent had no control versus complete control in choosing shock intensities to administer.

These outcomes underscore the deficiencies in reflection and planning associated with intoxication, and the corresponding insensitivity to potentially threatening or punishing consequences. Those under the influence of alcohol seemed inclined to put themselves in harm's way in the service of their apparent desire to react to the immediate situation and execute the most dominant and immediately gratifying response. Such action, of course, is not unlike that seen in individuals with trait antisociality and may reflect similar underlying processes.

5. Integration: Antisociality and Alcohol Intoxication

Our summary of recent research on affective modification of the startle reflex in psychopathic and normal intoxicated individuals was developed with three principal themes in mind. First, there may be different subtypes of chronically antisocial individuals in whom apparent deficits in normal fear-mediated inhibition of behavior can likely be attributed to different underlying causes. Second, alcohol intoxication may promote disinhibited behavior, not through direct dampening of subcortical fear centers, but through its impact on higher cognitive systems that normally interact with these centers to modulate behavior. Third, our understanding of both phenomena – antisociality and intoxication – stands to benefit from a more variegated conceptualization of emotional reactivity that considers affective processing at different neuropsychological levels.

5.1. Deconstructing Psychopathy

Cleckley (1976) hypothesized that the reckless, irresponsible behavior of psychopaths is a by-product of a core emotional deficit. Our research on affective modification of startle and temperament-related personality traits in criminal psychopaths (Patrick et al., 1993; Patrick, 1994) is consistent with this view. It indicates that there is a distinct subgroup of repetitive offenders, characterized by traits such as glib insouciance and callous exploitation of others (Cleckley, 1976), who are deficient in their reactivity to explicit fear cues. Furthermore, it appears that this affective deviation, in the absence of counteracting protective influences such as heightened intelligence or advantaged family circumstances, is associated with an enhanced risk of criminally deviant behavior (Patrick, Zempolich, & Levenston, 1997). However, this subtype accounts for only a portion of persistently antisocial individuals (Hare, Hart, & Harpur, 1991; Lykken, 1995).

One factor thought to account for persistent antisociality in the absence of a fearless temperament is defective socialization. Lykken (1995) postulated that the root cause of many "antisocial personalities" is inadequate parenting. Work by Wootton, Frick, Shelton, and Silverthorn (1997) supports this notion in that conduct disorder symptoms in children without psychopathic ("callous–unemotional") traits were found to be significantly related to ineffective parenting practices, whereas children exhibiting these traits to a high degree exhibited conduct problems *regardless* of the quality of parenting they received. In analyzing these and other relevant results, Frick (in press) concluded that fearless temperament and improper parenting probably constitute separate pathways to delinquency.

However, there is considerable evidence that other factors besides poor parenting can predispose one to antisocial deviance, even in the absence of a "psychopathic" temperament. Raine (1993) summarized data suggesting links between antisocial deviance and a variety of neuropsychological abnormalities. The prefrontal cortex and left temporal lobe were two brain regions highlighted in this review. Regarding the former, Raine concluded that "there is some evidence linking frontal dysfunction to antisocial and violent behavior in general, though the findings specifically for psychopathy are inconsistent. Frontal dysfunction may represent a general feature of antisocial behavior per se rather than being specific to a subtype of criminals such as psychopaths" (p. 113). This assertion is noteworthy because the prefrontal cortex projects to limbic structures, including the hippocampus and the amygdala, and is thought to play a role in abstraction, planning, emotional regulation, and behavioral inhibition (Fuster, 1989).

We argue for the probable existence of a significant subgroup of antisocial offenders who are analogous to intoxicated normal individuals, but distinct from "primary" psychopaths, in their proneness to antisocial acting-out. They exhibit deficiencies in higher information-processing systems that are essential to normal cognitive–emotional interactions, which in turn mediate behavioral inhibition in complex cuing contexts. Data relevant to this hypothesis were reported by Patrick et al. (1994). This study involved the same sample of criminal offenders who participated in the Patrick et al. (1993) study, classified into nonpsychopathic, simple antisocial, and detached-antisocial subgroups on the basis of PCL-R factor scores. Physiological responses (heart rate, skin conductance, and corrugator EMG activity) were recorded during a text-processing task in which subjects recalled and imagined descriptions of neutral and frightening situations when prompted by cue tones.

The principal finding of this study was that *both* antisocial groups showed diminished heart rate and skin conductance reactivity when processing fear material, although their performance of the task was normal in all other respects. The results of this study suggest an interesting dissociation between the reactions of simple antisocial offenders in a task involving processing of emotional language versus one involving presentation of explicit, pictorial representations. Only in the former instance, where emotional response was cued by semantic, linguistic processing, was there evidence of attenuated fear reactivity.

We believe that a more refined taxonomy of antisocial deviance is needed and should be based not merely on self-reported characteristics or traits inferred from overt behaviors but also on consideration of psychological processes subjected to assessment in a manner that permits inferences about underlying brain systems and pathways. Progress in our understanding of disinhibited antisocial behavior has been impeded by a lack of diagnostic specificity and a failure to appreciate critical differences in neural substrates and psychological processing involved in procedures such as simple conditioning, aversive anticipation, and passive avoidance learning. The available evidence argues for a more differentiated view of psychopathy, and of the methods used to assess emotional reactivity in antisocial and psychopathic individuals.

5.2. Alcohol Intoxication and Cognitive–Emotional Processing

Our research on ethanol and affect-related startle modification is quite relevant to the foregoing in that it suggests that alcohol intoxication can serve as a model of how disturbances in cognitive functioning can interfere with fear processing and behavioral inhibition in complex or conflictual cuing contexts. In two separate studies (Stritzke et al., 1995; Curtin et al., 1997), we found no evidence that alcohol diminished reactivity to simple, explicit aversive stimuli. However, in the latter study we found that alcohol blocked startle potentiation when a potent distracter was presented simultaneously with a threat cue. This result is consistent with an extensive literature indicating that alcohol interferes with higher cognitive operations including associative memory and attention, and that its effects on negative emotional reactivity may be secondary to these influences (Stritzke et al., 1996).

In animals it has been demonstrated that ethanol impairs spatial learning and memory (Matthews, Simson, & Best, 1995; Vandergriff, Matthews, Best, & Simson, 1995), functions that depend heavily on the hippocampus (Mayford, Bach, Huang, Wang, Hawkins, & Kandel, 1996). Even more pertinent to the present analysis, Melia, Corodimas, Ryabinin, Wilson, and LeDoux (1994) demonstrated a selective effect of ethanol on fear learning.

These investigators examined explicit cue conditioning and contextual conditioning in rats administered low and moderate doses of ethanol. The drug impaired learning of the association between the environmental context and noxious stimulation (shock), but did not affect conditioning to a tone cue that was paired explicitly with the shock. Although this study examined the effects of ethanol only on the acquisition of context-related fear, one would expect that if spatial memory and processing of contextual fear cues are related phenomena (Matthews, Best, White, Vandergriff, & Simson, 1996), ethanol might also interfere with the expression of contextual aversive learning.

These findings are in accord with the hypothesis that alcohol diminishes sensitivity to fear cues through interference with higher cognitive processing, rather than by direct dampening of subcortical defensive systems. The hippocampus may be one key site at which alcohol exerts such effects. Consistent with this, it appears that pathways from the hippocampus to the amygdala are critical for contextual, but not explicit, fear learning (LeDoux, 1995).

It is important to note, however, that this may be only one mechanism through which alcohol influences emotion and behavioral inhibition. Alcohol has well-documented effects on other cognitive processes, including attention (Lamb & Robertson, 1987; Zeichner, Allen, Petrie, Rasmussen, & Giancola, 1993; Holloway, 1994), that may reflect its impact on other neural systems besides the hippocampus. In addition, Davis and colleagues (Davis, Walker, & Lee, in press; Chapter 5) have recently presented evidence that the bed nucleus of the stria terminalis comprises the core of an anxiety system analogous to the amygdaloid fear system. A comprehensive theory of alcohol and emotion will undoubtedly need to incorporate these new findings. Furthermore, although our review has focused on the effects of ethanol on fear and negative affect, it is important to consider the possibility that alcohol might also promote disinhibition through its effects on the appetitive motivational system. For example, in their study of alcohol and fear, Curtin et al. (1997) used pleasant arousing pictures as distracters, raising the possibility that the stress-reducing effects of alcohol might be most evident in "conflict" situations where aversive stimuli are accompanied by competing appetitive cues.

5.3. Conclusion

The present analysis suggests that achieving greater specificity in the delineation of fear-processing deficits underlying disinhibited behavior in antisociality and intoxication will depend upon the deployment of task paradigms that provide valid indices of cognitive–emotional processing along different neural pathways. Through the combined efforts of cognitive, clinical, and neuroscientists, it should be possible to develop a taxonomy of cognitive–emotional processing pathways, indexed by different learning or performance tasks (e.g., explicit cue vs. contextual learning), which can illuminate deviations underlying pathological disinhibition. As a measure of affective responding explicitly tied to subcortical motive systems, startle reflex modification should prove to be an extremely valuable tool in this pursuit.

ACKNOWLEDGMENTS

Preparation of this chapter was supported by grants MH48657 and MH52384 from the National Institute of Mental Health.

CHAPTER ELEVEN

Schizophrenia Spectrum Disorders

KRISTIN S. CADENHEAD AND DAVID L. BRAFF

ABSTRACT

Disorders of the inhibitory control of attention have long been noted in schizophrenia spectrum patients. Operational, behavioral techniques were first applied to the construct of impaired sensory filtering in schizophrenia in the 1970s. Braff et al. (1978) noted Frances Graham's (1975) observation of short lead interval inhibition in normal subjects, and hypothesized, then demonstrated, that schizophrenia patients have diminished short lead interval inhibition reflecting impaired gating. Although originally thought to reflect an automatic, preattentive sensorimotor gating function, Dawson et al. (1993) demonstrated that short lead interval inhibition is modulated by attention and may represent a state-independent vulnerability marker for schizophrenia. The findings of impaired short lead interval inhibition in schizotypal subjects (Cadenhead et al., 1993), in conjunction with confirmation of a theoretical link between impaired short lead interval inhibition and thought disorder in schizophrenia patients (Perry & Braff, 1994), added further support to the notion that impaired short lead interval inhibition reflects a trait-linked deficit in sensorimotor gating in schizophrenia spectrum individuals. The neural basis of sensorimotor gating deficits in rats is now better understood, allowing the study of proposed brain abnormalities in schizophrenia patients in animal models. Future directions in application of short lead interval inhibition techniques to schizophrenia spectrum research will continue to include parallel animal model research in conjunction with studies of medication effects, gross and specific psychopathology, gender, laterality, family studies, and attentional manipulation in schizophrenia spectrum populations.

1. Overview of Attention, Information Processing, and Inhibition in Schizophrenia

Descriptions of impaired attention as a central feature of the pathology in schizophrenia spectrum disordered patients have been noted for most of the

Michael E. Dawson, Anne M. Schell, and Andreas H. Böhmelt, Eds. *Startle modification: Implications for neuroscience, cognitive science, and clinical science.* Copyright © 1999 Cambridge University Press. Printed in the United States of America. All rights reserved.

231

past century. Kraepelin (1921) described normal sensory registration but deficient active, sustained, or directed attention in dementia praecox patients. Bleuler (1911/1950) suggested that "acute attention is lacking" in schizophrenia patients. Beginning in the 1940s and 1950s, scholars (Cameron, 1944; Chapman, Freeman, & McGhie, 1959) began to advance the view that a cognitive disorder was primary and that other aspects of the schizophrenia patient's symptomatology were secondary to attentional and perceptual difficulties. The thought disorder of schizophrenia was postulated to result from a breakdown in the selective-inhibitory control of attention and the subsequent flooding of consciousness with incoming sensory data (Arieti, 1955; McKellar, 1957; Payne, Mattussek, & George, 1959; McGhie & Chapman, 1961; Maher, McKean & McLaughlin, 1966).

2. Sensory Gating in Schizophrenia

Operational, behavioral techniques were first applied to the construct of impaired sensory filtering in schizophrenia in the 1970s and early 1980s (Gottschalk, Haer, & Bates, 1972; Oltmanns & Neale, 1975; Nuechterlein & Dawson, 1984; Schneider, Dumais, & Shiffrin, 1984). Braff, Callaway, and Naylor (1977) used a self-stimulation P300 event-related potential (ERP) paradigm to assess the proposed time linkage of information-processing deficits in chronic and acute schizophrenia inpatients. In this study, subjects released a key and then received a stimulus after a variable delay. Since the subject "knew" that the stimulus was coming, the P300 amplitude was relatively diminished. Schizophrenia patients had relatively larger P300 magnitudes in the 250-msec delay condition, suggesting greater uncertainty that the stimulus was arriving. Braff and colleagues proposed that schizophrenia patients had difficulty with "very short term memory" and preattentive stimulus processing that could lead to information overload. Shagass (1977) observed that chronic schizophrenia patients had decreased somatosensory-evoked potential "recovery curves" at interstimulus intervals of 20 msec or less in a two-stimulus, "conditioning/testing" paradigm that yielded data he believed could be explained by an underactivation of cortical filtering. Freedman, Adler, Waldo, Pachtman, & Franks (1983) built on the work of Shagass and used the term "gating" to describe the normal inhibition of the second auditory stimulus-evoked P50 wave in a conditioning-testing paradigm. In many studies (Adler et al., 1982; Franks, Adler, Waldo, Alpert, & Freedman, 1983; Freedman et al., 1983; Judd, McAdams, Budnick, & Braff, 1992; Clementz, Geyer, & Braff, 1997), schizophrenia patients and their relatives have been shown to have increased P50 ERP magnitude to the second stimulus, suggesting a lack of the normal inhibition or sensory gating. Impaired P50 ERP gating has also been reported in clinically unaffected relatives of schizophrenia patients (Siegel, Waldo, Mizner, Adler, & Freedman, 1984). Lack of the normal inhibition of the P50 ERP in schizophrenia patients and their relatives suggests that impaired sensory gating may be a phenotypic marker for schizophrenia spectrum disorders.

3. Startle Inhibition as a Means of Measuring Sensorimotor Gating

Frances Graham (1975) demonstrated that a lead stimulus preceding a startle stimulus could inhibit or facilitate the eyeblink component of the human startle response depending on the temporal duration of the lead stimulus. In Graham's (1975) experiments, a continuous "prestimulus" 70-dB(A) tone was followed by a 104-dB(A) burst of white noise that was 50 msec in duration. Graham noted that while maximal magnitude inhibition occurred at lead intervals of 60–120 msec, maximal latency facilitation occurred at 30–60 msec, suggesting that two different processes are occurring (Graham, 1975). Graham's (1975) early observations have been noted in many species and across multiple sensory modalities (Hoffman & Ison, 1980; Ison & Hoffman, 1983; see Chapter 3). Graham (1975, 1992) proposed the protection-of-processing theory and suggested that the phenomenon of short lead interval inhibition may prevent disruptions during the initial stages of perceptual analysis. According to this view, low-intensity sensory stimulation evokes a "transient detecting reaction" that automatically triggers sensory gating mechanisms that allow complete perceptual analysis by preventing or attenuating startle reactions.

Graham's protection-of-processing theory has been supported by two lines of evidence. The first involves studies that examine the perceived intensity of the startle stimulus (Hoffman, Cohen, & Stitt, 1981; Perlstein, Fiorito, Simons, & Graham, 1993; see Chapter 3). In these studies, when the magnitude of the eyeblink response was reduced, so was the perception of the intensity of the startle-eliciting stimulus. The second line of evidence in support of the protection-of-processing hypothesis involved studies that examined the subjects' perception of the lead stimulus (Perlstein et al., 1993; Filion & Ciranni, 1994; Norris & Blumenthal, 1994). Filion and Ciranni (1994) and Perlstein et al. (1993) found that the lead stimulus was perceived as louder when it was paired with a startle-eliciting stimulus, a phenomenon called loudness assimilation. Correlational analyses in this study revealed that those participants with the greatest short lead interval inhibition had the most accurate perception of the lead stimuli (least loudness assimilation). Norris and Blumenthal (1994) noted that subjects more accurately identified one of three tone pitches used as lead stimuli on those trials that produced the most inhibition of the startle response.

4. Short Lead Interval Inhibition in Schizophrenia Patients

Braff et al. (1978) replicated Graham's findings of startle diminution with short lead interval effects in control subjects and hypothesized that schizophrenia patients would have decreased inhibition of the eyeblink magnitude at lead intervals between 30 and 120 msec, reflecting deficiencies in gating. In this study, 12 acute and chronic schizophrenia inpatients were compared with 20 control subjects on a startle paradigm that utilized a 1000-Hz, 71-dB(A) continuous tone as a lead stimulus and a 104-dB(A), 50-msec burst of white noise as the startle stimulus. As predicted, schizophrenia patients showed decreased short lead interval inhibition, as measured by potentiometer in the 60-msec lead interval condition. Schizophrenia patients also showed less shortening of the latency of the response compared with normal controls. These results were thought to represent a preattentive filtering dysfunction of schizophrenia patients, which could lead to information overload and cognitive disruption.

The original findings of impaired short lead interval inhibition in schizophrenia patients (Braff et al., 1978) have been supported by three other studies (Braff, Grillon, & Geyer, 1992; Grillon, Ameli, Charney, Krystal, & Braff, 1992; McDowd, Filion, Harris, & Braff, 1993) and not replicated by one (Bolino et al., 1994). Braff et al. (1992) confirmed and extended their original findings of impaired short lead interval inhibition in schizophrenia patients using a facial EMG/orbicularis occuli method of measuring the blink reflex of the human startle response. In this study, Braff et al. compared 39 medicated schizophrenia inpatients with 37 controls using both acoustic and tactile startle stimuli to assess short lead interval inhibition of the startle response. White noise of 70 dB(A) was used as background and stimuli included an 85-dB(A) discrete noise burst (20 msec in duration) as a lead stimulus that was followed 30, 60, or 120 msec later by a 116-dB(A) noise burst (40 msec) or 120 msec by a 30-psi air puff (40 msec) as a startle stimulus. By demonstrating impaired short lead interval inhibition in schizophrenia patients in both sensory modalities (see Fig. 11.1), Braff et al. suggested that the phenomenon is a more global and general dysfunction that is not limited to the acoustic pathways. Additionally, schizophrenia patients demonstrated normal startle latency facilitation at the 30-msec lead interval in this study, suggesting that schizophrenia patients detected the stimuli normally but failed to produce normal magnitude inhibition.

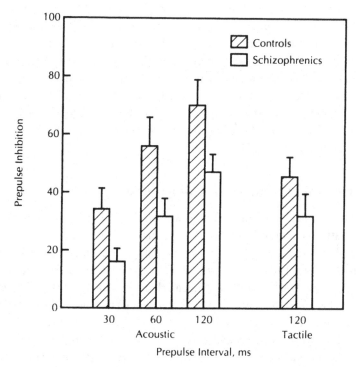

Figure 11.1. Lead stimulus (prepulse) inhibition presented as difference scores in the first acoustic and tactile blocks in 27 schizophrenic patients and 26 controls (Braff et al., 1992).

Grillon et al. (1992) utilized an acoustic startle paradigm that included four different lead stimulus intensities to determine whether the short lead interval inhibition reported by Braff et al. (1978, 1992) was due to schizophrenia patients' inability to detect weak lead stimuli or reflected a more general impairment of inhibitory functions. In their study, Grillon et al. compared 14 inpatients diagnosed with schizophrenia or schizoaffective disorder to 14 controls using a 106-dB(A) (40 msec) white-noise startle stimulus and a discrete (20 msec) white-noise burst as a lead stimulus. The lead interval was 120 msec and lead stimulus intensities were 75, 80, 85, and 90 dB(A) against a 70 dB(A) white-noise background. Schizophrenia patients demonstrated orderly short lead interval inhibition across all the lead stimulus intensities, indicating a response to the lead stimulus. When compared with controls, the schizophrenia patients had deficits in sensorimotor gating at all lead stimulus intensities, indicating that the impairment in short lead interval inhibition is a more general inhibitory impairment that is independent of the intensity of the lead stimulus. Grillon et al. used a 120-msec lead interval in their study and did not include a brief lead interval (i.e., 30 msec) that would have demonstrated a facilitation of startle latency if the subject was indeed detecting the lead stimulus. It could be argued that no independent measure of the subject's ability to detect the lead stimulus was used in this study, but if the lead stimulus acts automatically at a preattentive level of information processing, it is possible the subjects would not be consciously aware of the stimulus they are responding to physiologically.

5. Attentional Allocation and Schizophrenia

Impaired short lead interval inhibition was originally hypothesized to reflect an automatic, preattentive, sensorimotor gating function in normals (Graham, 1975) and a corresponding automatic processing deficiency in schizophrenia patients (Graham, 1975, 1979, 1980; Braff et al., 1978, 1992; Braff & Geyer, 1990; Dawson, Hazlett, Filion, Nuechterlein, & Schell, 1993). To better understand whether the sensorimotor gating deficits of schizophrenia patients were related to attentional factors, Dawson et al. (1993) utilized a short lead interval inhibition paradigm that was modulated by selective attention (see Chapter 7). In this study, 15 recent-onset, relatively asymptomatic schizophrenia patients were compared with 14 controls in a startle paradigm that included both "to-be-attended" and "to-be-ignored" continuous lead stimuli. In contrast to previous short lead interval inhibition studies in schizophrenia patients (Braff et al., 1978, 1992; Grillon et al., 1992), Dawson et al. used continuous 800- or 1200-Hz, 70-dB(A) tones as lead stimuli, then a 100-dB(A) startle stimulus (50 msec) against environmental background noise. Startle eyeblink magnitude was measured by EMG from the left eye consistent with the methods used by Grillon et al. (1992). In contrast, Braff et al. (1978, 1992) used right eye recording (see Section 9). Dawson et al. (1993) demonstrated that recent-onset, relatively asymptomatic schizophrenia patients have deficits in attentional modulation of short lead interval inhibition. Specifically, controls had enhanced short lead interval inhibition in the "to-be-attended" condition compared with the "to-be-ignored" condition, while schizophrenia patients did not show this effect. In the "to-be-ignored" condition, which was thought to reflect predominantly automatic attentional processes, the schizophrenia patients did not differ from controls, but there were significant differences between groups in the 120-msec lead interval "to-be-attended" condition. Dawson et al. suggested that asymptomatic schizophrenia patients are not abnormal in the automatic sensorimotor gating mechanism but do show abnormalities in the controlled attentional modulation of gating. It is unclear whether the "to-be-ignored" stimulus truly represents an automatic process given that stimulus discrimination was involved, but in this initial study, the response to this stimulus was not sensitive to the information-processing deficits of schizophrenia patients. In contrast, the lack of attentional modulation of short lead interval inhibition in asymptomatic schizophrenia patients suggests a trait-like impairment at the cortical level that is perhaps a state-independent vulnerability marker for schizophrenia.

Noting similarities between the performance of asymptomatic schizophrenia patients (Dawson et al., 1993) and normal older adults (Filion & McDowd, 1991) on the attentional modulation paradigm (Dawson et al., 1993), McDowd et al. (1993) performed a preliminary study in late-life schizophrenia patients and normal controls using an attentional version of Braff et al.'s (1992) paradigm that utilized 85-dB lead and 116-dB white-noise startle stimuli at lead intervals of 30, 60, and 120 msec to identify similarities and differences in inhibitory functioning between groups. McDowd et al. compared eight older early-onset schizophrenia patients to 10 normal controls first in a "noninstructed" phase, then in an "instructed" phase in which subjects were asked to press a key each time a lead stimulus was detected. In this paradigm, late-life schizophrenia patients had significantly diminished short lead interval inhibition when compared with elderly controls in the "instructed" condition and, like asymptomatic schizophrenia patients (Dawson et al., 1993), did not show the normal modulation of gating by the attention task. The pattern of results observed by McDowd et al. was thought to suggest that the inhibitory dysfunction of late-life schizophrenia patients may have both automatic and controlled components, and this area needs to be explored further.

6. Is Short Lead Interval Inhibition Trait-Related in Schizophrenia Spectrum Disorders?

6.1. Schizotypal Personality Disorder

The current thinking regarding the schizophrenia spectrum is that it is most likely a continuum of illnesses ranging from the more severe "Kraepelinean" schizophrenia to schizophrenia-related personality disorders and the relatively mild symptoms observed in family members of schizophrenia patients (Siever, 1991). Schizotypal personality disorder was empirically defined based on symptoms of individuals with a genetic relationship to schizophrenia (Spitzer, Endicott, & Gibbon, 1979) and may be a more common phenotypic expression of a schizophrenia-related diathesis than is schizophrenia itself (Kendler, Gruenberg, & Kinney, 1994). Because schizotypal personality disordered patients do not typically have the confounding effects of a chronic illness, long-term hospitalization, or chronic neuroleptic treatment, they are ideal for the study of the proposed trait-related gating deficits in schizophrenia spectrum individuals.

Cadenhead, Geyer, and Braff (1993) compared 16 nonhospitalized schizotypal personality disordered patients with 22 normal control subjects using the short lead interval inhibition task of Braff et al. (1992). Like schizophrenia patients, the schizotypal personality-disordered patients had deficits in acoustic short lead interval inhibition when compared with controls (see Fig. 11.2) but did not show deficits in the tactile component of the paradigm that had previously been noted in schizophrenia patients (Braff et al., 1992). One possible explanation for the lack of short lead interval inhibition deficits in the schizotypal personality-disordered patients may be that the tactile paradigm is less sensitive to the effect of more subtle psychopathology. The schizotypal personality-disordered patients had normal latency-to-peak startle response and demonstrated latency facilitation at 30 and 60 msec like the control subjects, implying normal detection of stimuli. The finding of impaired sensorimotor gating in a group of mostly unmedicated (14 of 16) schizotypal personality patients suggests that the observed short lead interval inhibition deficits in schizophrenia spectrum individuals are not secondary to antipsychotic medication or the effects of chronic illness and are likely trait- rather than state-related.

6.2. "Psychosis Prone" Subjects

Many investigators have screened general college populations to find individuals at risk for psychosis. Students who score high on psychochometric scales that were developed to measure psychotic-linked traits have been compared with those who score low on the scales in a variety of short lead interval inhibition studies (Simons & Giardina, 1992; Blumenthal & Creps, 1994; Schell, Dawson, Hazlett, & Filion, 1995; Cadenhead, Kumar, & Braff, 1996). Simons and Giardina (1992) used the Perceptual Aberration and Physical Anhedonia Scales (Chapman & Chapman, 1978) to select college students who scored high (greater than 2 standard deviations above the mean) on the scales as "psychosis prone" subjects to compare with controls, who scored low on the scales in a sensorimotor gating paradigm. Students who had high scores on the Perceptual Aberration Scale ($n = 18$) had impaired inhibition of startle magnitude when compared with controls ($n = 20$) and students with high scores on the Physical Anhedonia Scale ($n = 19$). The critical lead interval in this paradigm was 120 msec. A continuous, 70-dB, 1000-Hz tone was

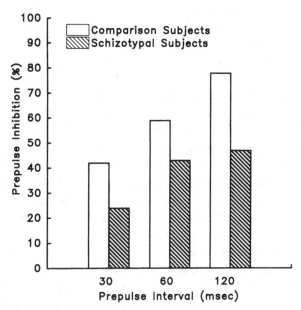

Figure 11.2. Percentage of lead stimulus (prepulse) inhibition in the first acoustic block in 12 patients with schizotypal personality disorder and 13 normal comparison subjects (Cadenhead et al., 1993).

the lead stimulus and a 50-msec, 102-dB burst of white noise was the startle stimulus (Simons & Giardina, 1992). These results were interesting because students who endorsed such symptoms as "sounds sometimes seem unusually loud" had impaired short lead interval inhibition, giving some face validity support to the concept of short lead interval inhibition being a measurement of sensorimotor gating (Simons & Giardina, 1992).

Schell et al. (1995) used similar selection methods to identify individuals who scored high on the Perceptual Aberration/Magical Ideation and Physical Anhedonia Scales and compared them with controls in an attentional modulation startle paradigm. Individuals who scored high on the scales did not demonstrate deficits in short lead interval inhibition in a nonattended condition, but, like schizophrenia patients (Dawson et al., 1993; McDowd et al., 1993), they failed to show normal attentional modulation of startle inhibition at 120 msec (Dawson et al., 1993; Schell et al., 1995). Individuals who scored high on the Perceptual Aberration/Magical Ideation Scale did show an effect of attention at the 240-msec lead stimulus interval, rather than at 120 msec, perhaps reflecting slower automatic or controlled processing (Schell et al., 1995).

Two other investigations (Blumenthal & Creps, 1994; Cadenhead, Perry, &

Braff, 1996) have attempted to replicate the findings of impaired short lead interval inhibition in individuals who score high on the Perceptual Aberration Scale (Simons & Giardina, 1992). Blumenthal and Creps (1994) used a startle paradigm with two different discrete lead stimuli (55 or 70 dB, 20 msec duration) and two startle stimuli (85 or 100 dB, 50 msec duration) to compare high scorers on the Perceptual Aberration/Magical Ideation and Physical Anhedonia Scales with controls. Cadenhead et al. (1996) used the same methods to select subjects and compared the groups in a short lead interval paradigm using a discrete lead stimulus (85 dB(A), 20 msec) and an acoustic (116 dB(A), 50 msec) or tactile (30 psi, 40 msec, air puff) startle stimulus. Neither of these studies was able to replicate the findings of Simons and Giardina (1992), consistent with the results of Schell et al. (1995), who did not find differences between groups in short lead interval inhibition to nonattended stimuli.

In many ways, the startle inhibition data of college students who score high on psychometric scales are difficult to interpret. Clinical evaluations (Chapman & Chapman, 1987; Cadenhead et al., 1996) and long-term follow-up (Chapman, Chapman, Kwapil, Eckblad, & Zinser, 1994) of individuals with inflated scale scores do not support the notion that these individuals as a group are prone to psychosis, meet criteria for schizotypal personality disorder, or belong in the schizophrenia spectrum. There do appear to be increased levels of psychopathology in some of the identified students with evidence of mild psychotic, affective, and anxiety symptoms (Chapman & Chapman, 1987; Lenzenweger, 1991; Cadenhead et al., 1996) as well as various personality disorder traits (Cadenhead et al., 1996). Chapman and Chapman (1987) state that methods need to be found to distinguish individuals who are prone to psychosis from those who are prone to affective disorder and never suggest the entire group of selected students are psychosis-prone or schizotypal. Sensorimotor gating deficits are not specific to individuals with schizophrenia spectrum illness but appear to be present in individuals who experience intrusive and irrelevant sensory, cognitive, or motor information (Swerdlow, Caine, Braff, & Geyer, 1992; Swerdlow, Benbow, Zisook, Geyer, & Braff, 1993). In this context, deficits in sensorimotor gating appear to be related to the experience of perceptual aberration, in some paradigms, whether it is part of a schizophrenia spectrum, affective, anxiety, personality, or neurological disorder.

7. Sensorimotor Gating and Thought Disorder

The original theories regarding sensorimotor gating deficits and schizophrenia suggested that because of a defective filtering mechanism, schizophrenia patients were bombarded by irrelevant stimuli, which resulted in cognitive fragmentation and thought disorder (Arieti, 1955; McKellar, 1957; Payne et al., 1959; McGhie & Chapman, 1961; Maher et al., 1966; Gottshalk et al., 1972; Braff et al., 1978; Braff et al., 1992). Impaired inhibition of internal stimuli could also lead to an increased awareness of preconscious material such as alternative meanings of words or interpretations of events (Frith, 1979). Auditory hallucinations might result from misinterpreted sounds and the intrusion of preconscious logogens (Frith, 1979; Morton, 1979). In the same way, efforts to interpret misperceived information could lead to delusional beliefs (Frith, 1979; Butler & Braff, 1991).

The theoretical link between impairment in short lead interval inhibition, sensorimotor gating, and thought disorder was better characterized by Perry and Braff (1994). These investigators used the Ego Impairment Index human experience variable, a performance measure of thought disorder derived from the Rorschach. Perry and Braff (1994) demonstrated significant correlations between poor responses (more thought disorder) and impaired short lead interval inhibition in 39 schizophrenia patients. The Ego Impairment Index provides an objective means of studying many components of thought disorder such as reality testing, reasoning, and quality of object relations, making it a sensitive measure of thought disorder in schizophrenia spectrum individuals (Perry, Viglione, & Braff, 1992; Cadenhead et al., 1996; Cadenhead, Perry, & Braff, 1996). Perry and Braff (1996) subsequently used a simultaneous startle and computerized Rorschach paradigm in 20 schizophrenia patients to extend their previous findings. In this study a strong relationship was again demonstrated between short lead interval inhibition and disturbed thought as measured by the Ego Impairment Index human experience variable. The association between thought disorder and short lead interval inhibition is also supported by the recent work of Docherty and Hebert (1996), who found a correlative relationship between the Communication Disturbances Index and impaired sensorimotor gating in 15 schizophrenia patients. The link between thought disorder and a behavioral measure of sensorimotor gating, with known neural circuitry (Swerdlow, Braff, Taaid, & Geyer, 1994; see Chapter 6), provides insight into the pathophysiology of disrupted cognitive processes and schizophrenia (Perry & Braff, 1994; see Chapter 13).

8. Animal Models of Sensorimotor Gating Deficits in the Schizophrenia Spectrum

Our understanding of the pathophysiology of schizophrenia spectrum disorders has been advanced with the use of animal models of specific schizophrenia-related deficits. The neural basis of sensorimotor gating deficits in rats is now thought to involve limbic system and basal ganglia interactions (Swerdlow et al., 1992; see Chapter 6). With increased understanding of the neural circuitry of short lead interval inhibition, models of proposed brain abnormalities in schizophrenia that modulate the circuit can be tested (Swerdlow et al., 1994). Lesions and neurotransmitter manipulations at various levels of the cortico–striato–pallido–pontine circuit can modulate inhibition of startle (Mansbach, Geyer, & Braff, 1988; Davis, Mansbach, Swerdlow, Braff, & Geyer, 1990; Geyer, Swerdlow, Mansbach, & Braff, 1990; Rigdon, 1990; Schwarzkopf, Mitra, & Bruno, 1992; Swerdlow et al., 1992; see Chapter 6). Specifically, increased dopamine activity and D_2 but not D_1 stimulation in the nucleus accumbens causes a decrease in sensorimotor gating that is reversed by antipsychotic medication (Swerdlow, Braff, Masten, & Geyer,1990). Adult rats with lesions of the medial prefrontal cortex and ventral hippocampus demonstrate reduced short lead interval inhibition when administered a mixed dopamine agonist (Swerdlow et al., 1995). Swerdlow et al.'s (1995) data support the hypothesis that cell damage of the frontal and temporal cortices, coupled with dopamine receptor activation, may lead to the observed sensorimotor gating deficits of schizophrenia patients. In support of neurodevelopmental theories of schizophrenic neuropathology, Lipska et al. (1995) found that post- but not prepubertal rats who had had neonatal excitotoxic damage to the ventral hippocampus had reduced short lead interval inhibition that was further exaggerated by a dopamine agonist.

9. Future Directions

In coming years, schizophrenia spectrum disordered subjects will be studied in both thematic and novel experimental designs. Thematic studies will incrementally pursue traditionally important areas of research utilizing measures of startle plasticity. These will include medication effects, gross and specific psychopathology (state variables), gender, laterality, family studies (trait variables), and attentional manipulation.

1. Studies of *medication effects* will examine startle plasticity measures as predictors of outcome. Do symptomatic individuals who show the normalization of startle inhibition during acute and/or chronic antipsychotic medication treatment also show differential clinical improvement? If so, what are the likely underlying neurobiological events that may be used to predict such a normalizing effect?

2. Do gross and/or specific *psychopathological factors* co-vary with startle inhibition deficits? In general, it appears that positive symptoms have significant

but low-order correlations with inhibitory deficits. When more sensitive measures of thought disorder are employed (e.g., Perry & Braff, 1994), this level of correlation increases significantly. It appears that more refined neuropsychological test probes and measures of thought disorder will need to be used in the future as functional correlates of startle inhibition deficits.

3. Since Swerdlow et al. (1993; Swerdlow, Hartson, & Auerbach, 1997) reported that normal men show higher levels of prepulse inhibition than do women, the *gender* variable needs to be more carefully examined in future studies of schizophrenia spectrum subjects. Since female subjects have lower levels of startle inhibition and since these levels fluctuate throughout the menstrual cycle, it appears that startle inhibition may be much more difficult to examine in female schizophrenia spectrum patients (Swerdlow, Hartman, & Auerbach, 1997).

4. The traditionally important issue of *laterality* has been one that has been largely overlooked in studies of schizophrenia spectrum populations. Right and left eye measures have been chosen based on poorly elucidated rationales. In the future, it will be important for this issue to receive greater scrutiny.

5. In an attempt to assess issues of *trait-related* vulnerability and as a prelude to molecular genetic approaches, family studies will undoubtedly be more prevalent in the coming years. Until now, gating studies in unaffected family members of schizophrenia patients have largely focused on P50 suppression rather than startle inhibition. These studies have identified trait-linked deficits in P50 suppression among family members of schizophrenia patients (Freedman et al., 1997). This molecular approach will undoubtedly be repeated using startle inhibition in addition to P50 suppression.

6. Studies of the *attentional* manipulation of startle inhibition have been reported (Dawson et al., 1993; McDowd et al., 1993; Schell et al., 1995). Since the techniques discussed above and in this book offer a means of assessing resource allocation in schizophrenia spectrum populations, increasingly sophisticated and inventive techniques will be utilized to assess how the allocation of attention to the prepulse increases the observed inhibition deficits.

In addition, a number of *novel approaches* are currently under way in research on startle inhibition in schizophrenia spectrum populations. These studies employ new combinations of techniques that utilize startle inhibition. For example, a traditional approach to understanding the neurobiological basis of cognitive and psychophysiological deficits in schizophrenia patients has been to correlate functional deficits with brain imaging-derived structural shifts observed in schizophrenia patients. This structural brain-imaging work still needs to be accomplished in conjunction with studies of startle inhibition. Experiments will also examine the differential neural activity in critical brain areas during startle testing. Functional magnetic resonance imaging studies offer enough flexibility to allow for the simultaneous measurement of startle inhibition and brain activity, allowing us to explore the neurobiology of startle inhibition. In advancing animal model studies, the use of dialysis probes (Humby, Wilkinson, Robbins, & Geyer, 1996), neurodevelopmental manipulations (Lipska et al., 1995), and genetic knock-out animals (Dulawa, Hen, Scearce, & Geyer, 1996) will increase our basic scientific knowledge of the neurobiology of startle inhibition.

When family studies of the heritability and transmission of startle inhibition have been completed, the molecular biological basis of startle inhibition can be further explored. Currently, Freedman and associates (1997) have reported linkage between P50 suppression and the alpha-7 region of the nicotinic receptor. Parallel studies of startle inhibition may allow us to understand the genetically identified regions associated with startle inhibition. It may then be possible to identify the specific genetic contributions to startle inhibition deficits in schizophrenia patients. These studies would be simpler to conduct than investigations of the genetic contributions to the entire syndrome of schizophrenia, and would offer reasonable paths to explore the molecular genetics of functional deficits in the schizophrenia spectrum.

Thus, both incremental step studies and novel approaches will expand our understanding of startle inhibition deficits in schizophrenia spectrum subjects.

ACKNOWLEDGMENTS

This work was supported by National Institute of Mental Health grants MH-01124 and MH-42228.

CHAPTER TWELVE

Startle Modification in Children and Developmental Effects

EDWARD M. ORNITZ

ABSTRACT

The development of lead stimulus modification of startle is characterized by increasing inhibitory and decreasing facilitatory modification during the childhood years. Inhibitory lead stimulus modification of startle is particularly weak during a stage of neurophysiological development that involves increased reactivity to stimuli at both cortical and subcortical levels. This neurophysiological stage, occurring during the preschool years, coincides with the Piagetian stage of preoperational behavior. Lead stimulus modification of startle matures during a period of cortical remodeling and other structural brain changes in association with other neurophysiological changes suggestive of the maturation of both cortical and subcortical inhibitory processes. This neurophysiological stage, occurring during the grade-school years, coincides with the Piagetian stage of concrete operations.

In contrast to lead stimulus modification of startle, mature rates of habituation of startle are already achieved during the preschool years. P300 responses to startling stimuli in school-age children show mature lead stimulus modification and habituation, as does the startle response itself. Attentional and affective modification of startle is different in children than in adults, but the direction of differences is inconsistent and requires further study. Autonomic, myogenic, and electroencephalography activity accompanying startle habituation in children do not habituate; heart rate increases as startle habituates, suggesting a state of arousal accompanying startle habituation. These relationships have not been studied in adults.

1. Development of Startle Modification by Lead Stimulation

1.1. Background from Adult Studies

The magnitude of the startle-blink reflex in the human adult can be modified by nonstartling lead stimulation in at least three ways (Graham, 1975;

Michael E. Dawson, Anne M. Schell, and Andreas H. Böhmelt, Eds. *Startle modification: Implications for neuroscience, cognitive science, and clinical science.* Copyright © 1999 Cambridge University Press. Printed in the United States of America. All rights reserved.

Anthony, 1985). First, inhibitory modification of the startle response to an intense sudden stimulus follows brief (e.g., 20 msec), low-intensity, nonstartling stimuli presented at short lead intervals (30–240 msec) prior to the startling stimulus (Graham, 1975; Graham & Murray, 1977). At these short lead intervals, the same amplitude inhibition may (Graham & Murray, 1977) or may not (Blumenthal & Levey, 1989) occur when the lead stimulus is sustained continuously throughout the warning interval depending on the lead stimulus intensity and other experimental parameters (see Chapter 3). Second, facilitation of startle magnitude follows longer (greater than 1400 msec) lead stimuli that are sustained continuously throughout the interval preceding the startling stimulus (Graham, 1975; Graham, Putnam, & Levitt, 1975). Facilitation following these long, continuous lead stimuli can occur in experimental designs in which the lead interval is constant or is variable in duration (Graham, 1975; Graham et al., 1975; Anthony, 1985; Chapter 4). In contrast, a brief (20 msec) stimulus presented 2000 msec prior to the startling stimulus induces startle facilitation only in the context of variable lead intervals and not when the lead interval is constant (Graham, 1975; Graham et al., 1975). Because of the uncertainty associated with the variable lead intervals, the facilitating effect had been attributed to a general attentional–activational mechanism. Subsequent research has shown that, in the adult human, a third type of startle modification involving nonstartling lead stimuli is due to selective attention, and the effect can be facilitatory or inhibitory depending on whether attention is directed toward or away from either the lead stimulus or the startling stimulus (Anthony, 1985; Chapter 4).

1.2. Development of Inhibitory and Facilitatory Modification of Startle under Variable Lead Interval Conditions

Prior to 8 years of age, mature patterns of lead stimulus modification of startle do not occur. In full-term newborns, the startle-blink response to a glabellar tap was not modified when preceded by a 90-dB tone at lead intervals of 75, 150, 300, and 600 msec or by a glabellar tap at 200 msec (Hoffman, Cohen, & English, 1985). Even when the lead stimulus (a glabellar tap) was of sufficient intensity itself to elicit a startle response, there was no startle response modification to the second tap at 300 msec (Hoffman, Cohen, & Anday, 1987). However, when lead intervals were increased to 600, 900, and 1200 msec, small (about 14–25 percent) but significant response inhibition was induced by these very strong lead stimuli (Hoffman et al., 1987; Anday, Cohen, Kelley, & Hoffman, 1989). Even at the longer lead intervals, startle-eliciting lead stimuli failed to inhibit the startle response to a second glabellar tap in preterm neonates (Hoffman et al., 1987; Anday et al., 1989). Using

84-dB lead stimuli and 109-dB startle stimuli, Graham, Strock and Zeigler (1981) found nonsignificant startle amplitude inhibition to be only 25 percent in 2- to 6-month-old infants at a lead interval of 200 msec. In 15-month-old infants, using similar stimuli and lead intervals of 125 and 225 msec, Balaban, Anthony, and Graham (1989) found nonsignificant startle amplitude facilitation and significant onset latency facilitation (shorter latencies on lead stimulus trials).

Studies of the maturation of lead stimulus-induced modification of startle comparing 3- to 8-year-old children and young adults have demonstrated significant effects of age on both startle magnitude and onset latency, (Ornitz, Guthrie, Kaplan, Lane, & Norman, 1986; Ornitz, Guthrie, Sadeghpour, & Sugiyama, 1991). In these studies, startle was evoked by 104-dB(SPL), 50-msec bursts of white noise, and the amplitude and onset latency of the blink reflex were measured after integration of the orbicularis oculi electromyogram (EMG). The children watched silent cartoons or movies while receiving the auditory stimuli in order to elicit their cooperation and minimize hand and eye movements. Lead intervals varied from 120 to 2000 msec and included intervals of 250 and 800 msec. Lead stimulation with 75-dB, 1000-Hz tones resulted in pronounced inhibition of both amplitude (75%) and latency in 18- to 20-year-old men when 20-msec tones preceded the startling stimuli by 120 or 250 msec. Following continuous lead stimulation for 2000 msec, these adults showed modest nonsignificant response facilitation. Eight-year-old boys showed mature inhibitory and facilitatory startle amplitude modification, but significantly less inhibition and more facilitation of onset latency compared with the men. Preschool boys showed significantly less amplitude and latency inhibition and more facilitation than the 8-year-olds and adults. In response to lead stimulation 120 msec before the startling stimuli, the preschool boys actually showed significant latency facilitation (Ornitz et al., 1986).

A similar study of the maturation of lead stimulation-induced modification of startle in 4- to 8-year-old girls and young women demonstrated significant effects of age on both startle amplitude and onset latency modification. Lead stimuli induced strong inhibition of both amplitude and latency of the startle-blink reflex in adult women when 25-msec tones preceded the startling stimuli by 120 or 250 msec. Following continuous lead stimulation for 2000 msec, the women showed weak nonsignificant response facilitation. Eight-year-old girls showed mature inhibitory startle amplitude modification, but significantly less inhibition of onset latency compared with adults. Preschool girls showed significantly less amplitude and latency inhibition and more facilitation than the 8-year-olds and adult women (Ornitz et al., 1991). These findings in female subjects were very similar to those obtained by Ornitz et al. (1986) in male subjects. Gender differences were limited to the 8-year-old age group. The 8-year-old girls showed significantly less startle amplitude inhibition than 8-year-old boys following the 120- and 250-msec lead stimulation intervals and less latency facilitation following 2000 msec of continuous lead stimulation.

In summary (Fig. 12.1), relatively little lead stimulus inhibition of startle at short lead intervals occurs prior to 8 years of age. Between early infancy and 5 years of age, startle amplitude inhibition does not exceed 30 percent and nonsignificant facilitation has been reported in 15-month- and 4-year-olds. Adult level response inhibition (50–75%) does not develop until 8 years of age (data are not available on 6- and 7-year-olds), at which time there are mild gender differences. In contrast, lead stimulus facilitation at long lead intervals is more prominent in preschool children than in 8-year-olds and adults. Modification of startle by lead stimulation is mediated by brain-stem neuronal networks (see Section 5.3.3 and Chapters 5 and 6 for the functional neuroanatomy). These findings suggest that brain-stem mechanisms that mediate startle response modification undergo development during early childhood and do not mature until about 8 years of age. A similar ontogenetic sequence of the development of lead stimulus inhibition of startle in the immature rat (Parisi & Ison, 1979) attests to the biological significance of inhibitory lead modification of startle and the development of brain-stem mechanisms that mediate it. The phylogenetic demonstration of lead stimulus inhibition of startle in the locust (Riede, 1993) further suggests an evolutionary significance that may encompass both the protection of sensory processing from disruptive motor responses and energy depletion from excessive startling in noisy environments.

1.3. Development of Facilitatory Modification of Startle under Constant Lead Interval Conditions

Startle responses to a 104-dB(SPL), 50-msec burst of white noise were facilitated by nonstartling tones sustained for 2000 msec prior to the startling stimulus in 3-, 4-, 5-, and 8-year-old boys and young men (Ornitz, Guthrie, Lane, & Sugiyama, 1990). Both startle amplitude and onset latency showed significantly greater facilitation in the preschool children than in the 8-year-olds and adults. The results of this experiment, which used a constant lead interval, were compared with those of Ornitz et al. (1986), in which the lead interval was varied. The maturational changes in startle facilitation in response to the 2000-msec lead interval were similar in both experiments. Hence the maturational effect on startle facilitation was independent of the uncertainty (as to when the startling stimulus would be given), which might be associated

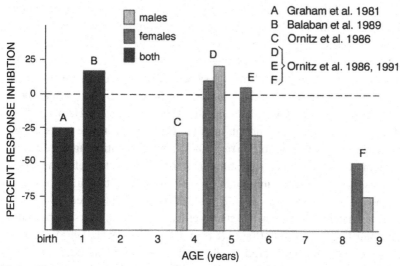

Figure 12.1. Maturation of inhibitory lead stimulus modification of startle amplitude. Inhibitory startle modification is weak or absent until 8 years of age. (A: Graham et al., 1981; B: Balaban et al., 1989; C: Ornitz et al., 1986; D–F: Ornitz et al., 1986, 1991.)

with variable lead intervals. These findings suggest that the neuronal mechanisms that mediate startle facilitation undergo development during early childhood and mature at about 8 years of age, and that this maturational sequence is relatively independent of attentional effects.

1.4. Developmental Changes in Startle Modification by Pairing of Equal Intensity Strong Electric Shocks to the Supraorbital Nerve in Neonates

Startle modification by lead stimuli, as described earlier in this section, is predicated on the assumption that the lead stimulus itself is weak and below the threshold for inducing startle. If the "lead stimulus" is of the same intensity as the startling stimulus, then the effect of the first of two "paired" startling stimuli on the second of the pair may involve refractory effects rather than lead stimuli effects even though the results may appear to be the same, usually inhibitory to the response to the second startle stimulus at relatively short interstimulus intervals. Such effects are often referred to as the recovery cycle. There have been a few studies in which startle-eliciting equal-intensity paired electric shocks to the supraorbital nerve (Hatanaka, Yasuhara, & Kobayashi, 1990) or glabellar taps (Hoffman et al., 1987; Anday et al., 1989) were used to elicit startle blinks in pre- and full-term neonates. The minimal startle modification induced in neonates when one startle-eliciting glabellar tap preceded another has been described in Section 1.2. In contrast, when one intense supraorbital nerve shock precedes another, marked startle modification occurs (Hatanaka et al., 1990) and follows the same U-shaped recovery function with respect to the interval between conditioning and test stimuli as had been reported earlier in adults with paired electric shocks (Kimura & Harada, 1976). In both studies, significant inhibition of the R2 response to the test stimulus was maximal (85–90% inhibition) at 100–250 msec conditioning-to-test stimulus intervals, suggesting a lead stimulus startle modification effect in which neonates showed a mature inhibitory response. However, the failure of the R2 response to the test stimulus to fully recover by 800–1000 msec (3000 msec for the neonates), as occurs when startle-eliciting electric shocks are preceded by nonstartling lead stimuli (Sanes & Ison, 1979; Rossi et al., 1995), suggests that the equal-intensity paired-shock stimulus experiments confound lead stimulation and recovery cycle (refractory effects) modification of startle.

2. Development of Startle Modification by Habituation

There have been two investigations of the development of startle modification by habituation. Ornitz, Russell, Yuan, and Liu (1996) described the habituation of the startle blink response in normal 7- to 11-year-old boys. In comparison with normal young adults, previously studied under identical experimental conditions (Ornitz & Guthrie, 1989), the major characteristic of the habituation, a significant linear decline in startle amplitude in response to 40 startle stimuli presented every 23–25 s, was similar, suggesting mature levels of startle modulation by habituation in this age group, as is the case for startle modulation by lead stimulation (Ornitz et al., 1986, 1990, 1991).

Ornitz, Russell, and Hirano (1997) have compared the habituation of startle in 56 normal 3- to 5-year-old and 61 normal 7- to 11-year-old boys. There was highly significant amplitude and latency habituation of startle. In contrast to the maturational effects described earlier for startle modification by lead stimuli, there were no age effects on either amplitude or latency habituation. Unlike lead stimulus modification of startle, maturation of startle habituation seems to be fully achieved during the preschool period of development.

Startle habituation may be mediated by mechanisms that are intrinsic and/or extrinsic to the stimulus-response pathway; intrinsic mechanisms are considered part of the reflex pathway itself, while extrinsic mechanisms tend to be components of modulatory systems (Davis & File, 1984). In the rat, lesion (Leaton, Cassella, & Borszcz, 1985), stimulation (Davis, Parisi, Gendelman, Tischler, & Kehne, 1982) and neuropharmacological studies (Kehne & Davis, 1984; Koch & Friauf, 1995) suggest that short-term (within session) habituation of startle is mediated by intrinsic mechanisms (see also Chapters 5 and 6). It can be postulated that the lack of any developmental effects on startle habituation reflects the very early maturation of intrinsic mechanisms within the stimulus–response pathway. In contrast, the robust developmental effects on lead stimulus modification of startle reflect early immaturity of mechanisms extrinsic to the stimulus–response pathway. Such extrinsic mechanisms have been demonstrated to reside in a lateral tegmental pathway in the brainstem (described in Section 5.3.3, below).

3. Developmental Aspects of Attentional Modification of Startle at Long Lead Intervals

Studies of the development of attentional modification of startle have been conducted under conditions of both passively and actively induced attention. Studies in the former group have been predicated on the assumption that a startle response will be enhanced when attention is passively directed to the startling stimulus by presenting it in the same sensory modality as an attention-eliciting background. Conversely, the startle response should be reduced when the startling stimulus is presented against the background of a contrasting sensory modality. The assumption is that a match between stimulus and background modality (e.g., a burst of noise presented during music) should enhance the startle response, while a mismatch (e.g., an intense light flash presented during the music) should reduce the startle response (Anthony & Graham, 1983, 1985; Balaban, Anthony, & Graham, 1985; Chapter 4). These studies have been limited to comparisons between 4-month-old infants and adults. When acoustic startle stimuli were presented after several seconds of acoustic stimulation, the startle response was enhanced; after several seconds of visual stimulation it was reduced, and reciprocal effects were induced with visual startle stimuli. Significant effects were limited to the 4-month-old infants (Anthony & Graham, 1983, 1985; Balaban et al., 1985) and did not occur in adults (Anthony & Graham, 1985; Balaban et al., 1985). The more interesting the background auditory or visual stimuli, the greater the enhancing effect of matching modalities and the greater the inhibiting effect of mismatched modalities in the infants (Anthony & Graham, 1983). An attentional effect, cardiac deceleration during the background visual or auditory stimulation, was documented for both the infants and the adults, but enhanced deceleration in response to "interesting" backgrounds (compared with "dull" backgrounds) occurred only in the infants (Anthony & Graham, 1985). Hence, it would seem that the startle response in 4-month-old infants reflects either a greater vulnerability to environmental influence than in adults or that the background stimulation used in these experiments simply did not engage the attention of adults to the same extent as the infants. Alternatively, the enhanced cardiac effects associated with the more "interesting" backgrounds in the infants suggest the possibility of an emotional effect underlying the attentional differences between the infants and adults (see Section 4.2). No comparable data exist for children older than 4 months of age.

There is one study of active attention in which the effects on startle in 5-year-old children are compared with adults (Anthony & Putnam, 1985). In this experiment, acoustic startling stimuli were presented during the 6-s warning interval of a reaction time task. Heart rate decelerated prior to the go signal (the offset of a 6-s mild vibrotactile stimulus) in both children and adults, indicating increased attention. While in adults, startle was severely attenuated when startle stimuli were presented just before the GO signal; in the 5-year-olds startle was facilitated. Anthony and Putnam (1985) interpreted these results in terms of a more diffuse attentional set in the 5-year-olds: The larger startle responses reflected processing of or attention to irrelevant as well as relevant sensory input. Since 5-year-olds show enhanced startle (relative to older children and adults) to lead stimuli at long lead intervals in startle modification by lead stimulation experiments (Ornitz et al., 1986, 1990, 1991), an alternative explanation of these findings is a nonspecific inability to inhibit in preschool children. Considering the fact that the developmental course of enhanced lead stimulus-induced startle facilitation at 5 years of age parallels deficient lead stimulus-induced startle inhibition at the same age (Ornitz et al., 1986, 1991), it may be that 5-year-olds can inhibit startle neither to protect sensory processing (short lead interval startle modification) nor to protect the integrity of a planned motor response (such as in the reaction time task). It would be of considerable interest to carry out the latter experiment across the childhood years to see to what extent the development course might parallel that of lead stimulus modification of startle.

4. Affective Modification of Startle

4.1. Background from Adult Studies

Lang and his colleagues (for reviews, see Lang, Bradley, & Cuthbert, 1990; Lang, Greenwald, Bradley, & Hamm, 1993; Chapter 8) have shown that the startle blink reflex, as a component of the startle response, a defensive or avoidance response to a sudden threat, is augmented when a startling stimulus is presented while the subject is in a highly aroused emotional state characterized by negative affective valence, for example, anger or fear. There is a "match" between the direction of affective valence and the defensive reflex. Conversely, the startle blink reflex is inhibited when there is a "mismatch," that is, when the subject is in a highly aroused emotional state characterized by positive affective valence, such as joy or lust (Lang et al., 1990). This differential effect occurs only when the arousal component of emotion is sufficiently high (Lang, 1995; Cuthbert, Bradley, & Lang, 1996). Experimentally, the effect of emotional state on startle is usually assessed by presenting startling stimuli while subjects watch pictures judged to be affectively valent (relative to neutral) and of low to high arousal potential (Lang et al., 1990).

4.2. Studies of Affective Modification of Startle during Childhood

In children, there is only one published investigation of affective influence on startle, and this study is limited to 5-month-old infants. To study infants, Balaban (1995) adapted the experimental techniques used to study affective modification of startle in adults by presenting photographic slides of human faces with happy, neutral, or angry expressions. When an acoustic startle stimulus was presented while viewing these pictures, the startle blink reflex was reduced while watching the happy expressions and increased while watching the angry expressions. From this single study it would appear that affective modification of startle is present during the first year of life. Alternatively, it is probable that, at 5 months of age, the infants in this study had less experience with angry than neutral or happy expressions, and hence directed more attention to the novel angry expressions, resulting in larger responses to startle probes presented concurrently (cf. Section 3 for attentional effects on startle in infants). Further investigation will be required to tease apart the attentional (Anthony & Graham, 1983, 1985) and affective (Balaban, 1995) components of startle modification in infancy.

Studies of toddlers, preschool, and school-age children will be required to determine whether affective and/or attentional modification of startle can be demonstrated during each of these developmentally unique periods of childhood. Such studies are just beginning and have appeared only in abstract form. McManis, Bradley, Cuthbert, and Lang (1995) were unable to demonstrate startle facilitation to pictures with negative affective valence in 7- to 10-year-old children and adolescents. However, when responses were segregated by gender, girls showed the expected (adult-like) facilitation of startle while viewing unpleasant pictures, whereas boys actually showed inhibition of startle (statistical significance of these trends was not stated). Cook, Hawk, Hawk, and Hummer (1995) also were unable to demonstrate the adult pattern of startle modification to affectively valent script-induced imagery in school-age children. Virtually identical startle magnitude was found during imagery designed to evoke feelings of pleasure, joy, sadness, fear, and anger. Further, the startle responses of children who scored higher on a fear survey schedule were smaller during unpleasant compared with pleasant imagery and were smaller in the "high fear" than in the "low fear" children. This significant affective valence by fear interaction was opposite to that found in adults (Cook, Hawk, Davis, & Stevenson, 1991). It is possible that in children, particularly boys (McManis et al., 1995) and more fear-prone children (Cook et al., 1995), greater attention to unpleasant pictures or imagery drew attentional resources away from the startling stimuli, resulting in smaller startle responses. Further investigation will be required to understand the relative contributions of attentional and emotional modification of startle and how their interactions might have different outcomes in infancy, childhood, and maturity. It is also possible that the distinction between attentional and emotional (particularly the arousal dimension of emotion) modification of startle might be less discrete than has been suggested in the literature of recent years (see, in this regard, the discussion of emotional modification of the startle-evoked P300 component of the event related potential in Section 5.3.4, below).

5. Autonomic, Myogenic, and Neurophysiologic Activity Accompanying the Startle Response during Childhood

One important unexplained feature of the human startle response is its extreme subject-to-subject (and within-subject) variability in the absence of modification. This variability has not been attributable to maturation, aging, emotional state, ethnicity, psychopathology, and so on, because, in all populations studied, investigators report excluding up to 10% of subjects who fail to show a startle response to very intense stimuli. The measured startle response is a motor response; autonomic, tonic myogenic, and electroencephalographic (EEG) changes and event-related potentials (ERPs) accompany the motor responses to startling stimuli. Several studies in children, motivated by interest in startle variability, have looked at possible associations between the magnitude of the startle blink and accompanying electrophysiological measures of autonomic state (heart rate), central nervous system activation (alpha activity), and muscle tone (tonic orbicularis oculi level) before and after startling and cognitive appraisal of the startling stimuli (P300 component of the ERP). These studies, described in the following sections, were conducted in the context of startle habituation (Ornitz et al., 1996) with the exception of one study of P300 and startle that was conducted in the context of lead stimulus modification of startle (Sugawara, Sadeghpour, de Traversay, & Ornitz, 1994).

5.1. Relationship to Individual Susceptibility to Startling

During a habituation study, Ornitz et al. (1996) found in 7- to 11-year-old boys an almost 30-fold variation in initial startle amplitude before habituation had developed. Could variations in startle amplitude or its habituation be "explained" by an association with either the initial amplitude or the changes in autonomic (heart rate), EEG (desynchronization), or myogenic (orbicularis oculi EMG) activity indexing activation or arousal accompanying the startle response to the repetitive startle stimulus? There were two major findings. First, the wide range of initial startle response amplitudes was independent of the tonic levels of the autonomic (heart rate), central nervous system (percent alpha), and facial muscular (orbicularis oculi EMG) activities that preceded and accompanied the startle responses to repetitive stimulation. Second, the autonomic, central nervous system, and myogenic responses to the startling stimuli each had its own unique type of change in response to repetitive stimulation, particularly in relation to habituation of the startle response itself. The tonic background orbicularis oculi EMG activity did not show significant habituation. Neither the pre- nor the poststartle percentage of alpha activity in the EEG showed significant change in tonic level with stimulus repetition. Significant alpha blocking waxed and waned as the startle response habituated, suggesting a fluctuating central state of awareness of external events, even though the motor response to the startling stimulus was becoming progressively smaller. Finally, the tonic levels of heart rate both before and after the startle stimulus, rather than habituating, showed significant linear increments that persisted over the course of 40 repetitions of the startle stimulus (see Section 5.2, below).

From these results, it can be concluded that the startle response to a sudden stimulus seems to be independent of the immediate physiological state at the time of stimulus presentation, to the extent that state is measured by tonic prestimulus central nervous system, autonomic, and myogenic activities. The individual subject's susceptibility to being startled appears to be an independent neurophysiological or psychophysiological function, the determinants of which remain to be explained.

5.2. Heart Rate Incrementation during Startle Habituation

As mentioned in the previous section, Ornitz et al. (1996) found that tonic levels of heart rate both before and after the startle stimulus, rather than habituating, showed significant linear increments that persisted throughout the course of startle habituation. Heart rate was measured during a 5-s epoch preceding (baseline) and two successive 5-s epochs immediately following each of 40 startle stimuli (poststimulus 1 and poststimulus 2). The most striking feature in Figure 12.2A was the increment in heart rate in the interval between the previous poststimulus 2 period and the subsequent baseline period of the next trial block. These between-trial heart rate increments were attributed to a heightened state of arousal persisting throughout the experimental session. The failure of the cardiac acceleration (the persistent increment in heart rate from the baseline period to poststimulus 1 seen in Fig. 12.2A) to habituate also suggests sustained arousal.

The concurrence of startle habituation and tonic heart rate increase may be understood in the context of the dual-process theory of habituation (Groves & Thompson, 1970; Thompson, Groves, Teyler, & Roemer, 1973; Thompson, Berry, Rinaldi, & Berger, 1979). In the dual-process theory, two independent processes of habituation and sensitization occur in response to repetitive stimulation. Habituation influences the stimulus–response pathway and is a decremental process; sensitization influences the state of the subject and is an incremental process (Groves & Thompson, 1970). State refers to the tonic level of excitation, activation, excitability, or arousal evoked by the repetitive stimulation (Groves & Thompson, 1970), "with arousal serving the role of sensitization of state" (Thompson et al., 1979). The startle-blink response reflected activity in the stimulus-response pathway and showed habituation (Fig. 12.2B). The facilitation of the cardiac activity (Fig. 12.2A) indexes the sensitization process, which is related to an induced state of tonic arousal, suggesting that the repetitive startling stimulation is inherently stressful even though the subjects appeared to ignore these sudden loud stimuli. As in the lead stimulus studies described above, the children's attention was directed to the ongoing silent movie.

5.3. P300 Accompanying Startle

Positive EEG deflections with the latency and scalp distribution characteristics of the P300 can be elicited automatically, in association with the startle blink, in response to loud auditory stimuli in a nontask context, that is, without target stimuli to which a response is required (Putnam & Roth 1987, 1990;

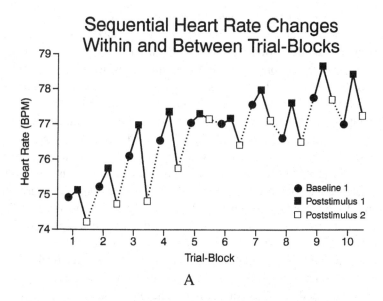

A

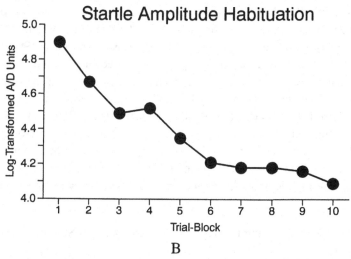

B

Figure 12.2. Tonic heart rate acceleration preceding (Baseline) and following (Post-stimulus 1 and Poststimulus 2) repetitive startling stimuli. *A* is contrasted with habituation of the startle response itself (*B*). Heart rates during the Baseline and Poststimulus periods (*A*) and amplitudes of orbicularis oculi EMG (*B*) are averaged for blocks of four trials into 10 successive trial blocks for 40 subjects. The dashed lines in *A* indicate the 5.0 period from the end of Poststimulus 2 of the prior trial to the beginning of the baseline period of the next trial, during which time data were not collected.

Ford & Pfefferbaum 1991; Chapter 14). In studies of the startle response in children (Sugawara et al., 1994; Hirano, Russell, Ornitz, & Liu, 1996), a prominent positive deflection at both Cz and Pz at a latency close to 300 msec on single trials in response to a 104-dB burst of white noise is readily observed. Averaging is not required to recognize this response on most trials, and in children it can frequently be identified in the raw EEG trace.

The automatic elicitation of P300 in a nontask situation (Putman & Roth, 1987, 1990; Ford & Pfefferbaum, 1991; Chapter 14) raises questions about the nature of P300, the amplitude of which usually increases with increasing relevance of a task associated with a stimulus and with decreasing probability (increasing uncertainty) that the stimulus will occur (Donchin, Karis, & Bashore, 1986; Donchin, Kramer, & Wickens, 1986). What, then, is the meaning of a P300 that occurs with the expected latency and scalp distribution, but as part of the startle response in a context in which there is no task and no uncertainty? Consideration of this question is complicated by the presence of P300 components of ERPs in response to relatively low-intensity nonstartling unattended task-irrelevant stimuli. These include the "passive auditory paradigm" (Polich, 1989), which may even generate a P300 response to rare tones in patients who are under anesthesia (Plourde, Joffe, Villemure, & Trahan, 1993) or comatose (Yingling, Hosobuchi, & Harrington, 1990), or the P300 response to auditory stimuli presented infrequently while subjects are engaged in preoccupying activities, such as working on puzzles or reading (Ritter, Vaughan, & Costa, 1968; Squires, Squires, & Hillyard, 1975; Polich, 1989). The attributes of the P300 component of the ERP evoked under these conditions have been compared to those of the orienting reflex (Ritter et al., 1968; Donchin, 1981; Pritchard, 1981). The P300 evoked in association with startle would appear to have much in common with the P300 evoked by nonstartling stimuli in nontask "passive" paradigms that may involve orienting.

5.3.1. P300 Accompanying Lead Stimulus Modification of Startle in Children

Sugawara et al. (1994) determined whether inhibitory and facilitatory lead stimuli would have effects on the P300 similar to those on the startle blink. Lead conditions were chosen to induce startle amplitude facilitation (4000-msec continuous tone), startle amplitude inhibition (120-msec lead interval), and startle onset latency facilitation (60-msec lead interval). In 93 7- to 11-year-old boys, there was significant startle amplitude and P300 amplitude facilitation following the 4000-msec tone, startle amplitude and P300 amplitude inhibition following the 120-msec lead interval, and startle onset latency and P300 peak latency facilitation (shorter latencies) following the 60-msec lead interval. Hence, the vertex-recorded P300 elicited by startling stimuli was modulated by nonstartling lead stimuli in a manner that paralleled that of modification of the brain stem-generated startle blink. Startle inhibition by lead stimuli is mediated by an inhibitory pathway in the mesopontine lateral tegmentum. This brain-stem circuitry has a similar effect on the P300 even though the latter may be generated in more rostral structures. Alternatively, this automatically elicited P300 may represent a limbic or cortical reflection of the sensory processing taking place in the brain stem. Either interpretation suggests a "bottom up" as contrasted with a "top down" mode of sensory processing. This P300 obeys the rules of startle modulation by brain-stem mechanisms rather than indexing cortical evaluation of stimuli for task relevance, stimulus probability, and prior uncertainty.

The inhibitory lead interval modification of P300 following startle found in children (Sugawara et al., 1994) has recently been reported in adults (Ford, Roth, Bell, Li, & Jain, 1996). Facilitatory lead modification did not occur, but it is noted that the lead interval of 600 msec is too short to expect facilitation.

5.3.2. P300 Accompanying Startle Habituation in Children

Hirano et al. (1996) determined whether habituation would have effects on the P300 similar to those on the startle blink. In 34 normal 7- to 11-year-old boys, startle blinks and P300 were recorded in response to 40 104-dB bursts of white noise presented at 23-s intervals while the boys watched a silent movie. Both startle and P300 amplitudes habituated toward asymptotic levels after the first 28 trials, suggesting that both startle and the subsequent cognitive evaluation of the startling stimulus, reflected in the P300 response, are modulated by a common neurophysiological mechanism extrinsic to the direct startle pathway and superimposed on intrinsic mechanisms of startle habituation. Analyses of the within-subject associations between startle and P300 initial amplitudes and rates of habituation showed that these parameters varied independently within the individual subject, suggesting that the P300 is not a component of the startle response. Rather, it reflects an evaluation of the startling stimulus, decreasing in amplitude as the surprising value of the startling stimulus decreases with habituation. The lack of significant within-subject association between the rates of habituation of startle and P300 amplitudes suggests the presence of other yet-to-be-defined factors influencing both the individual subject's reflex response (dependent on mechanisms intrinsic to the direct startle pathway) and the subsequent cognitive evaluation of stimulus and response.

The P300 peak latency showed a modest marginally significant positive correlation with the vertical electrooculogram (EOG) startle *peak* latency. The vertical EOG peak latency coincides with the termination of orbicularis oculi EMG activity and is a measure of the time of completion of lid closure. Since the P300 peak latency is proportional to and serves as a measure of the time required for stimulus evaluation (Kutas, McCarthy, & Donchin, 1977; and see reviews in Donchin, 1981; Pritchard, 1981; Howard & Polich, 1985), it seems that for this automatically elicited P300, a part of such evaluation may include the time for the completion of the reflex response (the startle blink). It is possible, then, that for sudden intense stimuli that evoke a reflex motor response, the P300 is indexing the evaluation not only of the stimulus but also of the subsequent reflex motor response to the stimulus. For strong sudden stimuli, capable of inducing large startles, the automatic P300 may reflect evaluation of the subject's own behavior in response to the stimulus. As the habituation process reflects the reduction of surprise induced by the startling stimulus when it occurs repetitively at a low rate of presentation in a context in which it is ignored and is not task-relevant, both the startle response itself and the subsequent mental evaluation of the importance of the startling stimulus (reflected in the P300) are reduced together to asymptotic levels at about the same time. The evaluation of the "importance" of the startling stimulus may also take account of and reflect the subject's reflex motor response to that stimulus.

5.3.3. Comparisons between Effects of Lead Stimulation and Habituation on Startle and P300

Startle inhibition by lead stimuli is a brain-stem function involving the early low-level processing of sensory input. This type of inhibition is mediated by an inhibitory pathway in the mesopontine lateral tegmental area as demonstrated by lesion (Leitner, Powers, Stitt, & Hoffman, 1981; Leitner & Cohen, 1985) and stimulation (Saitoh, Tilson, Shaw, & Dyer, 1987) studies in the rat. This pathway, which parallels the primary startle pathway in the brain stem (Lee, Lopez, Meloni, & Davis, 1996; Chapter 5), impinges on the latter at or prior to the medial pontomedullary reticular formation (Wu, Suzuki, & Siegel, 1988). It involves cholinergic transmission from the pedunculopontine tegmental nucleus to the nucleus reticularis pontis caudalis (Koch, Kungel, & Herbert, 1993). Hence, it seems likely that the mesopontine tegmental neuronal circuitry that mediates lead stimulus-induced inhibition of startle in the brain stem had a similar effect on the startle-evoked P300 (Sugawara et al., 1994).

The functional neuroanatomy of startle modification by habituation is not as specifically delineated as that underlying lead stimulation-induced inhibition of startle. Short-term habituation of startle, as studied by Hirano et al. (1996), is mediated primarily by mechanisms intrinsic to the direct startle pathway (see discussion in Section 2). However, extrinsic mechanisms may also be involved. Studies of the effects of human frontal lobe lesions on the habituation of awareness in peripheral vision (Troxler fading) suggest that frontal cortex increases habituation of attention to non-novel stimuli (Mennemeier, Chatterjee, Watson, Wertman, Carter, & Heilman, 1994). Hence, the similar course of habituation for both startle and P300 amplitudes suggests that both habituation processes may be modified by frontal cortex activity. Both the time course of habituation of the reflex motor (the startle blink) response to and the cognitive (the P300) evaluation of the repetitive startling stimulus could be modified by the same frontocortical activity.

In lead stimulus-induced modification of P300 and startle, Sugawara et al. (1994) postulated a "bottom up" mode of sensory processing in which the evaluation of the startling stimulus, indexed by P300 amplitude, obeyed the rules of startle modification by brain-stem mechanisms, that is, lead stimulus inhibition. In contrast, modification of P300 and startle by habituation may involve a "top down" modification by fronto-cortical mechanisms (Hirano et al., 1996).

5.3.4. Emotional Modification of P300 Accompanying Startle

Another type of "top down" modification involves the emotional state of the subject at the time of presentation of the startling stimuli. Experimentally, such state is usually manipulated by having subjects look at emotionally evocative pictures while startle stimuli are presented (as described in Section 4.1). Pictures rated unpleasant induce augmented startle amplitude, presumably because there is a "match" between the unpleasant aspects of the picture and the inherently unpleasant nature of the startling stimulus that evokes the startle response, an inherently defensive reflex (Lang et al., 1990). Rarely, subjects have been asked to rate the startling stimulus itself on the scales of affective valence and arousal used to rate their emotional reactions to pictures or other backgrounds to startle presentation (Bradley & Lang, 1994). In one study, children were asked to rate their emotional reactions to the startling stimuli at the end of a startle habituation study. Ratings of arousal and affective valence available from 21 of the 34 children in Hirano et al. (1996) revealed significant correlations between arousal (but not valence) and both magnitude and habituation of P300 but not of startle, reflecting the influence of one dimension of emotion on the cognitive evaluation of startle, but not on startle per se (Ornitz, 1996a).

Those children who rated the startling stimuli as having been more arousing had larger P300 responses to the startling stimuli. This finding is consistent with that of Schupp, Cuthbert, Bradley, Birbaumer, and Lang (1997), who presented startling stimuli to adults during presentation of affectively pleasant, neutral, and unpleasant pictures and found equally small P300 responses to startling stimuli in the presence of pleasant and unpleasant pictures relative to larger responses to neutral pictures. Attenuation of the P300 in the presence of affectively valent pictures is a consequence of allocating more attention to the pictures and less to the startling stimuli, "consistent with the idea that arousing stimuli draw more attentional resources" (Schupp et al., 1997). When startling stimuli are presented in the presence of only a neutral environment (e.g., watching a silent movie), then attentional resources are more available to the startling stimuli and individuals who are more aroused by such stimuli have larger startle responses. These results, consistent in adults and children, suggest a blurring of hard and fast distinctions between attention and arousal.

6. Developmental Aspects of Startle Modification in Relation to Brain Maturation and Neurophysiological Development

The most robust, and the most studied, developmental effects on startle modification have involved the maturation of startle inhibition induced by lead stimuli at relatively short lead intervals. Similar though less striking developmental changes involve startle facilitation induced by long lead intervals. In summary, prior to about 4 years of age, inhibitory startle modification is characterized by fluctuating weak inhibition (25% response inhibition in 2- to 6-month-olds (Graham et al., 1981)), nonsignificant facilitation (17% response increase in 15-month-olds (Balaban et al., 1989)), and, again, weak inhibition (23% response inhibition) in 3-year-old boys (Ornitz et al., 1986). In 4-year-old girls and boys there is nonsignificant startle amplitude facilitation (about 10% and 22%, respectively) 120 msec following lead stimulation. In 5-year-old boys, 30% response inhibition has developed. By 8 years, both girls and boys show strong significant response inhibition, 50% and 75%, respectively, approximating adult values. Facilitatory startle modification in response to prolonged continuous lead stimulation follows a similar developmental course (Ornitz et al., 1986, 1991). Both inhibitory and facilitatory startle modification show, respectively, significant peak losses in startle inhibition and peak gains in startle facilitation at about $4\frac{1}{2}$ years of age, followed by a progressive increase in inhibition and decrease in facilitation until 8 years of age, when mature values are obtained (Ornitz et al., 1986, 1990).

Inhibitory startle modification matures during the second of four maturational spurts in brain growth and neurophysiological change during childhood

(Ornitz, 1996b). This critical period of human neurologic growth and development takes place between 6 and 10 years of age and is characterized by many important structural brain and functional neurophysiological changes (Ornitz, 1996b). By the end of this second spurt in structural and functional brain development, at around 10 years of age, many significant subcortical functions have matured, and accelerated development of some measures of cortical activity have taken place (described in detail in Ornitz, 1996b). Many of the mature subcortical mechanisms are of an inhibitory nature, suggesting a relationship between the capacity to inhibit and the readiness for higher cognitive processes. During this period, there is an accelerated development of the ability to inhibit the retroactive interference of a second set of stimuli upon the recall of a prior set (Passler, Isaac, & Hynd, 1985). This is a frontal lobe function. It is suggested that the developing capacity to inhibit, which is requisite for frontal lobe-mediated cognition, may be linked to the development of subcortical inhibitory mechanisms.

All of these structural and functional changes occur during that period of childhood when children are able to engage meaningfully in learning and, in most cultures, are enrolled in school. This is approximately the Piagetian period of concrete operations (Inhelder & Piaget, 1958), during which time the child's concept of reality becomes less egocentric and less anthropomorphic, permitting the initial development of logical thinking. Hence the maturation of inhibitory mechanisms in the brain stem that damp the response to strong external stimuli and the reduction of excitation following continuous stimulation (sensory modulation) parallel the development of cortical (cognitive) processes that require the capacity of the child to separate effectively and conceptually from external objects and events, a capacity that would seem to require inhibitory functions.

Prior to the second maturation spurt in brain growth and change (i.e., between 3 and 5 years of age), there is an important period of neurophysiologic development characterized by a particular constellation of EEG, ERP, and startle physiology changes. Initiated around 4 years of age, this period is notable for a peak increment in ERP and a concurrent peak deficit in inhibitory startle modification. This stage of neurophysiologic development involving increased reactivity to stimuli at both cortical and subcortical levels, occurring between an earlier period of cortical maturation and a later period of cortical "remodeling" (Rabinowicz, 1986), coincides with the Piagetian stage of preoperational behavior. The neurophysiologic characteristics suggest the heightened awareness coupled with the inability to inhibit that characterize the preschool child.

An overview of these relationships between neurophysiologic development and behavior suggests two developmental stages that, not surprisingly, coincide with the preschool and school-age periods of childhood. Between 3 and 5 years, there is a neurophysiologic stage of increased receptivity coupled with disinhibition in response to environmental stimuli. Between 6 and 10 years, there is a neurophysiologic stage of increasing inhibition in response to stimuli, coupled with increasing development of neurophysiologic indices of information processing. In early adolescence, there is a third stage of development during which there is neurophysiologic evidence for further development of intracortical, particularly frontal, connectivity and final maturation of neurophysiological indices of information processing. These three neurophysiologic stages coincide with the Piagetian stages of preoperational behavior, concrete operations, and formal operations. Hence the developing neurophysiologic capacity to register, process, and extract information from stimuli, coupled with the increasing ability to inhibit responses to stimuli, appears to underlie the changing style of learning that progresses from the egocentric (preschool child) to the more objective but concrete (school-age child) and finally to abstract thinking (adolescent). Developmental changes in startle modification, particularly those involving inhibitory and facilitatory effects of lead stimulation, have been studied primarily in relation to the first two of these three stages of development (Fig. 12.3). Future investigation might reveal startle modification associations with the adolescent stage, as more detailed understanding of attentional, affective, and possible cognitive influence on startle modification occurs.

7. Summary

Startle modification in children is different from that in adults in some respects and similar in others. The most striking developmental effect involves lead stimulus modification of startle. There is a robust developmental effect on both inhibitory and facilitory lead stimulus modification of startle. Preschool children fail to show lead stimulus-induced startle inhibition and also show exaggerated lead stimulus-induced startle facilitation. Mature startle inhibition and facilitation are not achieved until about 8 years of age. This developmental effect has been attributed to neuronal pathways extrinsic to the direct startle pathway. In contrast, startle habituation, which is attributed to mechanisms intrinsic to the direct startle pathway, has already reached mature levels in 3- to 5-year-old children. Hence development appears to involve regulatory mechanisms extrinsic to the stimulus–response pathway rather than involving the stimulus–response pathway per se.

Lead stimulus-induced modification of startle matures (increasing inhibition and decreasing facilitation) during a period of structural brain changes in

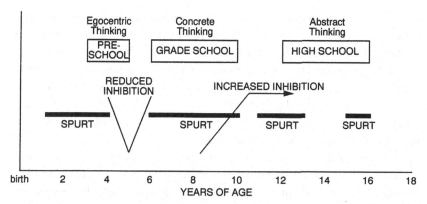

Figure 12.3. Stages of neuropsychological and cognitive development. A neurophysiological state characterized by reduced inhibition, including reduced inhibitory lead stimulus modification of startle, occurs between the first two spurts in brain maturation and neurophysiological development. It occurs during the preschool years and coincides with the Piagetian stage of preoperational behavior. A second state of increasing inhibition, including increased inhibitory lead stimulus modification of startle, begins during the grade-school years and coincides with the Piagetian stage of concrete operations. It develops during the second spurt in structural brain maturation and neurophysiological development.

association with multifold cortical and subcortical neurophysiological changes that are primarily inhibitory in nature. This maturational bias toward the development of inhibition during the primary school years follows a developmental stage characterized by a deficit in inhibition affecting not only lead stimulus modification of startle but also EEG and ERP activity. Hence, the extrinsic mechanisms that regulate lead stimulus modification of startle appear to be associated with developmental stages that coincide with the preschool and school-age periods of childhood. The former coincides with the Piagetian stage of preoperational behavior; its neurophysiological parameters suggest the preschooler's heightened awareness and receptivity coupled with the inability to inhibit. The latter coincides with the Piagetian stage of concrete operations; its neurophysiological parameters suggest the damping of response to strong external stimuli that is requisite to involvement in logical thinking and the learning process during the school years (see Fig. 12.3).

There are very few developmental studies of the influence of attention and emotion on startle. In both infants and 5-year-olds, experimental contexts that putatively heighten attention increased startle; adults did not show this effect. The same experimental parameters could have also induced arousal and/or startle facilitation to sustained lead stimuli, an effect to which preschool children are more susceptible. Limited studies of affective modification of startle suggest that school-age children fail to show the adult pattern of enhanced startle in the presence of pictures or imagery characterized by negative affective valence. In contrast, startle was increased while 5-month-old infants watched angry faces and decreased while they watched happy faces, effects analogous to those found in adults in response to pictures with negative and positive affective valence. At present there is no clear explanation for the results of these very preliminary studies.

The magnitude of the startle response shows great subject-to-subject and within-subject variability in normal populations both during childhood and in adulthood. In children, this variability cannot be explained by the immediate neurophysiological or autonomic state preceding startle stimulus presentation nor is there any association between the startle response and the heart rate change, alpha blocking, or P300 response evoked by the startling stimulus. These potential associations have not been studied in adult populations. Habituation and inhibitory lead interval modification of the P300 response to the startling stimulus appears to be similar in the mid-childhood years and adulthood. In school-age children, there is a tonic heart rate increase in the presence of startle response habituation, an effect suggesting the sensitization of state postulated in dual-process theory of habituation. This effect is yet to be studied in adult populations. It suggests the development of a tonic state of arousal during the repetitive presentation of startling stimuli, an effect compatible with the positive association between arousal ratings of the startling stimuli and magnitude of the startle-evoked P300 in the same children.

ACKNOWLEDGMENTS

The author's work cited in this chapter was funded by National Institutes of Health grant HD-14193 and the generous support of the Alice and Julius Kantor Charitable Trust.

PART V

Relationships with Other Paradigms and Measures

CHAPTER THIRTEEN

Behavioral Analogies of Short Lead Interval Startle Inhibition

DIANE L. FILION, KIMBERLE A. KELLY, AND
ERIN A. HAZLETT

ABSTRACT

Short lead interval startle inhibition is widely viewed as reflecting a low-level inhibitory/sensorimotor gating mechanism that serves to protect the processing of a lead stimulus from the potentially disruptive impact of a startle-eliciting stimulus. However, despite the acceptance of this view, it has received little empirical attention, and hence the significance of startle inhibition for cognition is not well understood. This chapter explores the cognitive significance of startle inhibition by comparing it with five behavioral cognitive/clinical measures that have an "inhibition-based" theoretical interpretation: attentional blink, negative priming, backward masking, perseverative responding on the Wisconsin Card Sorting Test, and thought disorder as reflected by the Ego Impairment Index. In each case, we explore the possibility that the behavioral and startle measures reflect a common underlying inhibitory process, comparing each measure to startle inhibition in terms of similarities and differences relating to experimental procedures, time course, critical stimulus characteristics, and patterns of response in normal and pathological subject groups.

1. Introduction

One reason for psychology's increasing interest in startle modification measures is their hypothesized reflection of cognitive processing, particularly in the case of the short lead interval measures. As reviewed earlier in this book (Chapters 3, 7, and 11), the dominant theoretical interpretations of short lead

Michael E. Dawson, Anne M. Schell, and Andreas H. Böhmelt, Eds. *Startle modification: Implications for neuroscience, cognitive science, and clinical science.* Copyright © 1999 Cambridge University Press. Printed in the United States of America. All rights reserved.

interval startle inhibition are (1) that it reflects a low-level inhibitory mechanism protective of lead stimulus processing (e.g., Graham, 1975, 1980) and (2) that it also reflects a more general inhibitory process, termed sensorimotor gating, a critical component of intact cognitive processing that involves the ability to filter or screen out irrelevant sensory, motor, or cognitive information in the early stages of information processing (e.g., Braff & Geyer, 1990; Geyer, Swerdlow, Mansbach, & Braff, 1990; Cadenhead, Geyer, & Braff, 1993). To date, the strongest evidence supporting these interpretations comes from two sources, studies examining startle effects on lead and startle stimulus perception (reviewed in Chapter 3), and findings documenting reduced startle inhibition in clinical populations characterized by deficits in the ability to regulate sensory stimulation (reviewed in Chapter 11). Although this evidence suggests a relationship between startle modification and cognitive processing, there is a great deal to be learned regarding the nature of this relationship.

The purpose of this chapter is to explore the cognitive significance of startle modification measures by examining their relationship to other cognitive/clinical measures that share a similar theoretical interpretation. This chapter will focus exclusively on *behavioral* measures of cognition (the event-related potential (ERP) correlates of startle modification are reviewed in Chapter 14) and their relationship to *short lead interval* startle inhibition (behavioral analogies and correlates of long lead interval effects have received little empirical attention to date). This chapter will review five cognitive/clinical measures that have an "inhibition-based" theoretical interpretation: attentional blink, negative priming, backward masking, perseverative responding on the Wisconsin Card Sorting Test, and thought disorder as reflected by the Ego Impairment Index. In each case, we will explore the possibility that the behavioral and startle measures reflect a common underlying inhibitory process, share a common neurophysiological basis, or both. As will be discussed in detail in the following sections, the attentional blink, backward masking, and negative priming measures are thought to reflect relatively low-level inhibitory processes lasting a few hundred milliseconds and occurring over a time course quite similar to startle inhibition. In contrast, the Wisconsin Card Sorting Test and the Ego Impairment Index are thought to reflect relatively high-level inhibitory processes that occur over a much broader range of time intervals. We will provide a brief description of each measure and then discuss the theoretical interpretation of the measure and how it compares to startle inhibition in terms of similarities and differences relating to experimental procedures, time course, critical stimulus characteristics, and patterns of response in normal and pathological subject groups.

2. Attentional Blink

When visual stimuli such as letters, digits, words, or pictures are presented in rapid succession to the same location, there are certain conditions in which the processing of one item in the stimulus stream results in a momentary deficit in the processing of subsequent items (e.g., Reeves & Sperling, 1986; Broadbent & Broadbent, 1987; Weichselgartner & Sperling, 1987). For example, when participants perform a task requiring the processing of at least two targets from among a stream of rapidly presented visual stimuli (typically 10–12 items per second), such as to name two letters that appear within a stream of digits, or to name two white letters that appear within a stream of black letters (see Fig. 13.1 for an illustration of this type of task), the result is a reliable reduction in the probability of detecting the second target stimulus when it is the second, third, or fourth item following the first target (see Fig. 13.2). This momentary reduction in the detectability of the second target has come to be known as the "attentional blink" (Raymond, Shapiro, & Arnell, 1992).

2.1. Theoretical Interpretation

Although it has been discovered only recently and is not well understood, a number of theoretical models have been proposed to explain the attentional blink. The inhibition model is based on active inhibitory processes theoretically similar to those hypothesized to underlie startle inhibition. According to the inhibition model, the rapid appearance of the +1 item immediately after the first target produces the potential for perceptual confusion (inadequate processing or inappropriate conjoining of letter names) during target identification processes. This potential confusion elicits inhibition of subsequently presented stimuli so that further potential confusion may be minimized (Raymond et al., 1992). The suggestion that the +1 item is critical in triggering the inhibition is based on findings that the attentional blink is abolished when the +1 item is removed from the stream. In this model, presentation of the first target initiates an attentional episode (or opens an "attentional gate"), allowing the processing of that item and, by virtue of its proximity, the +1 item as well. The potential for confusion among attributes between these two stimuli (the target and the +1 item) provokes an active inhibition of subsequent visual processing and thus produces the attentional blink.

In contrast to the inhibition model, two additional models, the interference model (Raymond, Shapiro, & Arnell, 1995) and the two-stage processing model (Chun & Potter, 1995), suggest that the attentional blink occurs because of capacity limitations and/or the second target being overwritten or

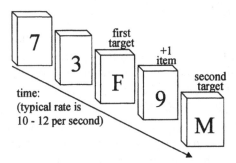

Figure 13.1. Illustration of a typical attentional blink paradigm. Visual stimuli are presented in rapid succession to a central location and participants are asked to identify target stimuli from among a stream on nontargets.

forgotten rather than because of an inhibition of the processing of the second target. These latter models are based on evidence suggesting that the similarity of the first and second targets interferes with successful retrieval of the second target (Shapiro, Raymond, & Arnell, 1994), as does similarity between the +1 item and the second target (Raymond, Shapiro, & Arnell, 1995). According to the two-stage model of attentional blink, stage 1 processing consists of rapid detection of relevant features for target identification for every item in the stream. Global discriminability between targets and nontargets affects the duration of stage 1 processing by determining the number of features that must be detected before stage 2 processing is triggered. The second stage reflects capacity-limited processing of the targets that occurs after detection. This processing is initiated by a transient attentional response triggered by target detection, and it is this processing that exceeds the duration of the target stimulus and therefore also encompasses the first post-target stimulus. The degree of local discriminability between the target and the +1 item affects the amount of processing required. When the second target occurs before stage 2 processing of the first target is complete, it must wait for processing capacity to become available, and the limited duration of the representation generated by stage 1 is subject to erasure by later stimuli in the stream, thus producing a detection deficit that decreases across interitem intervals but does not include the first post-target stimulus.

2.2. Comparison with Startle Inhibition

From the preceding sections, one can see an obvious similarity between the inhibition model of the attentional blink and the protection-of-processing

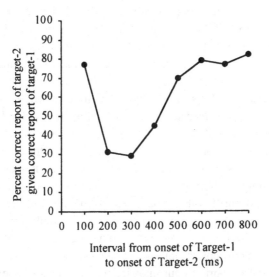

Figure 13.2. Typical results from an attentional blink experiment. Plotted values represent percent correct reports of a target-2 given that target-1 was correctly identified as a function of time between target-1 and target-2.

view of startle inhibition; both suggest that processing of subsequent stimuli is attenuated until perceptual processing of an initial stimulus is complete. In addition, the time course of the attentional blink is similar to the time course of startle inhibition. What is striking is not only the overlapping intervals at which the effects appear, but also the similar nonmonotonic U-shaped functions that describe the development, peak, and subsequent decline of inhibition over time. In attentional blink experiments, the processing of the +1 post-target item is unaffected by target processing, as is the processing of the +5 and later post-target items. Given the typical presentation rates of 10–12 stimuli per second, we can infer from existing attentional blink experiments that the attentional blink occurs between approximately 100 and 450 msec following onset of the first target, with maximal inhibition occurring between approximately 200 and 300 msec. The window for startle inhibition falls between approximately 30 and 800 msec, with maximal inhibition occurring at approximately 120 msec.

Despite these similarities, it is important to note that there are also several differences between the startle inhibition and attentional blink measures. First, the attentional blink is dependent on the requirement that participants actively attend to the first target; if participants are not required to attend to the first target stimulus, the attentional blink is abolished (Raymond et al.,

1992, 1995; Shapiro et al., 1994). In contrast, startle inhibition occurs reliably regardless of whether participants are required to attend to the lead stimulus (see Chapter 3). Second, the attentional blink appears to be dependent on the presence of the +1 post-target item; if that item is omitted from the stream, the attentional blink is abolished (Raymond et al., 1992). In contrast, there is nothing comparable to the +1 post-target item in the startle inhibition paradigm, there is simply the lead stimulus followed by the startle-eliciting stimulus. Third, because the attentional blink is a relatively newly discovered phenomenon, the generality and neurophysiological basis of the effect are not yet known. To date, for example, the attentional blink has been documented only for the processing of visual stimuli, and it remains to be seen whether the attentional blink occurs in other modalities. Startle inhibition has been documented with visual, auditory, and vibrotactile lead stimuli. Finally, as noted above, there are alternative theoretical accounts of the attentional blink that do not involve the concept of inhibition, and these models have received significant empirical support. To our knowledge, no studies have examined the attentional blink and startle modification in the same participants, nor has the attentional blink been studied in clinical populations that exhibit reduced startle inhibition. However, the remarkable similarities between these effects suggests that this may be an interesting and informative direction for future research.

3. Backward Masking

In a typical backward-masking paradigm, a target stimulus is followed by a masking stimulus, so-called because the presentation of the masking stimulus interferes with (or masks) processing of the target stimulus. Typically, masking is quantified as the performance degradation in target identification associated with presenting the masking stimulus at a particular lead interval (or stimulus onset asynchrony in masking terms, the interval between the onset of the target and the mask). The extent and nature of this masking effect depends on the particular experimental procedures and stimuli employed (e.g., Kahneman, 1968; Felsten & Wasserman, 1980). Backward masking has been shown to occur in both the auditory (Loeb & Holding, 1975) and visual modalities, but the literature most relevant to startle inhibition has involved visual backward masking, which will be the focus of this section. The two main categories of visual masking effects are integration effects (participants perceive an integration of the target and mask stimuli), which occur at lead intervals less than 20 msec, and interference effects (participants misperceive the target or report seeing only the mask), which occur at lead intervals between approximately 20 and 70 msec (e.g., Green, Nuechterlein, & Mintz, 1994). At lead intervals longer than approximately 70 msec, the target is identifiable because the mask has little or no effect.

3.1. Theoretical Interpretation

Interference effects in visual backward masking are thought to occur because processes elicited by the masking stimulus interfere with the processing of the target stimulus already in progress (Green et al., 1994). According to Breitmeyer and colleagues (e.g., Breitmeyer & Ganz, 1976; Breitmeyer, 1984), visual backward masking is the result of an interaction between transient and sustained processes initiated by the target and masking stimuli. According to this view, the "coarse" aspects of a visual stimulus (onset, offset, etc.) first initiate a transient processing episode, which is then followed by a shift to a sustained processing of the "fine" details of the stimulus (shape, etc.) necessary for identification. This interpretation suggests that when the transient processing associated with the masking stimulus interferes with the ongoing sustained processing of the target stimulus, target identification is disrupted.

3.2. Comparison with Startle Inhibition

As discussed by Braff, Sacuzzo, and Geyer (1991), support for the notion that backward masking and short lead interval startle inhibition reflect a common underlying inhibitory process stems primarily from the fact that both phenomena are hypothesized to be due to the interaction of transient and sustained processes. As reviewed in Chapter 3, startle inhibition is viewed as a measure of the suppression of a second stimulus during the initial processing of a first stimulus, and hence is a measure of processing protection, or *successful inhibition*. Visual backward masking is a measure of the disruption to sustained processing of a first stimulus produced by the transient processing of a second, and hence is a measure of processing-interference, or a *failure of inhibition*. If these views are accurate, it is reasonable to hypothesize that individuals exhibiting *reduced* startle inhibition (reflecting a reduced ability to protect sustained processing) would also be expected to exhibit *increased* masking interference.

Consistent with this prediction, abnormalities on both measures have been observed in various psychopathological disorders, particularly the schizophrenia spectrum disorders. For example, there are several reports that schizophrenia patients exhibit reduced startle inhibition (see review in Chapter 11) as well as increased masking interference (e.g., Green et al., 1994) relative to control participants. In addition, there is neuropharmacological evidence suggesting that dopamine overactivity is related to both reduced startle inhibition and backward-masking deficits observed in schizophrenia patients (Braff et al., 1991). Inducing dopamine overactivity pharmacologically produces deficient startle inhibition (Swerdlow, Braff, Geyer, & Koob, 1986), whereas patients on antipsychotic medications (which act as dopamine antagonists), show reduced masking deficits relative to unmedicated patients (Braff & Sacuzzo, 1982).

Despite this suggestive evidence, only one published study to date has investigated backward masking and startle inhibition in the same schizophrenia patients (Perry & Braff, 1994), and because this study was primarily concerned with correlations between these measures of information processing and tests of thought disorder, data were not presented on the relationship between backward masking and startle inhibition per se. Both measures were, however, found to be significantly correlated with thought disorder (as assessed by the Ego Impairment Index, Perry & Viglione, 1991, see below), suggesting that deficits in backward masking and startle modification may reflect similar processes. Clearly the comparison of backward masking and startle modification patterns within the same participants is an important direction for future research.

4. Negative Priming

Negative priming tasks are a special category of selective attention tasks in which, on a given trial, participants are required to attend to a target stimulus while ignoring a distractor stimulus presented simultaneously. On a subset of the trials, the to-be-attended target stimulus is the stimulus that served as the distractor on the immediately preceding trial. For example, in a task in which participants are to name which of a pair of letters comes first in the alphabet, one trial might involve presentation of the letters M and R (the participant would respond "M" and inhibit the letter name "R"), and the following trial might involve presentation of the letters "R" and "U." In this case, the correct response is "R," so the participant must respond by saying the letter name that was inhibited on the preceding trial. "Negative priming" refers to the significant slowing of response times that is reliably observed on these distractor-becomes-target trials compared with trials in which there is no relationship between the current target and the previous distractor. Negative priming occurs across a wide time course, but is typically studied at intervals ranging from 100 to 3000 msec, gradually diminishing as the interval lengthens.

Although negative priming is usually studied in the visual modality, there have been demonstrations of negative priming in the auditory modality as well (e.g., Banks, Roberts, & Ciranni, 1995).

4.1. Theoretical Interpretation

The theoretical interpretation of negative priming is that it reflects a transient inhibition of the representation of the distractor stimulus; the more strongly the distractor is inhibited, the more response time will be slowed when that stimulus is re-presented as the target (e.g., Tipper, 1985).

4.2. Comparison with Startle Inhibition

Based on the fact that startle inhibition and negative priming are both thought to reflect transient inhibitory processes, two studies have examined the relationship between these measures on a within-participant basis, with inconsistent results. Swerdlow, Filion, Geyer, and Braff (1995) found no significant correlation between startle inhibition and negative priming in a group of college student participants. In contrast, Filion and McDowd (1992) reported a significant correlation between these measures, observing the relationship in groups of both college-age and elderly participants. In this latter study, startle inhibition was measured within a task in which participants were to attend to certain lead stimuli and ignore others, whereas in the Swerdlow et al. study participants were not given a task to perform during the startle testing. The correlations that were observed between startle inhibition and negative priming in the Filion and McDowd study were observed exclusively with the startle inhibition scores from the attended-lead stimulus trials. For those trials, individuals who exhibited the most startle inhibition also tended to exhibit the most negative priming. Together, these results provide limited support for the notion that startle inhibition and negative priming might reflect a common underlying inhibitory process, but they suggest that the inhibition measured in negative priming tasks may be most closely associated with controlled attentional modulation of startle inhibition. Perhaps more convincing than the mixed results from these within-participant studies is the fact that abnormally reduced negative priming has been reported in several clinical disorders that also are associated with reduced startle inhibition. These disorders include schizophrenia (Beech, Powell, McWilliam, & Claridge, 1989), schizotypal personality disorder (Beech & Claridge, 1987; Beech, Baylis, Smithson, & Claridge, 1989), and obsessive–compulsive disorder (Enright & Beech,

1993a, b). One interesting direction for future research will be to examine the relationship between startle inhibition and negative priming within these clinical populations.

5. The Wisconsin Card Sorting Test

The Wisconsin Card Sorting Test (WCST) is a widely used neuropsychological measure of abstract reasoning and problem-solving that involves achieving abstract sets, maintaining these sets, and then changing them (Grant & Berg, 1948). The standard WCST consists of 128 cards, each of which contains geometric figures that may vary along several dimensions (e.g., color, form, number). Participants are instructed to place each card below one of four target or key cards using some principle to guide them. Although they are not informed of the correct principle, feedback is given after each card placement. The initial sorting principle is to match according to color, then once ten cards are correctly sorted, the principle is changed, although the participant is not informed of this change. The test proceeds until the participant has completed six sorting categories of ten cards each or has sorted all 128 cards, whichever occurs first. A number of different types of error scores can be calculated, but the most commonly used is a perseveration score reflecting the number of times a participant continued to use a previous rule after a new rule was in effect.

5.1. Theoretical Interpretation

In the WCST, the rules for card sorting constantly change, so the participant must inhibit a response that was previously correct in order to adapt to the new rules. Individuals who exhibit high perseverative error scores are thought to have difficulty inhibiting prior responses and shifting their strategies or cognitive sets.

5.2. Comparison with Startle Inhibition

Given the description above, it seems unlikely that the WCST and startle inhibition measures reflect a common underlying inhibitory process, especially given the vastly different time frames involved in these measures. In startle inhibition, the time course for the inhibitory process occurs very quickly, between 30 and 800 msec after the onset of the lead stimulus. In contrast, it takes several seconds for a participant to sort ten WCST stimulus cards into a correct category. Once this is achieved, the "inhibitory" processing begins and the participant must shift his or her cognitive set from "color" of the stimulus card to, for instance, the "number" of shapes on the card. However, despite these differences, there are significant reasons for hypothesizing a relationship between these two measures. In addition to sharing an inhibition-based theoretical interpretation, the primary link between the WCST and startle inhibition is the possibility that these measures share a common underlying neurophysiological basis.

The brain regions that modulate short lead interval startle inhibition are being well delineated using animal models (Chapter 6), and one cortical region that is known to modulate startle inhibition in rats is the medial prefrontal cortex (Bubser & Koch, 1994a; Koch & Bubser, 1994). This same brain region is implicated in WCST performance, based on the combination of several studies reporting that patients with schizophrenia show high perseverative error scores on the WCST compared with normal individuals (e.g., Fey, 1951; Malmo, 1974) and more recent studies showing that schizophrenia patients fail to exhibit the normal pattern of increased cerebral blood flow in the frontal lobe during WCST performance (e.g., Berman, Illowsky, & Weinberger, 1988; Weinberger, Berman, & Illowsky, 1988). Thus, there is considerable evidence that patients with schizophrenia perform poorly on this test, and that patients who perform poorly have abnormal frontal lobe functioning. Taken together, this evidence suggests that the WCST may be a useful measure of frontal lobe integrity.

Based on the suggestion that both WCST and startle inhibition may depend on frontal lobe function, Butler, Jenkins, Geyer, and Braff (1991) tested the hypothesis that schizophrenia patients who exhibit increased perseverative errors on the WCST would exhibit reduced startle inhibition. All of the participants were administered the standard WCST and underwent a startle modification paradigm. The results of this study confirmed that the patients exhibited significantly more perseverative error responses on the WCST compared with the normal controls. When the patients were subdivided into two subgroups, impaired and nonimpaired WCST performers, the impaired group consistently exhibited less startle inhibition compared with the nonimpaired group. However, as noted by the authors, this was true only for tactile-elicited startle, and statistical confirmation of this finding was deferred as the subgroup sample sizes were quite small. Although this finding is indirect and tentative, it provides additional support for the notion that startle inhibition and WCST share a common underlying neurophysiological basis, and leaves open the possibility that these measures may reflect a common underlying inhibitory process as well.

6. Behavioral Measures of Thought Disorder ("Ego Impairment Index")

The Ego Impairment Index is a measure of thought disorder derived from the Rorschach Inkblot Test. This index was developed by Perry and Viglione (1991) to assess ego impairment and disorganized thinking ("formal thought disorder") without relying on patients' accurate self-report and description of their behavior. As pointed out by Perry and Viglione (1991), it is often difficult to assess thought disorder in schizophrenia because to do so patients must be willing to openly discuss their thoughts. Thus, these authors argue it is useful to employ several assessment instruments to evaluate both thought process and content in order to best characterize thought disorder.

6.1. Theoretical Interpretation

The Ego Impairment Index yields six variables, with the variable of greatest interest for the present discussion being the "human experience variable." The responses on the human experience variable are labeled "good" and "poor" based on an extensive literature pertaining to typical subjects' Rorschach responses (see Perry & Viglione, 1991, for an overview). It is important to point out that "good" or "poor" does not imply any ethical value judgment, it is simply a comparison to normative responding. An example of a good human experience response might be, "two people lifting something, two people dancing . . . two insects trying to pull a stick" (Exner, 1986, cited in Perry & Viglione, 1991). In contrast, an example of a poor human experience response is, "Siamese twins, you can see the blood flowing between them." Poor responses on the Ego Impairment Index are hypothesized to reflect a loss in the normal ability to inhibit or gate intrusive or irrelevant cognitive or emotional information.

6.2. Comparison with Startle Inhibition

As discussed earlier (see also Chapter 11), deficits in startle inhibition are thought to reflect a deficit in sensorimotor gating, the ability to inhibit or gate intrusive or irrelevant sensory, motor, or cognitive information. This deficit is in turn hypothesized to render schizophrenic patients vulnerable to cognitive fragmentation, which in turn may lead to thought disorder and other signs and symptoms characteristic of the schizophrenia spectrum of disorders (Braff & Geyer, 1990). If this view is accurate, there should be a relationship between startle inhibition and thought disorder such that greater reductions in startle inhibition should be associated with more severe levels of thought disorder.

To examine this issue, Perry and Braff (1994) examined the relationship between startle inhibition and several measures of thought disorder including the Ego Impairment Index described above. The results showed that in schizophrenia patients, thought disorder, as assessed by the Ego Impairment Index, was indeed correlated with short lead interval startle inhibition. That is, schizophrenia patients who exhibited poor human experience responses on the Ego Impairment Index showed less startle inhibition than patients exhibiting less thought disorder. Moreover, of all of the variables included in this study, the startle inhibition measure was the single best predictor of thought disorder on the Ego Impairment Index (accounting for 18% of the total variance in the poor responses). More recently, Perry and Braff (1996) have reported correlations between the Ego Impairment Index and startle inhibition measured concurrently in a new cohort of schizophrenia patients (correlations range between −.54 and −.85). These preliminary findings provide additional support for the suggestion that the inhibitory deficits reflected by reduced startle inhibition might be responsible for a patient's inability to screen irrelevant sensory stimuli and thoughts from intruding into consciousness

7. Conclusion

As noted in the introduction to this chapter, increasing our understanding of the cognitive significance of startle modification represents an important direction for future research, and one fruitful strategy for this research lies in the examination of relationships between startle modification and other measures that share similar theoretical interpretations. This chapter focused on the relationship of short lead interval startle inhibition to three cognitive measures: attentional blink, negative priming, and visual backward masking; a neuropsychological measure, the Wisconsin Card Sorting Task; and a thought-disorder measure, the Ego Impairment Index. For each measure we attempted to evaluate the similarities and differences across time course, task characteristics, and clinical findings, to explore the possibility that the behavioral and startle measures reflect a common underlying inhibitory process, share a common neurophysiological basis, or both.

Review of the evidence regarding the relationship of startle inhibition measures to the attentional blink, negative priming, and backward-masking measures reveals several intriguing similarities as well as several important differences. The hypothesized inhibitory processes reflected by each of the behavioral measures occurs over a time window remarkably similar to the window for short lead interval startle inhibition. Moreover, for two of these measures, negative priming and backward masking, there are clinical findings to parallel those obtained with startle inhibition measures; clinical populations who exhibit reduced startle inhibition exhibit response patterns on backward masking and negative priming tasks that are consistent with reduced inhibition. Such parallels have yet to be tested for the attentional blink measures.

Despite these similarities, the differences among these measures weaken the suggestion that they may reflect a common underlying inhibitory process. One important difference is the fact that the behavioral measures reviewed appear to be primarily visual phenomena (particularly with respect to attentional blink and negative priming), whereas startle inhibition occurs regardless of stimulus modality. A second critical difference is the fact that startle inhibition is viewed as a low-level, automatic process that occurs regardless of attention or resource availability, whereas all of the behavioral measures require controlled attentional processes because participants must generate a voluntary verbal or manual response. Although attention can clearly increase startle inhibition, indicating an influence of controlled attentional processing on startle inhibition, controlled processing is not required for inhibition to occur (Chapters 3 and 7).

Despite these differences, it is important to note that even if the behavioral measures do not reflect precisely the same inhibitory processes as do the startle inhibition measures, they may still contribute significantly to our understanding of startle inhibition. For example, these measures provide support for the existence of low-level inhibitory processes and suggest that such processes play an important role in both simple and complex information processing. Our understanding of the cognitive significance of startle inhibition can benefit significantly from the knowledge gained about these behavioral measures, each of which is currently receiving a great deal of empirical attention, and the role they play in information processing.

In terms of the relationship between startle inhibition and the two clinical measures, the significance of the evidence reviewed is twofold. First, the evidence relating startle inhibition and the WCST provides further support for the hypothesis that these measures share a common underlying neurophysiological basis, dependent on the frontal lobes. Second, the correlational findings in schizophrenia patients relating startle inhibition to WCST and startle inhibition to thought disorder on the Ego Impairment Index constitute the clearest link to date between the low-level inhibitory process reflected by startle and higher level cognition. As reports of clinical populations with deficient startle inhibition continue to accumulate, finding and understanding such links becomes increasingly important. To this end, the findings reviewed in this chapter underscore the importance of interrelating startle inhibition measures with a variety of other cognitive and/or clinical measures to increase our understanding of the implications of both normal and aberrant startle inhibition for everyday cognition.

CHAPTER FOURTEEN

Event-Related Potential Components and Startle

JUDITH M. FORD AND WALTON T. ROTH

ABSTRACT

This chapter considers how the P50, N1, and P300 components of the auditory event-related brain potential (ERP) are related to startle. Although both blink and ERPs can be elicited by startling noises, blinks are muscular and ERPs are neural. Comparing startle blinks and ERPs reveals at what point the neural processes supporting them diverge. Each ERP component is evaluated against variables known to affect startle-stimulus intensity, stimulus rise time, habituation, and leading stimuli presented at both short and long lead intervals. ERPs recorded in startle modification paradigms suggest that the relationship between startle blinks and ERPs is weak. P50, N1, and P300 are all inhibited by short lead intervals, but with different time courses from startle; only the fronto-central P300 is facilitated with long lead intervals.

1. Introduction

Psychophysiologists tend to specialize. Those who study event-related brain potentials (ERPs) usually do not study startle, perhaps because startle produces tremendous blinks and muscle contraction "artifacts" on the scalp, often much larger than ERPs. Yet startling stimuli elicit ERPs, and by comparing blinks and ERPs elicited by startling stimuli, we will learn about the dependence and interdependence of the neural pathways that support these two responses.

1.1. Developments Encouraging Study of Startle with ERPs

Two developments have encouraged looking at ERPs in conjunction with startle. First, parallels have been observed between startle modification and

Michael E. Dawson, Anne M. Schell, and Andreas H. Böhmelt, Eds. *Startle modification: Implications for neuroscience, cognitive science, and clinical science.* Copyright © 1999 Cambridge University Press. Printed in the United States of America. All rights reserved.

suppression of P50; schizophrenics have been found to differ from normals in both startle inhibition by lead stimuli at short lead intervals and P50 suppression (Chapter 11). Second, although blinks generate broad positive electrical fields that decrease in amplitude from the front to the back of the head, investigators have begun to use mathematical subtraction algorithms to remove the artifactual effects of blinks and eye movements from scalp-recorded ERPs (see Gratton, Coles, & Donchin, 1983; Miller, Gratton, & Yee, 1988; Brunia, Mocks, & van den Berg-Lenssen, 1989). The positive startle blink field peaks at about 100 msec, just when the N1 component of the ERP peaks. Without removal of blink artifacts, the positive voltages of the blink and the negative voltages of N1 can cancel each other out at the scalp.

1.2. Possible Relationships between Startle and ERP

In this chapter we will consider how three commonly studied auditory ERP components, P50, N1, and P300, are related to startle by evaluating each against variables known to affect startle. A strong relationship would be demonstrated if a certain ERP component is always present when startle occurs and always absent when startle does not occur. That is, parameters that determine startle should determine the amplitude of the ERP component. Also, the ERP component should be associated with startle rather than with an orienting or defensive response to the startle stimulus. A weaker relationship would be demonstrated if an ERP component parallels startle only under certain circumstances. These relationships are best demonstrated when both blinks and ERPs are measured simultaneously.

A strong relationship is unlikely between startle and any of the three ERP components we have chosen to investigate because all of them can be elicited by auditory stimuli whose intensity is far below the startle threshold. Yet each has been thought to be similar to startle in certain ways. P50 is affected similarly by lead stimuli (e.g., Freedman, Adler, & Waldo, 1987), N1 reacts similarly to tone rise time (e.g., Putnam & Roth, 1990), and P300 becomes obligatory (see below) at stimulus intensities above the startle threshold (e.g., Roth, Dorato, & Kopell, 1984). These partial parallels may reveal something about processes that are associated with startle.

Few studies have simultaneously recorded ERPs and startle. First, few ERP experiments have employed stimuli intense enough to elicit startle, even on the first stimulus presentation. Second, until recently, trials on which startle was elicited were routinely discarded as "contaminated" by blink. Third, the emphasis on the cognitive correlates of ERP components have diverted investigators away from experiments where "simple" stimulus parameters relevant to startle were manipulated. By necessity, we will include in our review studies where startle was not measured, and probably not elicited, but in which parameters affecting startle were varied (Chapter 2).

2. Parameters Affecting Startle

In brief, stimulus intensity (generally greater than 70 dB) and stimulus rise time (generally less than 45 msec) are important determinants of startle. Also, with even one repetition of the stimulus, startle tends to habituate. Lead stimuli have complex effects, with inhibition at short lead intervals (~100 msec; Chapter 3) and facilitation or inhibition with longer intervals (approximately 2–4 s; Chapter 4). Because startle modification occurs with crossmodal stimuli, it cannot be the result of simple neural refractory effects, receptor fatigue, or homosynaptic depression (Graham & Murray, 1977).

3. How Startle Parameters Affect ERP Components

ERPs are time-locked changes in the brain's electrical activity as observed in the electroencephalogram (EEG). ERPs allow a continuous, millisecond-to-millisecond assessment of brain activity related to sensory, cognitive, and motor processing. The progression of processing can be ascertained by inspection of the various peaks and valleys (components) in the ERP waveform. The peaks and valleys are named according to polarity and latency. For example, P50 is a positive peak occurring 50 msec poststimulus. When stimuli are presented close together, their ERPs can overlap. However, a subtraction technique makes it possible to remove components of the ERP to the first stimulus (S1) from the ERP to the second stimulus (S2). ERPs to the S1 in isolation, or unpaired, are subtracted from the ERP to the same stimulus when paired (for a more elaborate application of this methodology, see Woldorff, 1993).

ERP evidence relevant to lead stimulus effects often comes from paradigms where stimulus intensities are equal, and stimuli are given in trains rather than in pairs separated by much longer intervals. The P50 component of the ERP is an exception, since it has been studied extensively in paired click presentation. N1, however, is more often elicited to stimuli presented in trains with the length of the lead interval being varied across blocks. Davis, Mast, Yoshie, and Zerlin (1966) found that for N1-P2 amplitude,[1] the effects

---

[1] N1 is often measured relative to a subsequent positive peak, P2, and called N1-P2.

of lead intervals in paired stimuli were comparable to the effects of constant stimulus onset asynchrony. Cardenas, McCallin, Hopkins, and Fein (1997) compared P50 amplitudes elicited by clicks in pairs and in repetitive trains and found that lead interval length had the same magnitude of effect when clicks were presented in clicks or in trains. We will refer to stimulus onset asynchrony as lead interval, even in paradigms using repetitive trains.

4. The P50 Component

P50 is a positive-going component that peaks about 50 msec after the onset of an auditory stimulus. It should not be confused with P30 which is not affected by lead stimuli (Perlstein, Fiorito, Simons, & Graham, 1993). Although it may depend on subcortical structures for its elicitation (Woods, Clayworth, Knight, Simpson, & Naeser, 1987; Bickford-Wimer et al., 1989), P50 is probably generated in superficial temporal sites (Knight, Scabini, Woods, & Clayworth, 1988; Reite, Teale, Zimmerman, Davis, Whalen, & Edrich, 1988). It is largest at the vertex, or central midline scalp site (Cz).

4.1. Stimulus Intensity

P50 amplitude increases with stimulus intensity from 60, 77, and 95 dB (Kaskey, Salzman, Klorman, & Pass, 1980). From 75 to 110 dB, there appears to be a four-fold increase in P50 (Table 6 in Perlstein et al., 1993).

4.2. Stimulus Rise Time

Kodera, Hink, Yamada, and Suzuki (1979) showed P50 amplitude decreases with increases in rise times of 5, 10, and 20 msec.

4.3. Habituation

Polich, Aung, and Dalessio (1988) delivered 30-, 50-, and 70-dB tones at interstimulus intervals of 1, 3, and 5 s, in four blocks of 16 tones each. They reported "only minor changes across the four trial blocks" for either amplitude or latency of N1 or P50,[2] which they called P1.

---

[2] Investigators using repetitive trains of stimuli have called P50 P1, although it is most likely the same component (Erwin & Buchwald, 1986).

4.4. Lead Stimulus Effects

The P50 response to S2 is smaller than the P50 to S1 of a pair, which is referred to as P50 suppression. P50 suppression is obtained with a tactile stimulus as S1 and a startling tone as S2, suggesting that P50 suppression, like startle-blink modification, is not simply due to refractory effects (Simons & Perlstein, 1996).

4.4.1. Short Lead Intervals

P50 suppression has been reported at various intervals. Nagamoto, Adler, Waldo, and Freedman (1989) compared P50 suppression with 75-, 125-, and 500-msec lead intervals and showed a direct relationship between P50 amplitude and lead interval, suggesting that simple refractory effects could be operating. However, arguing against simple refractory effects are data from other studies showing nonmonotonic relationships between P50 amplitude and lead intervals. In a later study, Nagamoto, Adler, Waldo, Griffith, and Freedman (1991) failed to find greater suppression with a 100- than a 500-msec lead interval (see their fig. 3). Additionally, a more recent study extended the lead interval down to 60 msec, and instead of finding greater suppression with a 60- than a 360-msec lead interval, the authors found just the opposite (Simons & Perlstein, 1996).

Pilot data from ten young subjects studied in our own laboratory also suggest that P50 suppression is not simply a refractory effect. We recorded ERPs during a startle modification paradigm described in Figure 14.1. Apparent in Figure 14.2 is a tendency for P50 to be suppressed with the 500-msec ($p < .10$, two-tailed) but not with the 120-msec lead interval at Cz ($p < .75$). This is weak support for other reports showing a nonmonotonic relationship between lead interval and amplitude.

4.4.2. Long Lead Intervals

The effect of long lead intervals on P50 amplitude is important in determining whether P50 behaves like startle. We are not aware of any published data showing an enhancement of P50 amplitude with long lead intervals, like startle blink. Adler, Pachtman, Franks, Pecevich, Waldo, and Freedman (1982) compared P50 amplitudes at lead intervals of 500, 1000, and 2000 msec and found more P50 suppression at a 500-msec lead interval than at 1000- and 2000-msec lead intervals, but there was no evidence of response enhancement with a 2-s lead interval. Our pilot data mentioned above, and shown in Figure 14.2, are ambiguous; at Fz, P50 appears larger when the noise is preceded by the 4-s continuous tone than when presented alone, but not at Cz. P50 should not be

Events

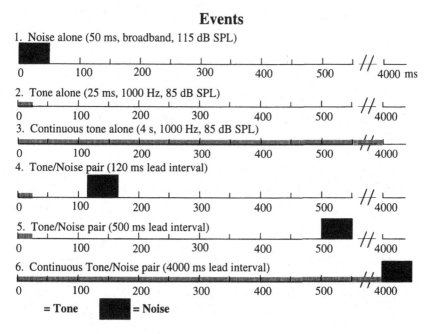

Figure 14.1. Schematic of paradigm indicates that there were six event types: noise alone, tone alone, 4-s continuous tone alone, noise preceded 120 ms by the tone, noise preceded 500 msec by the tone, and noise preceded by the continuous tone. These event types occurred in a pseudo-random sequence, with 14- to 18-s interevent intervals.

affected by any increase in alertness resulting from the long lead interval because alertness does not affect P50 (Adler et al., 1982). Involving subjects in discrimination tasks also does not affect P50 to unpaired clicks (Guterman, Josiassen, & Bashore, 1992) or to S1 clicks (Jerger, Biggins, & Fein, 1992). A discrimination or motor task may (Guterman et al., 1992) or may not (Jerger et al., 1992) reduce the amount of P50 suppression to S2. In any case, unlike startle, attention does not *increase* the amplitude of P50 at long lead intervals.

4.5. Studies Comparing P50 Suppression and Blink Modification

Other investigators have taken a different approach to the question of whether P50 suppression is similar to startle modification by recording both P50 and startle blink in the same experiment. Schwarzkopf, Lamberti, and Smith (1993) studied the effects of lead stimuli on startle blinks and P50 in the same subjects but not with the same stimulus intervals; that is, for startle-blink modification, they used the lead interval that is typically used (120 msec), and for

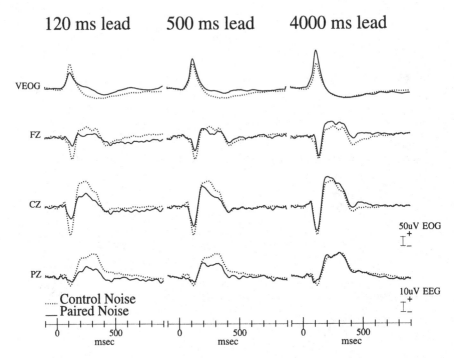

Figure 14.2. Grand average waveforms are shown for responses to noises when presented alone (dotted line) or when preceded by a leading stimulus with a 120-, 500-, or 4000-msec lead interval. The leading stimulus for the shorter lead intervals was a 25-msec tone, and for the long lead interval it was a 4000-msec continuous tone. Blinks seen in the VEOG tracing have been mathematically removed from the recordings from the frontal (Fz), central (Cz), and parietal (Pz) sites. Positivity is plotted up.

P50 suppression, they also used the lead interval that is typically used (500 msec). They reported only a weak within-subject positive association between the amount of startle blink inhibition and the amount of P50 suppression, an association that disappeared when P50 amplitude to S1 was factored out. Instead, they reported the amount of decrement in startle response over the course of the experiment was related to the amount of P50 suppression. P50 amplitude, not P50 suppression, was related to startle modification such that large P50 amplitudes were related to larger amounts of startle modification.

Although Perlstein et al. (1993) were not explicitly studying the relationship between P50 suppression and startle-blink modification, their study does allow some comparison of these physiological responses. They recorded P50 suppression and startle-blink inhibition in the same subjects, but used a 120-msec lead interval in one group of subjects and a 500-msec lead interval in another. S1 was always low-intensity (75 dB) and S2 could be either low- or high- (110 dB) intensity. Unlike Schwarzkopf et al. (1993), Perlstein et al. (1993) used both eye-movement correction procedures and component overlap subtraction procedures. To the high-intensity tones, startle-blink amplitude was reduced by 66% with the 120-msec lead interval and 24% with the 500-msec lead interval; P50 amplitude appeared to be reduced equivalently at both lead intervals. Although the amount of P50 suppression was not statistically compared with the amount of startle-blink inhibition, it would appear that with the two lead intervals used, the amount of modification of P50 and startle blink is different.

Our pilot study with ten subjects mentioned above directly compares P50 and blink amplitudes with different lead intervals. In these subjects, blink was inhibited at 120 but not 500 msec. Conversely, P50 was suppressed at 500 but not at 120 msec. Although these data are preliminary, they suggest that P50 suppression and startle-blink inhibition behave very differently. Furthermore, the amount of P50 suppression at 500 msec and the amount of startle modification at 120 msec were not positively or significantly correlated in these ten subjects.

4.6. Summary

P50 suppression must be a very distant cousin of startle modification, if related at all. P50 amplitude suppression is like that of startle in that it occurs with crossmodal stimulation, but the effective lead intervals for inhibiting blink and P50 are very different. Unfortunately, data on P50 enhancement with long lead intervals are incomplete. If startle enhancement with long lead intervals results from enhanced alertness, these effects may not occur with P50, which has been shown to be unaffected by alertness. The most damaging results for arguments identifying P50 suppression with startle-blink inhibition are reports of no within-subject relationship between P50 suppression and startle-blink inhibition.

The lack of close association between P50 suppression and startle modification is hardly surprising given the different stimulus characteristics (usually clicks vs. noises), different responses (cortical vs. muscular), and different optimal lead intervals (120 vs. 500 msec). Even when elicited by the same stimuli using the same lead intervals, P50 suppression and startle-blink modification do not appear to be related (Perlstein et al., 1993). Our pilot study suggests that P50 suppression and startle modification are not related when recorded from the same subjects, to the same stimuli, with the same lead intervals, in a task-free paradigm.

5. The N1 Component

In their review of N1, Näätänen and Picton (1987) concluded that at least six different cerebral processes can contribute to N1, all occurring between 50 and 150 msec poststimulus onset. Because they overlap, they are usually not distinguished in experimental studies. According to Näätänen and Picton, it is most likely the first and third subcomponents of the N1 that are affected by lead interval, but in different ways.[3] Component 1 peaks at 100 msec and is maximal fronto-centrally, is affected by intensity, and is fast-recovering, that is, it has a relative refractory period of 4 s or slightly longer. It is considered to be relatively modality-specific, emanating from primary auditory cortex. Component 3 is maximal centrally, is most easily elicited by intense sounds, and is slow-recovering, that is, it has a relative refractory period of 30 s. It is considered to be relatively modality-nonspecific, emanating from widespread generators that involve diffuse polysensory cortical systems. Simons and Perlstein (1997) suggest that component 1 is like P30 and is directly related to lead interval, while component 3 is like P50 and sensitive to leading stimuli.

5.1. Stimulus Intensity

A fast-recovering N1 component that fails to grow in amplitude with increasing loudness is probably component 1. A slow-recovering component that does grow with increasing loudness is probably component 3 (Näätänen & Picton, 1987). In the Perlstein et al. (1993) study described above, both P50 and N1 to high-intensity tones mirrored loudness, but P50 and N1 to low-intensity tones did not.

5.2. Stimulus Rise Time

Like startle, the amplitude of component 3 peak is sensitive to rise time, being larger to sounds with faster rise times (Kodera et al., 1979; Loveless & Brunia, 1990; Putnam & Roth, 1990).

5.3. Habituation

N1 amplitude to intense noises appears to habituate over 60 trials, broken into four blocks of 15 each when presented at a constant interstimulus interval of

---

[3] Component 2 is best recorded over temporal regions of the scalp and is biphasic with a positive element followed by a larger negativity between 120 and 165 msec. This component is not relevant to this discussion.

8.4 s (Putnam & Roth, 1990). This is in contrast to the report of Polich et al. (1988) for N1s recorded to 70-dB tones, using interstimulus intervals of 1, 3, and 5 s. Perhaps component 3 was elicited by Putnam and Roth, and component 1 by Polich et al. Based on the habituation curves and responsiveness to rise time, Putnam and Roth (1990) concluded that N1 was similar to startle.

5.4. Lead Stimulus Effects

Like startle blink and P50, component 3 of N1 to startling noises is modified by both ipsi- and crossmodal lead stimuli (Simons & Perlstein, 1996). All other studies mentioned below involved only ipsimodal stimuli.

5.4.1. Short Lead Intervals

Many studies showing monotonic associations between lead interval and N1 amplitude used nonstartling noises and did not remove component overlap (e.g., Davis et al., 1966; Schall, Schön, Zerbin, Effers, & Oades, 1996), although monotonic relationships have also been seen when component overlap was removed and when startling tones (Perlstein et al., 1993) or noises were used (our pilot data in Fig. 14.2). Furthermore, nonmonotonic relationships are also seen when startling tones were used and component overlap is removed. Simons and Perlstein (1996) found a nonmonotonic relationship using startling tones: larger N1s at the short (60 msec) than at the long (360 msec) lead interval. Budd and Michie (1994) have also shown N1 amplitude to be nonmonotonically related to lead interval. They presented subjects with 80-dB tones at lead intervals varying randomly from 100 to 1000 msec and found that N1 was enhanced at lead intervals less than 300 msec, intervals where blink is suppressed.

Reconciling findings of monotonic and nonmonotonic relationships between N1 amplitude and lead interval cannot hinge on the startle-eliciting stimulus properties or component overlap. Perhaps differences are related to how the stimuli were presented and perceived. Budd and Michie presented moderate-intensity tones in a continuous though uneven train, perhaps resulting in "perceptual streaming" of tones occurring very close together. This would make meaningful comparisons difficult between the Budd and Michie data and data collected in pairs or regular repetitive trains.

5.4.2. Long Lead Intervals

Except for our pilot studies, none of the studies mentioned above was designed to observe response facilitation of N1 with long lead intervals. As can be seen in Figure 14.2, unlike blink amplitude, N1 amplitude was not facilitated with the 4-s continuous tone. This is especially interesting considering that the 4-s continuous tone is an alerting stimulus, and N1 has been repeatedly shown to be affected by arousal and alertness (Näätänen & Picton, 1987). Possibly N1 elicited by startling noises, in contrast to N1 elicited by innocuous tones, is completely obligatory and cannot be affected by attention.

5.5. Direct Comparisons of N1 and Startle-Blink Modification

In our pilot study, we found that, unlike blinks, N1 was reduced at both 120- and 500-msec lead intervals, and was significantly more reduced at the shorter interval (Fig. 14.2).

5.6. Summary

N1 amplitude has a number of similarities to startle blink. It increases with increases in loudness, it decreases with increases in stimulus rise time, and its course of habituation is similar to startle. When elicited by substartle threshold sounds, it is affected by the direction of attention. In these ways N1 is a close cousin of startle blink, as proposed by Putnam and Roth (1990). The effects of lead stimuli on N1, however, suggest it is quite different from startle. Although N1 is inhibited by crossmodal lead stimuli, the effects of lead interval length on N1 and startle are very different. Blink is not suppressed at 500-msec lead intervals but N1 is. The studies reported by Budd and Michie (1994) and Simons and Perlstein (1996) report curvilinear relationships between lead interval and N1, with the break in the lead-interval function occurring at 300 msec in the Budd and Michie study and between 60 and 360 msec in the Simons and Perlstein study. If the break is at 300 msec, as suggested by the Budd and Michie study, we would have to conclude that N1 is not inhibited at the same lead intervals as startle blink; if the break is at 120 msec, then we would conclude that it is. Without finer gradations in paired stimulus paradigms, we cannot know where the inhibition is maximal for N1. Our pilot data suggest that unlike startle blink, N1 is not facilitated with long lead intervals.

6. The P300 Component

Although P300 is often defined by its reliance on attention (Donchin & Coles, 1988; Verleger, 1988), it can be elicited in passive situations when no task is assigned (Ford, Roth, & Kopell, 1976), especially by salient stimuli such as loud noises. Some investigators divide P300 into a parietally maximal P3b, elicited during active attention, and a more frontally distributed P3a, elicited in passive situations. Although the P300 elicited by startling noises could be P3a, it also shares some characteristics with the classical P3b. First, both are augmented by attention (Roth et al., 1984; Ford, Roth, Isaacks, Tinklenberg, Yesavage, & Pfefferbaum, 1997). Second, the amplitude of a noise-elicited P300 has the same scalp distribution as a tone-elicited P300 in paradigms requiring an active button-press response (Ford et al., 1996).

Possibly P3a and P3b are both activated when a salient stimulus is given target status. P3a might be elicited by any salient stimulus, and P3b might be added when that stimulus is task-relevant. Neuroanatomical data support the P3a/P3b distinction: A noise stimulus that is irrelevant to the task elicits a P300 whose amplitude depends on the volume of the gray matter in the frontal lobes, while a noise stimulus that is relevant to the task elicits a P300 whose amplitude depends on the volumes of both the frontal and parietal lobe gray matter (Ford, Sullivan, Marsh, White, Lim, & Pfefferbaum, 1994).

Because we are not certain whether a startling noise elicits P3a or P3b or both, we choose to remain agnostic in this chapter and refer to the noise-elicited late positive component as P300.

6.1. Stimulus Intensity

Parietal P300 amplitude increases with stimulus intensity (Roth et al., 1984) and duration (Putnam & Roth, 1990). Because blink showed a steady rise with durations ranging from 3, 10, 30, and 90 msec and P300 showed an abrupt rise from 30- to 90-msec durations, Putnam and Roth concluded that parietal P300 does not reflect the same processes as startle blink.

6.2. Stimulus Rise Time

Putnam and Roth (1990) also found that P300 at Pz did not obey the same rise-time function as blink. While blink increased in amplitude with decreases in rise time from 45, 30, 15, to 3 msec, P300 amplitude did not. This was one more piece of evidence suggesting that P300 and startle blink are different.

6.3. Habituation

Putnam and Roth (1990) recorded responses to intense noises in four blocks of 15 trials each. P300 amplitude decreased from the first to the second block and then partially recovered for the third and fourth block. Startle blink showed a strong linear trend, decreasing across blocks. Again, P300 and startle blink diverge.

6.4. Lead Stimulus Effects

Because noise-elicited P300s have both exogenous and endogenous features, its modulation by a brain-stem circuit (Chapter 5) is especially interesting.

6.4.1. Short Lead Intervals

Using a paired-stimulus paradigm with nonstartling tones, Schall and Ward (1996) presented target and nontarget stimuli that were preceded 500 or 100 msec by a click. Although the authors did not report a statistical comparison of the P300s elicited in these pairings, the waveforms in their Figure 2 suggest that P300 was inhibited equally with the 100- and 500-msec lead intervals. Sugawara, Sadeghpour, de Traversay, and Ornitz (1994) compared the effects of 60- and 120-msec lead intervals on ERPs to startling noises in normal 9-year-old boys. P300 recorded at Cz was not inhibited with the 60-msec lead interval, but was with 120 msec. In the pilot study mentioned above, we compared the effects of 120- and 500-msec lead intervals on P300s to startling noises in adults at frontal (Fz), central (Cz), and parietal (Pz) sites. Especially at Pz (see Fig. 14.2), there was more reduction at the 120- than at the 500-msec interval, as would be expected if refractory period effects are operating.

Woods and Courchesne (1986) studied the recovery period of the target P300. Each trial contained three tones (high- and low-pitch) within a 2-s period; the interval between the first and second tones could be 500, 1000, and 1500 msec. Subjects were asked to press a button to either the high- or low-pitch tones. The remarkable finding in this study was that three P300s could be elicited in a 1500-msec period, suggesting that P300 generators had very short refractory periods. The P300 elicited with a 500-msec lead interval was smaller than those elicited with the 1000- and 1500-msec intervals, which resulted in equivalent P300s[4] suggesting a very fast psychological refractory period for P300. Not known is whether three startle stimuli presented in rapid succession would all elicit a P300.

6.4.2. Long Lead Intervals

To demonstrate response facilitation in 9-year-old boys, Sugawara et al. (1994) delivered a 4000-msec continuous tone before presenting the noise with no silence between the tone and the noise. They found that P300 at Cz was facilitated by the 4000-msec tone. Our pilot data suggest a similar trend for Fz and Cz, but not for Pz. Given the sensitivity of the parietal P300 to attention, alert-

---

[4] It is noteworthy that N1 and P2 needed longer lead intervals to recover than did P300, suggesting that P300 is associated with high-speed cognitive operations, being fully recovered by 1000 msec.

ness, and arousal (Polich & Kok, 1995), it is surprising that we are not finding that P300 amplitude is enhanced by the long lead interval stimulus.

6.5. Direct Comparisons of P300 and Startle Modification

The work of Sugawara et al. and our work allow the direct comparison of P300 and startle modification, and both laboratories report some important dissociations. Sugawara et al. reported that startle blink was inhibited with both 60- and 120-msec lead intervals, but P300 was inhibited only with the 120-msec lead interval. We showed that blinks were reduced with the 120-msec lead interval but not the 500-msec interval, and that P300 amplitudes at Fz, Cz, and Pz were reduced at both intervals. Dissociations are seen between startle and P300 modification at Pz with 4-s continuous lead stimuli in adults: Blink is enhanced, but P300 is not.

6.6. Summary

P300 is not affected by experimental variables in the same way as startle. Putnam and Roth (1990) concluded that the parietal P300 is similar to startle in its relation to loudness, less similar in terms of habituation, and dissimilar in being insensitive to stimulus rise time. The effects of lead interval are further evidence against their similarity. Startle and both frontal and parietal P300s do not respond to short lead intervals in the same way. Whether P300 is facilitated with longer lead intervals remains to be demonstrated in a larger group of adult subjects. Early evidence from our ten adult subjects suggests that P300 recorded at frontal and central sites is facilitated.

Attention toward the lead stimulus increases the amount of short lead interval inhibition of startle and increases long lead interval facilitation if the lead stimulus and startle stimulus are in the same modality. The effects of attention on P300 modification by a leading stimulus have not been studied. Such studies are needed to further explore the overlap between the processes responsible for startle and P300 modification by leading stimuli.

Table 14.1 outlines effects relevant to startle and summarizes the discussion of individual ERP components mostly elicited by noises.

7. Conclusion

The relationship between startle and ERPs is a weak one. While there are similarities, there are also dissimilarities. On the one hand, except for the fronto-central P300, none of the ERP components was significantly facilitated at

Table 14.1. *Similarities between Startle Blink and ERP Components*

Amplitude Effects	Blink	P50	N1	P300
Increase with loudness?	Yes[15,5a]	Yes[12]	Yes[14]	Yes[15]
Decrease with rise time?	Yes[14]	Yes[8]	Yes[14]	No[14]
Decrease with habituation?	Yes[14]	Yes[13]	Yes[14] No[13]	No[14]
Cross-modal inhibition?	Yes[12]	Yes[12]	Yes[12]	?
Inhibition by lead stimulus:				
Amplitude smaller with	Yes[12,5]	Yes[10]	Yes[4,12]	Yes[4]
shorter than longer lead intervals?		Yes[4,17,11]	Yes[2,17]	No[16]
Facilitation by lead stimulus:				
Amplitude greater with	Yes[5]	?	No[4]	Yes
long lead interval than unpaired?				(at Cz)[4,18]
Increase with attention or alertness?	Yes[5]	Yes[6]	Yes[9] No[1,7]	No[3,15]

[a] Numbers refer to the following reports: (1) Adler et al., 1982; (2) Budd and Michie, 1994; (3) Ford, et al., 1996; (4) Ford and Roth, pilot data presented in this chapter; (5) Graham, 1975; (6) Guterman et al., 1992; (7) Jerger et al., 1992; (8) Kodera et al., 1979; (9) Näätänen and Picton, 1987; (10) Nagamoto et al., 1989; (11) Nagamoto et al., 1991; (12) Perlstein et al., 1993; (13) Polich et al., 1988; (14) Putnam and Roth, 1990; (15) Roth et al., 1984; (16) Schall and Ward, 1996; (17) Simons and Perlstein, 1997; (18) Sugawara et al., 1993.

long lead intervals like startle. On the other hand, each component was inhibited at short lead intervals but with different time courses from each other and from startle blink. For example, while blink is maximally inhibited with a 120-msec lead interval, inhibition is maximal for P50 with a 500-msec lead interval and for N1 with an approximately 300-msec lead interval. The difference in time courses of inhibition does not follow the latency of the component; N1, which occurs after P50, is maximally inhibited at shorter lead intervals than in P50. Clearly, the neural paths that support startle-elicited blinks and ERPs diverge very early, perhaps by 50 msec.

Investigation of the relationship between startle and ERPs is still in a very early stage. A component specifically reflecting the firing of startle circuitry may be very small on the scalp compared with even P50, the smallest of the three components we considered. Yet well-designed and carefully analyzed experiments might be able to prove the existence of such a component at the scalp. Furthermore, the use of probe stimuli to assess direction of attention and the allotment of attentional resources before and after startle stimuli has yet to be exploited. Such probe experiments might shed light on the nature of the facilitation effects produced by continuous lead stimuli. Methodological advances in the artifact-free measurement of ERPs and their complementary magnetic counterparts will pave the way for future progress.

ACKNOWLEDGMENTS

Work on this project was supported by the Department of Veterans Affairs, the National Institutes of Health (MH30854), and the National Institute of Mental Health (MH40052).

CHAPTER FIFTEEN

Startle Modification during Orienting and Pavlovian Conditioning

OTTMAR V. LIPP AND DAVID A. T. SIDDLE

ABSTRACT

Startle modification at long lead intervals has been assessed during orienting to signal stimuli and during Pavlovian conditioning to investigate attentional and emotional processes in humans. The results obtained in studies of orienting are not consistent with the assertion that startle is inhibited if attentional resources are allocated to a modality that is different from the one in which the startle-eliciting stimulus is presented. Research in Pavlovian conditioning that focused on the effects of emotion on startle modification has replicated the fear-potentiated startle effect observed in nonhuman animals. Research in both realms provides strong evidence that attentional and emotional processes interact to affect startle.

1. Introduction

Research on associative learning has undergone considerable change during the last 30 years. The conceptual framework has shifted from the notion that associative learning, and particularly Pavlovian conditioning, involves the formation of new stimulus–response connections to a position that asserts that the conditioned response is an indication that the organism has acquired new information (Mackintosh, 1983). Within this information-processing framework, there is an emphasis on the unexpectedness of the unconditional stimulus (Rescorla & Wagner, 1972), the extent to which the conditioned and unconditioned stimuli are primed in a short-term memory store (Wagner, 1978), the relative predictive accuracy of all cues (Mackintosh, 1974), the type of processing (automatic or controlled) that is devoted to the conditioned stimulus (CS) (Pearce & Hall, 1980; Dawson & Schell, 1985), and the nature

Michael E. Dawson, Anne M. Schell, and Andreas H. Böhmelt, Eds. *Startle modification: Implications for neuroscience, cognitive science, and clinical science.* Copyright © 1999 Cambridge University Press. Printed in the United States of America. All rights reserved.

of the attentional process underlying the processing of conditioned and unconditioned stimuli (Öhman, 1983, 1992).

The emphasis on cognitive processes and the neglect of emotional processes in theories of Pavlovian conditioning is somewhat surprising considering that most of the data on which these theories are based were gathered in conditioning procedures that used aversive unconditioned stimuli (USs). One of the most frequently employed conditioning procedures, the conditioned emotional response paradigm, assesses conditioning as the disruptive effect of a Pavlovian conditioned fear response on instrumental behavior. Although changes in behavior that are indicative of strong emotional responses such as fear are measured as an indication of learning, emotional processes have not generally been included in the theoretical analysis (but see Konorski, 1967). Nevertheless, emotional responses to the conditioned stimulus can be treated as one facet of the behavioral changes that occur during conditioning.

Baeyens and his colleagues (Baeyens, Eelen, & Crombez, 1995) have proposed distinct learning systems for evaluative or affective and propositional or signal learning that are said to follow different rules. Evaluative learning, the learning of likes and dislikes, is said to be governed by the referential system, a rather primitive system that does not require the involvement of cognitive factors. Propositional learning is said to reflect an expectancy system, which involves higher cortical processes (for a potential neurophysiological underpinning of this distinction, see LeDoux, 1990). Baeyens et al. proposed that the referential system follows rules that are different from those that govern signal learning. Evaluative learning is said to occur without awareness of the fact that CS and US are paired, to be affected by stimulus contiguity, but not contingency, and to be resistant to the standard extinction procedures of CS-only presentation. Baeyens et al. have gathered some empirical support for their proposal using paired presentations of pictures or flavors. Changes in affective valence are usually assessed with questionnaire measures. These studies have been criticized for a number of methodological weaknesses such as lack of control for nonassociative processes and demand characteristics associated with the use of questionnaire measures (Shanks & Dickinson, 1990; Davey, 1994). Moreover, the use of pre- and post-pairing questionnaire measures of affective valence does not allow the observation of the time course of change in affective valence during conditioning and places constraints on the design of experiments.

An empirical test of the role of emotional processes in human Pavlovian conditioning requires a measure that permits the tracking of affective changes across trials of conditioning. Research on human Pavlovian conditioning has relied primarily on physiological changes such as electrodermal responses or heart rate changes to index the complex attentional and processing changes thought to underlie this phenomenon. Although autonomic responses are sensitive indicators of conditioning in a wide variety of situations (for a review, see Öhman, 1983), this is not always the case. For example, autonomic measures do not differentiate between positively and negatively valent stimuli (Lang, Bradley, & Cuthbert, 1990) or between aversive and nonaversive conditioning (Lipp & Vaitl, 1990).

The startle probe technique might provide a valuable addition to the array of measures used in research on Pavlovian conditioning and, in particular, in studies that seek to evaluate the role of emotional and attentional processes. Probe startle has been shown to be a sensitive indicator of affective processes (Chapter 8). Startle elicited at long lead intervals during aversive lead stimuli is enhanced compared with startle elicited during pleasant stimuli. Moreover, probe startle at long lead intervals is also sensitive to attentional processes (Chapters 4 and 7), which are at the very center of any contemporary theory of Pavlovian conditioning (Hall, 1995). Thus, the startle probe technique may aid in a more complete understanding of the attentional and emotional processes observed during Pavlovian conditioning in humans.

Before discussing studies of conditioning that utilize the startle probe technique, we will review findings derived from research on orienting. Some contemporary theories (e.g., Wagner, 1978) suggest that a single information-processing framework can account for Pavlovian conditioning and habituation, and there is some evidence to support this approach (Siddle, 1991). Although information-processing theories of habituation differ in detail, they share the assumption that attentional processes are of central importance for the elicitation of orienting and for the occurrence of habituation. The nature of the attentional processes ranges from passive attention, which is thought to be at least partially automatic, to active selective attention that involves controlled processing (Graham & Hackley, 1991). Which attentional process is involved depends on whether subjects are presented with a simple sequence of habituation stimuli in the absence of an explicit task instruction or whether they are asked to perform a task with the stimuli. In either case, orienting is said to be related to the attentional resources that are allocated to the stimuli, and habituation is a consequence of the fact that fewer attentional resources are required to process a repeatedly presented stimulus (Siddle, 1991). Discussion of the effects of orienting on startle modification will be restricted to studies that have employed signal stimuli, that is, stimuli that were made significant by instruction. Graham (1992) and Putnam and Vanman (Chapter 4) have reviewed studies concerned with orienting and startle modification.

2. Startle Modification and Orienting to Signal Stimuli

Early studies of startle modification indicated enhancement of startle elicited about 2 s after the onset of a lead stimulus. Graham (1975, 1992) suggested that the orienting reflex that accompanies the processing of the lead stimulus is reflected in this enhancement of probe startle. It was reasoned that the extent of startle modification can be used as an index of the extent of attentional processing of a lead stimulus. The use of signal stimuli in such investigations was prompted by the assumption that attentional processing of signal stimuli, as indexed by orienting, does not decline as quickly as does processing of nonsignal stimuli. A series of experiments reviewed by Putnam (1990) provides an example.

Different groups of subjects were presented with stimuli from the auditory, visual, or tactile modalities. Subjects were asked to perform a speeded motor response to the offset of the stimulus. Acoustic startle probes were presented at varying lead intervals during the stimuli and during interstimulus intervals. In comparison with startle responses elicited during stimulus-free periods, startle elicited during tone signals was facilitated, whereas startle elicited during visual or tactile stimuli was inhibited. The extent of blink modification was largest to probes presented late during the signal stimuli. Discounting alternative explanations such as interference from the motor response, the results were interpreted as supporting an attentional account of startle modification. According to this account, startle is enhanced if elicited while attentional resources are allocated to the modality in which the startle-eliciting stimulus is presented. Thus, acoustic startle will be enhanced during tone signals, but inhibited during visual or tactile signals.

More recent findings by Filion, Dawson, and Schell (1993, 1994) are consistent with these results. Subjects were asked to perform a discrimination task by counting the number of longer-than-usual presentations of one tone stimulus and ignoring presentations of a second tone. To encourage cooperation, subjects earned a monetary reward if they could report the correct number of longer-than-usual tones. Acoustic startle probes were presented during some of the tone stimuli and during intertrial intervals. Startle probes presented at a lead interval of 2000 msec after tone onset elicited larger responses than did probes presented during intertone intervals. Moreover, startle to probes presented during relevant stimuli was larger than to probes presented during irrelevant stimuli, a result that is consistent with attentional accounts.

Recent findings from our laboratory, however, do not seem to be consistent with a modality-specific attentional account (Lipp, Siddle, & Dall, 1997, 1998). In elaborating on a study that varied conditioned stimulus modality in a Pavlovian conditioning experiment, we employed the discrimination task used by Filion et al. (1993, 1994). Half the subjects performed the task with tone stimuli and half with pictures of a circle and an ellipse. An auditory startle probe was presented at lead intervals of 3500 and 4500 msec after stimulus onset during lead stimuli and during some intertrial intervals. Startle facilitation was larger in the tone group during to-be-counted than during to-be-ignored lead stimuli, a result that replicated the findings of Filion et al. Contrary to the predictions of modality-specific attentional accounts, however, the same pattern of results emerged in the group trained with visual lead stimuli. Figure 15.1 depicts the results of a replication study that also included a third group who were trained with vibrotactile stimuli. Again, there was more startle facilitation during to-be-counted visual stimuli. To complicate the picture even more, startle modification was not differentially affected by task instructions in the vibrotactile condition. This pattern of results was confirmed in a third study, which used different visual and tactile lead stimuli. Colored lights replaced the pictures of circles and ellipses, and tactile stimuli were presented to the left and the right hand instead of to different locations on one hand. Electrodermal responses in all experiments were larger during to-be-counted stimuli and task performance did not differ in the different modality groups.

The finding of enhanced acoustic startle during acoustic and visual task-relevant stimuli is difficult to reconcile with the notion that attention to a lead stimulus can facilitate startle if lead and startle stimulus are presented in the same modality, but will inhibit startle if they are in different modalities. Rather, the data indicate that startle is enhanced during attention-demanding stimuli regardless of stimulus modality. Graham (1992) proposed that startle facilitation at long lead intervals may reflect orienting to the lead stimulus. The finding that startle modification is larger during to-be-counted stimuli that elicited larger electrodermal orienting responses is consistent with this notion. It should be noted that we found some evidence for modality-specific startle modification. Startle responses elicited during acoustic lead stimuli were larger than during visual lead stimuli. However, this difference was not affected by task requirements. No effects of attention on startle modification were observed with tactile lead stimuli. This finding is currently not understood and requires further investigation.

The conditions under which attention effects on startle modification will be modality-specific or modality-nonspecific remain unclear. Differences in the procedures used in the studies reviewed by Putnam (1990) and in our studies may provide an explanation. In the studies reviewed by Putnam only one stimulus was presented and no discrimination was required up to the point

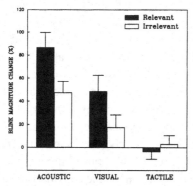

Figure 15.1. Mean change in blink magnitude during task-relevant and task-irrelevant lead stimuli in a discrimination task as a function of lead stimulus modality (vertical lines represent standard errors of the mean; unpublished data).

when the motor response was due, that is, after the presentation of the startle probes. In our work, discrimination between signal and nonsignal events occurred prior to the presentation of startle probes. Our task imposed a higher cognitive load requiring discrimination, duration estimates, and memory of the number of longer-than-usual stimuli. It may be that these task requirements trigger attentional processes that differ from those involved in the foreperiod of a reaction time task. Finally, every lead stimulus contained a probe in the Putnam studies, whereas only half of the stimuli were probed in our experiments; that is, probes were more predictable in the former studies. It may be that startle facilitation is reduced if the probe stimulus is highly predictable. Taken together, the procedural differences could well account for differences in results and require more parametric study.

Vanman, Boehmelt, Dawson, and Schell (1996) provided a first attempt to assess the effects of both attentional and emotional processes on probe startle in a discrimination task that used positively and negatively valent pictures as lead stimuli. Subjects were required to count the number of longer-than-usual picture presentations. Whether pictures were to-be-counted or to-be-ignored was signaled by a tone stimulus. Using four different lead intervals (250, 750, 2450, and 4450 msec) Vanman et al. found effects of emotion, that is, larger startle elicited by an auditory stimulus during negatively valent pictures, at 750, 2450, and 4450 msec. Attentional effects, that is, larger startle during to-be-counted lead stimuli, were found at 4450 msec. In a second experiment, one group of subjects counted the number of longer-than-usual positive slides, whereas a second counted longer-than-usual negative slides. Here, valence effects were found at probe positions of 250, 750, and 4450 msec.

Attentional effects were not evident during the stimuli, but were found at a probe position 950 msec after lead stimulus offset. The absence of attentional effects in the second experiment is not consistent with the results obtained when neutral visual stimuli are used (Lipp et al., 1997), and seem to indicate that emotional effects can override attentional effects.

Current research that investigates startle modification during signal stimuli seems to offer two exciting new directions of inquiry. First, findings from our laboratory suggest that modality-specific attentional accounts are not sufficient to explain attentional startle modification effects. There seems to be good evidence for modality-specific and -nonspecific attentional effects, and further research is required to determine the conditions under which they occur. Moreover, the work by Vanman et al. indicates that the discrimination task paradigm may provide a way to isolate attentional and emotional startle modification effects, which are frequently confounded in conditioning studies.

3. Startle Modification during Pavlovian Conditioning

3.1. Empirical Findings

Startle modification during human Pavlovian conditioning has been studied to investigate emotional processes such as conditioned fear. Although attentional processes feature prominently in current theories of conditioning (Hall, 1995), interpretations of startle potentiation during conditioning in terms of attentional processes have not yet been offered. This seems due mainly to the assumption that attention-related startle facilitation requires that the lead stimulus, that is, conditional stimulus, and startle probe be presented in the same modality. In the majority of the conditioning studies that have measured potentiated startle in humans, however, visual stimuli have been used as conditioned stimuli and acoustic stimuli as startle probes (Spence & Runquist, 1958; Ross, 1961; Grillon, Ameli, Merikangas, Woods, & Davis, 1993; Hamm, Greenwald, Bradley, & Lang, 1993; Hamm & Stark, 1993; Hamm & Vaitl, 1993; Lipp, Sheridan, & Siddle, 1994; Grillon & Davis, 1995; Hamm & Vaitl, 1996; Siddle, Lipp, & Dall, 1997; Lipp, Siddle, & Dall, 1998; but see Flaten & Hugdahl, 1991; Flaten, 1993). Traditional, modality-specific, attentional accounts predict that acoustic blink elicited during a visual conditional stimulus will be inhibited. However, facilitation of acoustic startle during a visual to-be-counted stimulus in a discrimination task seems to indicate that an attentional account of the "fear-potentiated startle" is feasible. This issue will be discussed in more detail after a brief review of the studies that have investigated startle modification during conditioning in humans.

Grillon and his colleagues examined the effect of threat of shock on startle modification. Although no CS-US pairings were presented in these studies, the processes that underlie responses observed in threat of shock procedures are thought to be similar to those that underlie conditioned responding. Participants were instructed that shock could be presented during some phases of the experiment, whereas other phases were safe. The different phases were signaled either by instruction (Grillon, Ameli, Woods, Merikangas, & Davis, 1991) or by a light stimulus (Grillon et al., 1993; Grillon & Davis, 1995). The phases lasted for about 60 s and acoustic startle probes were presented across these phases. One shock was presented about halfway through the experiment after several dangerous and safe phases had passed. The experiments yielded a similar pattern of results. Startle magnitude was larger and startle latency was shorter during dangerous phases than during safe phases. Enhanced startle was present during the first dangerous phase and did not change after presentation of the shock stimulus. Thus, anticipation of an aversive stimulus seems to be sufficient to enhance startle responses in comparison with those elicited when no such anticipation is present. Moreover, the anticipatory effect can be established by instruction and does not require presentation of an aversive stimulus.

The first human study that used a conventional conditioning procedure to investigate the effects of fear on blink reflexes was reported by Spence and Runquist (1958). Participants were trained with pairings of a light CS and a shock US at an interstimulus interval of 500 msec in either forward or backward pairings. Shock was not presented on some of the training trials, but blinks were elicited by an air-puff stimulus 500 or 4500 msec after onset of the CS. On trials with a lead interval of 4500 msec the CS was presented for the entire lead interval. Spence and Runquist found no differences between forward and backward groups at the 500-msec lead interval, but response magnitude at the 4500-msec lead interval was larger in the forward than in the backward group. These results are difficult to interpret. The assumption that backward conditioning can serve as a proper control condition in which no learning will occur has been questioned (for a review, see Spetch, Wilkie, & Pinel, 1981). Moreover, it is not clear whether the enhanced responses at 4500 msec reflected conditioned fear or enhanced orienting due to the prolongation of the CS. Ross (1961) investigated the effects of interstimulus interval during conditioning on blink reflex modification. Five groups of subjects were trained with pairings of a light CS that lasted for 250 msec and a shock US at different interstimulus intervals (−1, 0.5, 2, 5, or 10 s). The lead interval was varied within subjects and lasted 0.5, 2, 5, or 10 s. The US was replaced on test trials by an air puff. Ross reported larger blink responses at the 5- and 10-s lead interval in the 2- and 5-s interstimulus interval groups than in the −1- and 0.5-s interstimulus interval groups. Moreover, probe responses at lead intervals of 2, 5, and 10 s were larger than those at the 0.5-s lead interval in all but the backward control group. It is unclear, however, whether changes in blink modification reflected fear elicited by the CS or the orienting to the omission of the US, which preceded the presentation of the reflex probe in most cases.

The confounds that made an interpretation of the early studies difficult were avoided in more recent studies that have used long-lasting CSs, e.g., 8-s, in a delay conditioning design that allows presentation of probe stimuli prior to and unaffected by presentation of the US. Hamm et al. (1993) trained five groups of subjects in a differential conditioning design using CS pictures that differed between groups in emotional valence. Auditory reflex probe stimuli were presented at lead intervals of 3.5, 5.75, and 8 s after CS onset during habituation and during extinction. Startle magnitude facilitation and latency shortening were larger during CS+ than during CS− in the extinction phase. Moreover, blink magnitude was larger and blink latency was shorter during CS− than during the intertrial interval. Hamm and Stark (1993) also found differential modification of blink magnitude that remained unchanged throughout extinction. However, no difference was found between blink reflexes elicited during CS− and during intertrial intervals.

The difference in blink modification between probes presented during CS− and during the intertrial interval (Hamm et al., 1993) is difficult to reconcile with current theories of conditioning. It may be that the difference reflects attentional effects due to the requirement of stimulus discrimination that is part of differential conditioning. To avoid this problem, Lipp, Sheridan, and Siddle (1994) used a single-cue conditioning procedure. Half the subjects received paired presentations of a conditioned and an unconditioned stimulus (Conditioning group) whereas the other half received the stimuli in a random order (Control group). Within each group, the unconditional stimulus was an electric shock for half the subjects and an imperative stimulus for a speeded motor response for the other half (Lipp & Vaitl, 1990). The imperative stimulus was a tone in the first experiment and a tactile stimulus in the second. A visual stimulus presented for 8 s was used as the CS for all subjects, and acoustic startle probes were presented during some conditioned stimuli at lead intervals of 3 or 6 s, and during some intertrial intervals. Electrodermal conditioning was evident in both Conditioning groups regardless of the nature of the unconditional stimulus (see Fig. 15.2A). Potentiated startle, however, was observed only in the Conditioning group trained with an aversive US (see Fig. 15.2B). There was no startle potentiation during a stimulus that was uncorrelated with the occurrence of shock or a conditioned stimulus that predicted an imperative stimulus (see also Hamm & Vaitl, 1993, 1996). These results seem to indicate

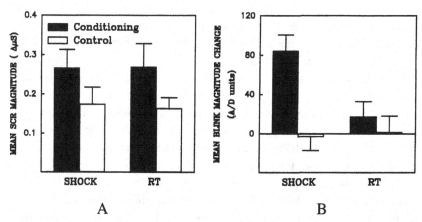

Figure 15.2. Mean electrodermal first-interval response magnitude (*A*) and mean change in blink magnitude (*B*) during single cue Pavlovian acquisition as a function of experimental condition and nature of the unconditional stimulus. (From Lipp, Sheridan, & Siddle (1994), Human blink startle during aversive and nonaversive Pavlovian conditioning, *Journal of Experimental Psychology: Animal Behavior Processes, 20*, 380–389. Copyright 1994 by the American Psychological Association. Reprinted with permission.)

that in a single cue conditioning design, startle modification is restricted to USs that might be expected to elicit emotional responses.

The failure to find significant startle modification during a CS that preceded a reaction time task is not consistent with results obtained in the stimulus discrimination task or the findings reported by Putnam (1990). However, our studies that used a nonaversive reaction time US, as well as the studies by Hamm and Vaitl, incorporated an explicit imperative signal in an S1–S2 paradigm. The discrimination task and the studies reviewed by Putnam did not use a second stimulus, but used the offset of the warning stimulus (S1) as the critical event. Moreover, the duration of the warning stimulus was longer in the conditioning studies (8 s) than in the discrimination task (5 s) or reaction time studies (6 s). At present it seems premature to speculate which of these differences may be responsible for the different results.

3.2. Processes Underlying Blink Modification during Pavlovian Conditioning

Although the failure to find blink modification in anticipation of an imperative stimulus does not imply that attentional processes cannot also affect startle modification during Pavlovian conditioning, conditions in which there is an interaction between attentional and emotional mechanisms have yet to be delineated. A recent series of studies from our laboratory that varied the modality of the US or the CS focused on this issue (Siddle, Lipp, & Dall, 1997; Lipp, Siddle, & Dall, 1998).

As mentioned above, Lipp et al. (1994, Experiment 1) found no potentiated startle during a visual stimulus that predicted the acoustic imperative signal for a speeded motor response. This result is inconsistent with predictions derived from a modality-specific attentional account of startle modification (Anthony, 1985). Modality-specific attentional accounts predict that while the visual warning stimulus is presented, attentional resources will be allocated to the auditory modality in anticipation of the imperative signal. Thus, acoustic startle elicited during the visual stimulus will be enhanced. This reasoning has been employed to explain enhanced acoustic startle responses observed during a tactile warning stimulus (Anthony & Putnam, 1980). Thus, startle potentiation observed during conditioning may be affected not only by the intensity of the unconditional stimulus, but also by its modality. We tested this prediction in a series of experiments that varied US modality (electrotactile vs. acoustic) and US intensity (weak vs. intense) in either a within- or a between-subject design (Siddle, Lipp, & Dall, 1997). Subjects were required to perform speeded motor responses to all USs to enhance attentional focus on the stimuli and to ensure conditioning with low-intensity stimuli. Acoustic startle probes were presented at lead intervals of 3.5 and 7.5 s after CS onset. The results (Fig. 15.3) indicate that unconditional stimulus intensity, but not modality, affects startle modification. Thus, it may have been the intensity (108 dB(A)) and not the modality of the acoustic stimulus that caused the startle facilitation reported by Anthony and Putnam (1980). The facilitated startle may have reflected conditioned fear and not attention.

To investigate the effects of attention to the CS on startle modification, we varied CS modality (Lipp, Siddle, & Dall, 1997). Previous research has shown that startle modification is larger during interesting, attention-commanding lead stimuli if lead stimuli and the startle-eliciting stimulus are presented in the same modality. If lead stimuli are presented in a different modality from the startle-eliciting stimulus, startle modification is larger during less interesting stimuli. Subjects were trained in a differential conditioning design with electric shock as the US. The CSs were tones for half the subjects and pictures for the other half, the same stimuli as used in the discrimination task described in the previous section. The CSs lasted for 8 s and startle probes were presented at lead intervals of 3.5 and 7.5 s.

Figure 15.4 summarizes the startle modification findings. In the group trained with tone CSs, startle magnitude was potentiated substantially and to

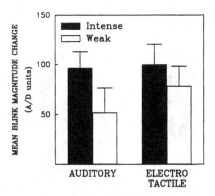

Figure 15.3. Mean change in blink magnitude during single cue Pavlovian acquisition as a function of unconditional stimulus modality and intensity. (Copyright 1997, Society for Psychophysiological Research. Reproduced with permission of the publisher and the authors from Siddle, Lipp, & Dall, 1997.)

the same extent during both conditioned stimuli (see Fig. 15.4B). Potentiation during CS+ was larger than during CS− in the group trained with visual stimuli. Startle elicited during the CS− was significantly larger than startle elicited during intertrial intervals, replicating previous findings (Hamm et al., 1993). The extent of startle latency shortening (Fig. 15.4A) differed between stimulus conditions in both modality groups, with latency shortening being larger during CS+ than during CS−. Differential skin conductance responding was evident in both modality groups. The difference in the extent of magnitude facilitation between the modality groups seems to provide evidence for the impact of attentional processes. It is difficult to see how either emotional mechanisms or nonspecific arousal could differ between the two groups. The lack of differential startle modification during CS+ and CS− in the group trained with tones may reflect a ceiling effect. It is possible that the modality-specific blink modification attributed to attentional factors was too large to allow differential effects of emotion to become apparent. This interpretation is supported by the results obtained for blink latency shortening where clear evidence for differential startle modification emerged in both groups. In previous studies, latency shortening and magnitude facilitation have yielded similar results; that is, more magnitude facilitation was associated with greater latency shortening and vice versa. It seems reasonable to assume that the same would hold for the present study if there were no ceiling effect.

The enhanced startle during a visual stimulus that predicts the absence of an aversive US is puzzling. Conditioning theories (e.g., Rescorla & Wagner,

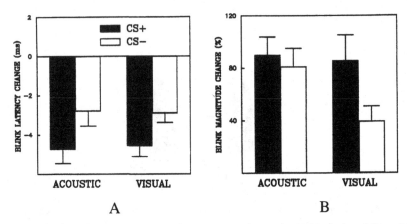

Figure 15.4. Mean change in blink latency (*A*) and magnitude (*B*) during differential Pavlovian acquisition as a function of conditional stimulus modality. (Copyright 1998, Society for Psychophysiological Research. Reproduced with permission of the publisher and the authors from Lipp, Siddle, & Dall, 1997.)

1972) predict that a CS− will become a safety signal that predicts the absence of the US. Thus, startle inhibition might be expected to probes presented during a CS−. The result cannot be attributed to nonspecific sensitization elicited by the intermittent presentations of the US. Lipp et al. (1994) found no enhanced startle during a visual CS that was presented in a random sequence with a shock US. It could be argued that incomplete discrimination and thus generalization of learning from the CS+ caused the enhanced startle. This seems unlikely in view of the fact that previous studies used more complex conditioned stimuli that were more easily discriminated (Hamm et al., 1993).

Greater startle modification during an auditory CS+ than a visual CS+ is inconsistent with findings from animal research. Falls and Davis (1994) trained different groups of rats with visual, auditory, or somato-sensory CSs and found no difference in the amount of modification of the acoustic startle reflex. Similarly, Campeau and Davis (1995a, b) found no difference in startle facilitation during visual or auditory CSs using either within- or between-subject conditioning designs. The finding that rats do not display different amounts of startle facilitation during CSs of different modalities matches another species difference obtained in research on the effects of attention on blink modification. In contrast to humans, rats do not display enhanced acoustic startle following a discrete acoustic lead stimulus if the lead interval is variable (Graham, 1975). It may be that attentional effects on startle modification that are found in humans do not emerge in rodents.

Taken together, studies that have investigated startle modification during conditioning indicate that affective valence can be changed for previously neutral stimuli regardless of whether threat paradigms or more traditional aversive conditioning paradigms are used. The role of attentional processes in startle modification during conditioning is as yet unknown, but there is evidence that attention allocated to the modality of the US does not affect the results. As in the discrimination task, overall startle modification during conditioning is influenced by conditioned stimulus modality, but this effect seems to be independent of the effects of emotional or attentional processes.

4. Conclusion

The use of probe startle provides opportunities to learn more about the processes involved in human Pavlovian conditioning. Attentional processes have been shown to be important in blink modification during simple signal stimuli. However, results from a discrimination task that employed acoustic, visual, or tactile stimuli seem to indicate that the assumption that blink facilitation requires a match between the modality of the signal and probe stimuli is overly simplistic. Current research in Pavlovian conditioning has focused mainly on emotional processes that are involved if a neutral CS is paired with an aversive US. However, no discussion of conditioning can ignore the role played by attentional processes. It is essential, therefore, that future investigation of startle modification during conditioning take attentional processes into account to reconcile the apparent contradictory findings obtained in discrimination tasks and differential nonaversive conditioning. It is difficult to explain why startle is facilitated during a visual task-relevant stimulus that is to be counted or a visual CS+ that predicts an aversive US, but not during a visual CS+ that predicts an imperative stimulus of a reaction time task. Studies of emotional processes during conditioning in humans will need to delineate the nature of the affective changes during conditioning and the mechanisms that mediate them. Startle modification will be an important measure in these efforts.

References

Acocella, C. M. & Blumenthal, T. D. (1990). Directed attention influences the modification of startle reflex probability. *Psychological Reports, 66,* 275–285.

Acri, J. B., David, E. M., Popke, E. J., & Grunberg, N. E. (1994). Nicotine increases sensory gating measured by inhibition of the acoustic startle reflex in rats. *Psychopharmacology, 114,* 369–374.

Adler, L., Pachtman, E., Franks, R., Pecevich, M., Waldo, M., & Freedman, R. (1982). Neurophysiological evidence for a defect in neuronal mechanisms involved in sensory gating in schizophrenia. *Biological Psychiatry, 17,* 639–654.

Adolphs, R., Tranel, D., Damasio, H., & Damasio, A. R. (1994). Impaired recognition of emotion in facial expressions following bilateral damage to the human amygdala. *Nature, 372,* 669–672.

Adolphs, R., Tranel, D., Damasio, H., & Damasio, A. R. (1995). Fear and the human amygdala. *Journal of Neuroscience, 15,* 5879–5891.

Aggleton, J. P. (1992). The functional effects of amygdala lesions in humans: A comparison with findings from monkeys. In J. P. Aggleton (Ed.), *The amygdala: Neurobiological aspects of emotion, memory and mental dysfunction* (pp. 485–503). New York: Wiley-Liss.

Aitken, C. J., Siddle, D. A. T., & Lipp, O. V. (1995). The effects of threat and nonthreat word lead stimuli on blink modulation [Abstract]. *Psychophysiology, 32* (Suppl. 1), S15.

Al-Amin, H. A. & Schwarzkopf, S. B. (1996). Effects of the PCP analog dizocipline on sensory gating: Potential relevance to clinical subtypes of schizophrenia. *Biological Psychiatry, 40,* 744–754.

Alheid, G., deOlmos, J. S., & Beltramino, C. A. (1995). Amygdala and extended amygdala. In G. Paxinos (Ed.), *The rat nervous system* (pp. 495–578). New York: Davis.

Allen, N. B., Trinder, J., & Brennan, C. (1997). *Affective startle modulation in clinical depression.* Manuscript submitted for publication.

Allen, N. B., Wong, S., Kim, Y., & Trinder, J. (1996). Startle reflex and heart rate responses during appetitive and aversive anticipation [Abstract]. *Psychophysiology, 33* (Suppl. 1), S18.

American Psychiatric Association (1994). *Diagnostic and statistical manual of mental disorders* (4th ed.). Washington, DC: Author.

Anday, E., Cohen, M. E., Kelley, N., & Hoffman, H. S. (1989). Sensory processing in the term and preterm infant: Use of reflex modification procedures. *Developmental Psychobiology, 22,* 211–219.

Anthony, B. J. (1985). In the blink of an eye: Implications of reflex modification for information processing. In P. K. Ackles, J. R. Jennings, & M. G. H. Coles (Eds.), *Advances in psychophysiology* (Vol. 1, pp. 167–218). Greenwich, CT: JAI Press.

Anthony, B. J., Butler, G. H., & Putnam, L. E. (1978). Probe startle inhibition during HR deceleration in a forewarned RT paradigm [Abstract]. *Psychophysiology, 15,* 285.

Anthony, B. J., & Graham, F. K. (1983). Evidence for sensory-selective set in young infants. *Science, 220,* 742–744.

Anthony, B. J., & Graham, F. K. (1985). Blink reflex modification by selective attention: Evidence for the modulation of "automatic" processing. *Biological Psychology, 20,* 43–59.

Anthony, B. J., & Putnam, L. E. (1980). Startle and cardiac indices of developmental differences in anticipatory attention [Abstract]. *Psychophysiology, 17,* 324–325.

Anthony, B. J., & Putnam, L. E. (1985). Cardiac and blink concomitants of attentional selectivity: A comparison of adults and young children. *Psychophysiology, 22,* 508–516.

Arieti, S. (1955). *Interpretation of schizophrenia.* New York: Brunner.

Arrindell, A., Emmelkamp, P. M. G., & van der Ende, J. (1984). Phobic dimensions: I. Reliability and generalizability across samples, gender and nations. *Advances in Behavior Research and Therapy, 6,* 207–253.

Baeyens, F., Eelen, P., & Crombez, G. (1995). Pavlovian associations are forever: On classical conditioning and extinction. *Journal of Psychophysiology, 9,* 127–142.

Bakshi, V. P., & Geyer, M. A. (1995). Antagonism of phencyclidine-induced deficits in prepulse inhibition by the putative atypical antipsychotic olanzapine. *Psychopharmacology, 122,* 198–201.

Bakshi, V. P., Swerdlow, N. R., & Geyer, M. A. (1994). Clozapine antagonizes phencyclidine-induced deficits in sensorimotor gating of the startle response. *Journal of Pharmacology and Experimental Therapeutics, 271,* 787–794.

Balaban, M. T. (1995). Affective influences on startle in five-month-old infants: Reactions to facial expressions of emotion. *Child Development, 66,* 28–36.

Balaban, M. T. (1996). Probing basic mechanisms of sensory, attentional, and emotional development: Modulation of the infant blink response. In C. Rovee-Collier & L. P. Lipsitt (Eds.), *Advances in infancy research* (Vol. 10, pp. 219–256). Norwood, NJ: Ablex Publishing Corporation.

Balaban, M. T., Anthony, B. J., & Graham, F. K. (1985). Modality-repetition and attentional effects on reflex blinking in infants and adults. *Infant Behavior and Development, 8,* 443–457.

Balaban, M. T., Anthony, B. J., & Graham, F. K. (1989). Prestimulation effects on blink and cardiac reflexes of 15-month-old human infants. *Developmental Psychobiology, 22,* 115–127.

Balaban, M. T., Losito, B. D. G., Simons, R. F., & Graham, F. K. (1986a). Offline latency and amplitude scoring of the human reflex eyeblink with Fortran IV [computer program abstract]. *Psychophysiology, 23,* 612.

Balaban, M. T., Losito, B. D. G., Simons, R. F., & Graham, F. K. (1986b). Offline latency and amplitude scoring of the human reflex eyeblink with Fortran IV. Unpublished user's guide.

Balaban, M. T., & Taussig, H. N. (1994). Salience of fear/threat in the affective modulation of the human startle blink. *Biological Psychology, 38,* 117–131.

Banks, W. P., Roberts, D., Ciranni, M. (1995). Negative priming in auditory attention. *Journal of Experimental Psychology: Human Perception and Performance, 21,* 1354–1361.

Bartemeier, L. H., Kubie, L. S., Menninger, K. A., Romano, J., & Whitehorn, J. C. (1946). Combat exhaustion. *Journal of Nervous and Mental Diseases, 104,* 358–389.

Bechara, A., Tranel, D., Damasio, H., Adolphs, R., Rockland, C., & Damasio, A. R. (1995). Double dissociation of conditioning and declarative knowledge relative to the amygdala and hippocampus in humans. *Science, 269,* 1115–1118.

Beck, A. T., Ward, C. H., Mendelsohn, M., Mock, J., & Erbaugh, J. (1961). An inventory for measuring depression. *Archives of General Psychiatry, 4,* 561–571.

Beech, A., Baylis, G. B., Smithson, P., Claridge, G. S. (1989). Individual differences in schizotypy as reflected in measures of cognitive inhibition. *British Journal of Clinical Psychology, 28,* 117–129.

Beech, A., & Claridge, G. (1987). Individual differences in negative priming: Relations with schizotypal personality traits. *British Journal of Psychology, 78,* 349–356.

Beech, A., Powell, T., McWilliam, J., & Claridge, G. S. (1989). Evidence of reduced "cognitive inhibition" in schizophrenia. *British Journal of Clinical Psychology, 28,* 109–116.

Beggs, A. L., Steinmetz, J. E., & Patterson, M. M. (1985). Classical conditioning of a flexor nerve response in spinal cats: Effects of tibial nerve CS and a differential conditioning paradigm. *Behavioral Neuroscience, 99,* 496–508.

Berg, K. M. (1973). Elicitation of acoustic startle in the human (Doctoral dissertation, University of Wisconsin, 1973). *Dissertation Abstracts International, 34,* 5217B–5218B.

Berg, K. M. (1985). Temporal masking level differences for transients: Further evidence for a short-term integrator. *Perception & Psychophysics, 37,* 397–406.

Berg, W. K., & Davis, M. (1985). Associative learning modifies startle reflexes at the lateral lemniscus. *Behavioral Neuroscience, 99,* 191–199.

Berman, K. F., Illowsky, B. P., Weinberger, D. R. (1988). Physiological dysfunction of dorsolateral prefrontal cortex in schizophrenia: IV. Further evidence for regional and behavioral specificity. *Archives of General Psychiatry, 45,* 616–622.

Bernstein, I. H., Rose, R., & Ashe, V. (1970). Preparatory state effects in intersensory facilitation. *Psychonomic Science, 19,* 113–114.

Berntson, G. G., Cacioppo, J. T., & Quigley, K. S. (1991). Autonomic determinism: The modes of autonomic control, the doctrine of autonomic space, and the laws of autonomic constraint. *Psychological Review, 98,* 459–487.

Bickford-Wimer, P. C., Nagamoto, H., Johnson, R., Adler, L. E., Egan, M., Rose, G. M., & Freedman, R. (1989). Auditory sensory gating in hippocampal neurons: A model system in the rat. *Biological Psychiatry, 27,* 183–192.

Bleuler, E. (1950). *Dementia praecox or the group of schizophrenias* (J. Zinkin, Trans.). New York: International University Press. (Original work published 1911.)

Bloch, R. M. (1972). *Inhibition and facilitation effects of a prepulse on the human blink response to a startle pulse.* Unpublished doctoral dissertation, University of Wisconsin, Madison.

Blumenthal, T. D. (1988). The startle response to acoustic stimuli near startle threshold: Effects of stimulus rise and fall time, duration, and intensity. *Psychophysiology, 25,* 607–611.

Blumenthal, T. D. (1994). Signal attenuation as a function of integrator time constant and signal duration. *Psychophysiology, 31,* 201–203.

Blumenthal, T. D. (1995a). Prepulse inhibition of the startle eyeblink as an indicator of temporal summation. *Perception and Psychophysics, 57,* 487–494.

Blumenthal, T. D. (1995b). Comparing three methods of quantifying eyeblink EMG magnitude [Abstract]. *Psychophysiology, 32* (Suppl. 1), S13.

Blumenthal, T. D. (1996). Inhibition of the human startle response is affected by both prepulse intensity and eliciting stimulus intensity. *Biological Psychology, 44,* 85–104.

Blumenthal, T. D. (1997). Prepulse inhibition decreases as startle reactivity habituates. *Psychophysiology, 34,* 446–450.

Blumenthal, T. D., Avendano, A., & Berg, W. K. (1987). The startle response and auditory temporal summation in neonates. *Journal of Experimental Child Psychology, 44,* 64–79.

Blumenthal, T. D., & Berg, W. K. (1986a). Stimulus rise time, intensity, and bandwidth effects on acoustic startle amplitude and probability. *Psychophysiology, 23,* 635–641.

Blumenthal, T. D. & Berg, W. K. (1986b). The startle response as an indicator of temporal summation. *Perception and Psychophysics, 40,* 62–68.

Blumenthal, T. D., Chapman, J. G., & Muse, K. B. (1995). Effects of social anxiety, attention, and extraversion on the acoustic startle eyeblink response. *Personality & Individual Differences, 19,* 797–807.

Blumenthal, T. D., & Creps, C. L. (1994). Normal startle responding in psychosis-prone college students. *Personality and Individual Differences, 17,* 345–355.

Blumenthal, T. D., & Gescheider, G. A. (1987). Modification of the acoustic startle response by a tactile prepulse: Effects of stimulus onset asynchrony and prepulse intensity. *Psychophysiology, 24,* 320–327.

Blumenthal, T. D., & Goode, C. T. (1991). The startle eyeblink response to low intensity acoustic stimuli. *Psychophysiology, 28,* 296–306.

Blumenthal, T. D., & Levey, B. J. (1989). Prepulse rise time and startle reflex modification: Different effects for discrete and continuous prepulses. *Psychophysiology, 26,* 158–165.

Blumenthal, T. D., Schicatano, E. J., Chapman, J. G., Norris, C. M., & Ergenzinger, E. R., Jr. (1996). Prepulse effects on magnitude estimation of startle-eliciting stimuli and startle responses. *Perception & Psychophysics, 58,* 73–80.

Blumenthal, T. D. & Tolomeo, E. A. (1989). Bidirectional influences of vibrotactile prepulses on modification of the human acoustic startle reflex. *Psychobiology, 17,* 315–322.

Boelhouwer, A. J. W., Frints, C. J. M., & Westerkamp, V. (1989). The effect of a visual prestimulus upon the human blink reflex [Abstract]. *Psychophysiology, 26,* S14.

Boelhouwer, A. J. W., Teurlings, R. J. M. A., & Brunia, C. H. M. (1991). The effect of an acoustic warning stimulus upon the electrically elicited blink reflex in humans. *Psychophysiology, 28,* 133–139.

Bogerts, B. (1993). Recent advances in the neuropathology of schizophrenia. *Schizophrenia Bulletin, 19,* 431–445.

Bogerts, B., Ashtari, M., Degreef, G., Alvir, J. M. J., Bilder, R. M., & Lieberman, J. A. (1990). Reduced temporal limbic structure volumes on magnetic resonance images in first episode schizophrenia. *Psychiatry Research and Neuroimaging, 35,* 1–13.

Bohlin, G., & Graham, F. K. (1977). Cardiac deceleration and reflex blink facilitation. *Psychophysiology, 14,* 423–430.

Bohlin, G., Graham, F. K., Silverstein, L. D., & Hackley, S. A. (1981). Cardiac orienting and startle blink modification in novel and signal situations. *Psychophysiology, 18,* 603–611.

Boehmelt, A. H., Dawson, M. E., Vanman, E. J., & Schell, A. M. (1996). Prestimulus modality and effects of attention on startle eyeblink modification [Abstract]. *Psychophysiology, 33* (Suppl. 1), S24.

Bolino, F., Di Michele, V., Di Cicco, L., Manna, V., Daneluzzo, E., & Cassachia, M. (1994). Sensorimotor gating and habituation evoked by electrocutaneous stimulation in schizophrenia. *Biological Psychiatry, 36,* 670–679.

Bolino, F., Manna, V., Di Cicco, L., Di Michele, V., Daneluzzo, E., Rossi, A., & Casacchia, M. (1992). Startle reflex habituation in functional psychoses: A controlled study. *Neuroscience Letters, 145,* 126–128.

Bonnet, M., Bradley, M. M., Lang, P. J., & Requin, J. (1995). Modulation of spinal reflexes: Arousal, pleasure, action. *Psychophysiology, 32,* 367–372.

Boulis, N., & Davis, M. (1989). Footshock-induced sensitization of electrically elicited startle reflexes. *Behavioral Neuroscience, 103,* 504–508.

Boulis, N. M., Kehne, J. H., Miserendino, M. J. D., & Davis, M. (1990). Differential blockade of early and late components of acoustic startle following intrathecal infusion of 6-cyano-7-nitroquinoxaline-2,3-dione (CNQX) or D,L-2-amino-5-phosphonovaleric acid (AP-5). *Brain Research, 520,* 240–246.

Bowditch, H. P., & Warren, J. W. (1890). The knee-jerk and its physiological modifications. *The Journal of Physiology, 11,* 25–64.

Bracha, S. H. (1987). Asymmetric rotational (circling) behavior, a dopamine-related asymmetry: Preliminary findings in unmedicated and never-medicated schizophrenia patients. *Biological Psychiatry, 22,* 995–1003.

Bradley, M. M., Cuthbert, B. N., & Lang, P. J. (1990). Startle reflex modification: Emotion or attention? *Psychophysiology, 27,* 513–522.

Bradley, M. M., Cuthbert, B. N., & Lang, P. J. (1991). Startle and emotion: Lateral acoustic probes and the bilateral blink. *Psychophysiology, 28,* 285–295.

Bradley, M. M., Cuthbert, B. N., & Lang, P. J. (1993). Pictures as prepulses: Attention and emotion in startle modification. *Psychophysiology, 30,* 541–545.

Bradley, M. M., Cuthbert, B. N., & Lang, P. J. (1995). Imagine that! Startle in action and perception [Abstract]. *Psychophysiology, 32* (Suppl. 1), S21.

Bradley, M. M., Cuthbert, B. N., & Lang, P. J. (1996a). Lateralized startle probes in the study of emotion. *Psychophysiology, 33,* 156–161.

Bradley, M. M., Cuthbert, B. N., & Lang, P. J. (1996b). Picture media and emotion: Effects of a sustained affective context. *Psychophysiology, 33,* 662–670.

Bradley, M. M., Cuthbert, B. N., & Lang, P. J. (1996c). *Affective norms for English words (ANEW). Technical manual and affective ratings.* Gainesville, FL: The Center for Research in Psychophysiology, University of Florida.

Bradley, M. M., Drobes, D., & Lang, P. J. (1996). A probe for all reasons: Reflex and RT measures in perception [Abstract]. *Psychophysiology, 33* (Suppl. 1), S25.

Bradley, M. M., Gianaros, P., & Lang, P. J. (1995). As time goes by: Stability of affective startle modulation [Abstract]. *Psychophysiology, 32* (Suppl. 1), S21.

Bradley, M. M., Greenwald, M. K., & Hamm, A. O. (1993). Affective picture processing. In N. Birbaumer & A. Öhman (Eds.), *The structure of emotion: Psychophysiological, cognitive, and clinical aspects.* Toronto: Hogrefe & Huber.

Bradley, M. M., & Lang, P. J. (1992, October). *Temperament and emotional reactivity: Sociability, fear, and restraint.* Paper presented at the Thirty-Second Annual Meeting of the Society for Psychophysiological Research, San Diego, California.

Bradley, M. M., & Lang, P. J., (1994). Measuring emotion: The self-assessment manikin and the semantic differential. *Journal of Behavioral Therapy and Experimental Psychiatry, 25,* 49–59.

Bradley, M. M., Lang, P. J., & Cuthbert, B. N. (1993). Emotion, novelty, and the startle reflex: Habituation in humans. *Behavioral Neuroscience, 107,* 970–980.

Bradley, M. M., & Vrana, S. R. (1993). The startle probe in the study of emotion and emotional disorders. In N. Birbaumer & A. Öhman (Eds.), *The structure of emotion* (pp. 270–287). Seattle: Hogrefe & Huber.

Bradley, M. M., Zack, J., & Lang, P. J. (1994). Cries, screams, and shouts of joy: Affective responses to environmental sounds [Abstract]. *Psychophysiology, 31* (Suppl. 1), S29.

Braff, D. L., Callaway, E., & Naylor, H. (1977). Very short-term memory dysfunction in schizophrenia. *Archives of General Psychiatry, 34,* 25–30.

Braff, D. L., & Geyer, M. A. (1990). Sensorimotor gating and schizophrenia: Human and animal studies. *Archives of General Psychiatry, 47,* 181–188.

Braff, D. L., Grillon, C., & Geyer, M. A. (1992). Gating and habituation of the startle reflex in schizophrenic patients. *Archives of General Psychiatry, 49,* 206–215.

Braff, D. L., Perry, W., Cadenhead, K. S., Swerdlow, N. R., & Geyer, M. A. (1995). Prepulse inhibitory deficits in schizophrenia: Gender effects. *Biological Psychiatry, 37,* 654.

Braff, D. L., & Sacuzzo, D. P. (1982). Effect of antipsychotic medication on speed of information processing in schizophrenic patients. *American Journal of Psychiatry, 139,* 1127–1133.

Braff, D. L., Sacuzzo, D. P., & Geyer, M. A. (1991). Information processing dysfunctions in schizophrenia: Studies of visual backward masking, sensorimotor gating, and habituation. In S. R. Steinhauer, J. H. Gruzelier, J. H., & J. Zubin (Eds.), *Handbook of schizophrenia, Vol. 5: Neuropsychology, psychophysiology and information processing* (pp. 303–334). Amsterdam: Elsevier Science Publishers.

Braff, D. L., Stone, C., Callaway, E., Geyer, M., Glick, I., & Bali, L. (1978). Prestimulus effects on human startle reflex in normals and schizophrenics. *Psychophysiology, 15,* 339–343.

Breitmeyer, B. (1984). *Visual masking: An integrative approach.* New York: Oxford University Press.

Breitmeyer, B., & Ganz, L. (1976). Implications of sustained and transient channels for theories of visual pattern masking, saccadic suppression, and information processing. *Psychological Review, 83,* 1–17.

Broadbent, D. E., & Broadbent, M. H. P. (1987). From detection to identification: Response to multiple targets in rapid serial visual presentation. *Perception & Psychophysics, 42,* 105–113.

Brooks, R. A. (1986). A robust layered control system for a mobile robot. *IEEE Journal of Robotics and Automation, 2,* 14–23.

Brooks, R. A. (1989). Fast, cheap and out of control: A robot invasion of the solar system. *Journal of the British Interplanetary Society, 42,* 478–485.

Brooks, R. A. (1991). New approaches to robotics. *Science, 253,* 1227–1232.

Brown, J. S., Kalish, H. I., & Farber, I. E. (1951). Conditioned fear as revealed by magnitude of startle response to an auditory stimulus. *Journal of Experimental Psychology, 41,* 317–328.

Brown, P. B., Maxfield, B. W., & Moraff, H. (1973). *Electronics for neurobiologists.* Cambridge, MA: MIT Press.

Brown, P., Rothwell, J. C., Thompson, P. D., Britton, T. C., Day, B. L., & Marsden, C. D. (1991). New observations on the normal auditory startle reflex in man. *Brain, 114,* 1891–1902.

Brunia, C. H. M., Mocks, J., & van den Berg-Lenssen, M. M. C. (1989). Correcting ocular artifacts in the EEG: A comparison of several methods. *Journal of Gerontology, 40,* 595–600.

Bubser, M., & Koch, M. (1994a). Haloperidol reduces the sensorimotor gating deficit that is induced by dopamine depletion in the medial prefrontal cortex of rats. *Society for Neuroscience Abstracts, 20,* 828.

Bubser, M., & Koch, M. (1994b). Prepulse inhibition of the acoustic startle response of rats is reduced by 6-hydroxydopamine lesions of the medial prefrontal cortex. *Psychopharmacology, 113,* 487–492.

Buckland, G., Buckland, J., Jamieson, C., & Ison, J. R. (1969). Inhibition of startle response to acoustic stimulation produced by visual prestimulation. *Journal of Comparative and Physiological Psychology, 67,* 493–496.

Budd, T. W., & Michie, P. T. (1994). Facilitation of the N1 peak of the auditory ERP at short stimulus intervals. *NeuroReport, 5,* 2513–2516.

Bunney, W. (1990). Dopamine glutamate interactions and schizophrenia. *American College of Neuropsychopharmacology, 60.*

Burke, J., & Hackley, S. A. (1997). Prepulse effects on the photic eyeblink reflex: Evidence for startle-dazzle theory. *Psychophysiology, 34,* 276–284.

Bushman, B. J., & Cooper, H. M. (1990). Effects of alcohol on human aggression: An integrative research review. *Psychological Bulletin, 107,* 341–354.

Buss, A. H., & Plomin, R. (1975). *A temperament theory of personality development.* New York: Wiley.

Buss, A. H., & Plomin, R. (1984). *Temperament: Early developing personality traits.* Hillsdale, NJ: Erlbaum.

Butler, R. W., & Braff, D. L. (1991). Delusions: A review and integration. *Schizophrenia Bulletin, 17,* 633–647.

Butler, R. W., Braff, D. L., Rausch, J. L., Jenkins, M. A., Sprock, J., & Geyer, M. A. (1990). Physiological evidence of exaggerated startle response in a subgroup of Vietnam veterans with combat-related PTSD. *American Journal of Psychiatry, 147,* 1308–1312.

Butler, R. W., Jenkins, M. A., Geyer, M. A., & Braff, D. L. (1991). Wisconsin card sorting deficits and diminished sensorimotor gating in a discrete subgroup of schizophrenic patients. In C. A. Tamminga & S. C. Schulz (Eds.), *Advances in neuropsychiatry and psychopharmacology, Volume 1: Schizophrenia research* (pp. 163–168). New York, NY: Raven Press, Ltd.

Cadenhead, K. S., Geyer, M. A., & Braff, D. L. (1993). Impaired startle prepulse inhibition and habituation in schizotypal patients. *American Journal of Psychiatry, 150,* 1862–1867.

Cadenhead, K. S., Kumar, C., & Braff, D. L. (1996). Clinical and experimental characteristics of hypothetically psychosis prone college students. *Journal of Psychiatry Research, 30,* 331–340.

Cadenhead, K. S., Perry, W., & Braff, D. L. (1996). The relationship of information-processing deficits and clinical symptoms in schizotypal personality disorder. *Biological Psychiatry, 40,* 853–858.

Caine, S. B., Geyer, M. A., & Swerdlow, N. R. (1991). Carbachol infusion into the dentate gyrus disrupts sensorimotor gating of the startle reflex in rats. *Psychopharmacology, 105,* 347–354.

Caine, S. B., Geyer, M. A., & Swerdlow, N. R. (1995). Effects of D3/D2 dopamine receptor agonists and antagonists on prepulse inhibition of acoustic startle in the rat. *Neuropsychopharmacology, 12,* 139–145.

Cameron, N. (1944). An experimental analysis of schizophrenic thinking. In J. S. Kasanin (Ed.), *Language and thought in schizophrenia.* California University Press.

Campeau, S., & Davis, M. (1995a). Involvement of the central nucleus and basolateral complex of the amygdala in fear conditioning measured with fear-potentiated startle in rats trained concurrently with auditory and visual conditioned stimuli. *Journal of Neuroscience, 15,* 2301–2311.

Campeau, S., & Davis, M. (1995b). Involvement of subcortical and cortical afferents to the lateral nucleus of the amygdala in fear conditioning measured with fear-potentiated startle in rats trained concurrently with auditory and visual conditioned stimuli. *Journal of Neuroscience, 15,* 2312–2327.

Campeau, S., Miserendino, M. J. D., & Davis, M. (1992). Intra-amygdala infusion of the N-methyl-D-aspartate receptor antagonist AP5 blocks acquisition but not expression of fear-potentiated startle to an auditory conditioned stimulus. *Behavioral Neuroscience, 106,* 569–574.

Cappell, H., & Greeley, J. (1987). Alcohol and tension reduction: An update on research and theory. In H. Blane & K. Leonard (Eds.), *Psychological theories of alcoholism* (pp. 15–54). New York: Guilford.

Cardenas, V. A., McCallin, K., Hopkins, R., & Fein, G. (1997). *A comparison of the repetitive click and conditioning-testing P50 paradigms.* Manuscript submitted for publication.

Carter, N. L., & Kryter, K. D. (1962). Masking of pure tones and speech. *Journal of Auditory Research, 2,* 66–98.

Cassella, J. V., & Davis, M. (1986). Habituation, prepulse inhibition, fear conditioning, and drug modulation of the acoustically elicited pinna reflex in rats. *Behavioral Neuroscience, 100,* 39–44.

Cassella, J., Hoffman, D., Rajachandran, L., Donovan, H., Bankoski, C., Lang, S., Johnson, A., Thurkauf, A., & Hutchison, A. (1994). The behavioral profile of NGD 94-1, a potent and selective dopamine D4 receptor antagonist. *Proceedings of the American College of Neuropsychopharmacology, 228.*

Castellanos, F. X., Fine, E. J., Kaysen, D., Marsh, W. L., Rapoport, J. L., & Hallett, M. (1996). Sensorimotor gating in boys with Tourette's syndrome and ADHD: Preliminary results: *Biological Psychiatry, 39,* 33–41.

Center for the Study of Emotion and Attention (CSEA-NIMH). (1997). The international affective picture system [photographic slides]. Gainesville: The Center for Research in Psychophysiology, University of Florida.

Chapman, L. J., & Chapman, J. P. (1978). The measurement of differential deficit. *Journal of Psychiatric Research, 14,* 303–311.

Chapman, L. J., & Chapman, J. P. (1987). The search for symptoms predictive of schizophrenia. *Schizophrenia Bulletin, 13,* 497–503.

Chapman, L. J., Chapman, J. P., Kwapil, T. R., Eckblad, M., & Zinser, M. C. (1994). Putatively psychosis-prone subjects ten years later. *Journal of Abnormal Psychology, 103,* 171–183.

Chapman, L. J., Chapman, J. P., & Raulin, M. L. (1978). Body-image aberration in schizophrenia. *Journal of Abnormal Psychology, 87,* 399–407.

Chapman, J., Freeman, T. F., & McGhie, A. (1959). Clinical research in schizophrenia – the psychotherapeutic approach. *British Journal of Medical Psychology, 32,* 2.

Chun, M. M., & Potter, M. C. (1995). A two-stage model for multiple target detection in rapid serial visual presentation. *Journal of Experimental Psychology: Human Perception and Performance, 21,* 109–127.

Clark, D. M. (1988). A cognitive model of panic attacks. In S. Rachman & J. D. Maser (Eds.), *Panic: Psychological perspectives* (pp. 71–89). Hillsdale, NJ: Erlbaum.

Clark, V., & Hillyard, S. A. (1996). Spatial selective attention affects early extrastriate but not striate components of the visual evoked potential. *Journal of Cognitive Neuroscience, 8,* 387–402.

Clarkson, M. W., & Berg, W. K. (1984). Bioelectric and potentiometric measures of eye blink amplitude in reflex modification paradigms. *Psychophysiology, 21,* 237–241.

Cleckley, H. (1976). *The mask of sanity* (5th ed.). St. Louis, MO: Mosby.

Clementz, B. A., Geyer, M. A., & Braff, D. L. (1997). P50 suppression among schizophrenia and normal comparison subjects: A methodological analysis. *Biological Psychiatry, 41,* 1035–1044.

Codispoti, M., Bradley, M. M., & Lang, P. J. (1996). Probing the mind's eye: Reflex modulation for briefly presented pictures [Abstract]. *Psychophysiology, 33* (Suppl. 1), S29.

Cohen, J. (1988). *Statistical power analysis for the behavioral sciences* (2nd ed.). Hillsdale, NJ: Lawrence Erlbaum.

Coles, M. G. H., Gratton, G., Bashore, T. R., Eriksen, C. W., & Donchin, E. (1985). A psychophysiological investigation of the continuous flow model of human information processing. *Journal of Experimental Psychology: Human Perception and Performance, 11,* 529–553.

Collins, D., Hale, B., & Loomis, J. (1995). Differences in emotional responsivity and anger in athletes and nonathletes: Startle reflex modulation and attributional response. *Journal of Sport & Exercise Psychology, 17,* 171–184.

Conger, J. (1956). Reinforcement theory and the dynamics of alcoholism. *Quarterly Journal of Studies on Alcohol, 17,* 296–305.

Conrad, A. J., Abebe, T., Austin, R., Forsythe, S., & Scheibel, A. B. (1991). Hippocampal pyramidal cell disarray in schizophrenia as a bilateral phenomenon. *Archives of General Psychiatry, 48,* 413–417.

Cook, E. W., III, & Berg, W. K. (1995). Startle blink measurement: Stimulus, response, and quantification issues [Abstract]. *Psychophysiology, 32* (Suppl. 1), S12.

Cook, E. W., III, Davis, T. L, Hawk, L. W., & Spence, E. L. (1992). Fearfulness and startle potentiation during aversive visual stimuli. *Psychophysiology, 29,* 633–645.

Cook, E. W., III, Davis, T. L., Hawk, L. W., Spence, E. L., & Gautier, C. H. (1992). Fearfulness and startle potentiation during aversive visual stimuli. *Psychophysiology, 29,* 633–645.

Cook, E. W., III, & Gautier, C. H. (1992, October). Emotion, startle, and individual differences: A dimensional analysis. In G. E. Bruder & R. J. Davidson (Chairs), *Psychophysiological studies of emotion and mood disorders.* Symposium conducted at the Thirty-Second Annual Meeting of the Society for Psychophysiological Research, San Diego, California.

Cook, E. W., III, Goates, D. W., Hawk, L. W., & Palmatier, A. D. (1996). Specificity of startle modulation revisited: Relationships of affective and prepulse modification to fearfulness and schizotypy [Abstract]. *Psychophysiology, 33* (Suppl. 1), S31.

Cook, E. W., III, Hawk, L. W., Davis, T. L., & Stevenson, V. E. (1991). Affective individual differences and startle reflex modulation. *Journal of Abnormal Psychology, 100,* 5–13.

Cook, E. W., III, Hawk, L. W., Hawk, T. M., & Hummer, K. (1995). Affective modulation of startle in children [Abstract]. *Psychophysiology, 32* (Suppl. 1), S25.

Cook, E. W., III, & Miller, G. A. (1992). Digital filtering: Background and tutorial for psychophysiologists. *Psychophysiology, 29,* 350–367.

Cook, E. W., III, Stevenson, V. E., & Hawk, L. W. (1993, September). Enhanced startle modulation and negative affectivity. In R. J. Davidson (Chair), *Psychophysiological approaches to affective and anxiety disorders.* Symposium conducted at the Annual Meeting of the Society for Research in Psychopathology, Chicago, Illinois.

Cook, E. W., III, & Turpin, G. (1997). Differentiating orienting, startle and defense responses: The role of affect and its implications for psychopathology. In P. J. Lang, R. F. Simons, & M. T. Balaban (Eds.), *Attention and orienting: Sensory and motivational processes* (pp. 137–164). Hillsdale, NJ: Erlbaum.

Corbetta, M., Miezin, F. M., Dobmeyer, G. L., Shulman, G. L., & Petersen, S. E. (1991). Selective and divided attention during visual discrimination of color, shape and speed. *Journal of Neuroscience, 11,* 2383–2402.

Corr, J. P., Wilson, G. D., Fotiadou, M., Kumari, V., Gray, N. S., Checkley, S., Gray, J. A. (1995). Personality and affective modulation of the startle reflex. *Personality and Individual Differences, 19,* 543–553.

Cowan, N. (1995). *Attention and memory: An integrated framework.* Oxford: Oxford University Press.

Cowey, A., & Stoerig, P. (1995). Blindsight in monkeys. *Nature, 373,* 247–249.

Cranney, J., & Cohen, M. E. (1985). The glabella startle reflex: Inhibition by frequency and intensity modulation. *Perception & Psychophysics, 37,* 28–34.

Crick, F. (1994). *The astonishing hypothesis.* New York: Scribner's.

Crofton, K. M., & Sheets, L. P. (1989). Evaluation of sensory system function using reflex modification of the startle response. *Journal of the American College of Toxicology, 8,* 199–211.

Cruccu, G., Ferracuti, S., Leardi, M. G., Fabbri, A., & Manfredi, M. (1991). Nociceptive quality of the orbicularis oculi reflexes as evaluated by distinct opiate- and benzodiazepine-induced changes in man. *Brain Research, 556,* 209–217.

Curtin, J. J., Lang, A. R., Patrick, C. J., & Stritzke, W. G. K. (1997). *Alcohol and fear-potentiated startle: The role of distraction in the stress-response dampening effects of intoxication.* Unpublished manuscript.

Cuthbert, B. N., Bradley, M. M., & Lang, P. J. (1996). Probing picture perception: Activation and emotion. *Psychophysiology, 33,* 103–111.

Cuthbert, B. N., Bradley, M. M., York, D., & Lang, P. J. (1990). Affective imagery and startle modulation [Abstract]. *Psychophysiology, 27,* S24.

Cuthbert, B. N., Schupp, H. T., Bradley, M. M., Birbaumer, N., & Lang, P. J. (1997). *Cortical potentials in emotional perception.* Manuscript submitted for publication.

Cuthbert, B. N., Schupp, H. T., Bradley, M. M., McManis, M. H., & Lang, P. J. (1997). *Probing affective pictures: Attended startle and tone probes.* Manuscript submitted for publication.

Cuthbert, B. N., Strauss, C., Drobes, D., Patrick, C. J., Bradley, M. M., & Lang, P. J. (1997). *Startle and the anxiety disorders.* Manuscript submitted for publication.

Dahlstrom, W. G., Welsh, L. E., & Dahlstrom, L. E. (1972). *An MMPI handbook* (Vol. 1). Minneapolis: University of Minnesota Press.

Davey, G. C. L. (1994). Is evaluative conditioning a qualitatively distinct form of classical conditioning? *Behavior Research and Therapy, 32,* 291–299.

Davidson, R. J. (1992). Anterior cerebral asymmetry and the nature of emotion. *Brain & Cognition, 20,* 125–151.

Davis, H., Mast, T., Yoshie, N., & Zerlin, S. (1966). The slow response of the human cortex to auditory stimuli: Recovery process. *Electroencephalography & Clinical Neurophysiology, 21,* 105–113.

Davis, M. (1974a). Sensitization of the rat startle response by noise. *Journal of Comparative and Physiological Psychology, 87,* 571–581.

Davis, M. (1974b). Signal-to-noise ratio as a predictor of startle amplitude and habituation in the rat. *Journal of Comparative and Physiological Psychology, 86,* 812–825.

Davis, M. (1979). Diazepam and flurazepam: Effects on conditioned fear as measured with the potentiated startle paradigm. *Psychopharmacology, 62,* 1–7.

Davis, M. (1980). Neurochemical modulation of sensory-motor reactivity: Acoustic and tactile startle reflexes. *Neuroscience Biobehavioral Reviews, 4,* 241–263.

Davis, M. (1984). The mammalian startle response. In R. C. Eaton (Ed.), *Neural mechanisms of startle behavior* (pp. 287–342). New York: Plenum Press.

Davis, M. (1986). Pharmacological and anatomical analysis of fear conditioning using the fear-potentiated startle paradigm. *Behavioral Neuroscience, 100,* 814–824.

Davis, M. (1992). The role of the amygdala in conditioned fear. In J. Aggleton (Ed.), *The amygdala: Neurobiological aspects of emotion, memory and mental dysfunction* (pp. 255–305). New York: John Wiley & Sons, Inc.

Davis, M., & Astrachan, D. I. (1978). Conditioned fear and startle magnitude: Effects of different footshock or backshock intensities used in training. *Journal of Experimental Psychology: Animal Behavior Processes, 4,* 95–103.

Davis, M., & File, S. E. (1984). Intrinsic and extrinsic mechanisms of habituation and sensitization: Implications for the design and analysis of experiments. In H. V. S. Peeke & L. Petrinovich (Eds.), *Habituation, sensitization, and behavior* (pp. 287–324). New York: Academic Press.

Davis, M., & Gendelman, P. M. (1977). Plasticity of the acoustic startle response in the acutely decerebrate rat. *Journal of Comparative and Physiological Psychology, 91,* 549–563.

Davis, M., Gendelman, D. S., Tischler, M. D., & Gendelman, P. M. (1982). A primary acoustic startle circuit: Lesion and stimulation studies. *Journal of Neuroscience, 2,* 791–805.

Davis, M., Gewirtz, J., & McNish, K. (1995). Effects of amygdala lesions vs. lesions of the bed nucleus of the stria terminalis on explicit cue vs. contextual fear conditioning. *Society for Neuroscience Abstracts.*

Davis, M., Hitchcock, J., & Rosen, J. (1987). Anxiety and the amygdala: Pharmacological and anatomical analysis of the fear potentiated startle paradigm. In G. H. Bower (Ed.), *Psychology of learning and motivation* (Vol. 21, pp. 263–305). New York: Academic Press.

Davis, M., Mansbach, R. S., Swerdlow, N. R., Campeau, S., Braff, D. L., & Geyer, M. A. (1990). Apomorphine disrupts the inhibition of acoustic startle induced by weak prepulses in rats. *Psychopharmacology, 102,* 1–4.

Davis, M., Parisi, T., Gendelman, D. S., Tischler, M. D., & Kehne, J. H. (1982). Habituation and sensitization of startle reflexes elicited electrically from the brainstem. *Science, 218,* 688–690.

Davis, M., Schlesinger, L. S., & Sorenson, C. A. (1989). Temporal specificity of fear-conditioning: Effects of different conditioned stimulus–unconditioned stimulus intervals on the fear-potentiated startle effect. *Journal of Experimental Psychology: Animal Behavior Processes, 15,* 295–310.

Davis, M., Walker, D. L., & Lee, Y. (in press). Amygdala and bed nucleus of the stria terminalis: Differential roles in fear and anxiety measured with the acoustic startle reflex. In L. Squire & D. Schacter (Eds.), *Biological and psychological perspectives on memory and memory disorders.* Washington, DC: American Psychiatric Press.

Dawson, M. E., Filion, D. L., & Schell, A. M. (1989). Is elicitation of the autonomic orienting response associated with allocation of processing resources? *Psychophysiology, 26,* 560–572.

Dawson, M. E., Hazlett, E. A., Filion, D. L., Nuechterlein, K. N., & Schell, A. M. (1993). Attention and schizophrenia: Impaired modulation of the startle reflex. *Journal of Abnormal Psychology, 102,* 633–641.

Dawson, M. E., & Schell, A. M. (1985). Information processing and human autonomic classical conditioning. In P. K. Ackles, J. R. Jennings, & M. G. H. Coles (Eds.), *Advances in psychophysiology* (Vol. 1, pp. 89–165). Greenwich, CT: JAI Press Inc.

Dawson, M. E., Schell, A. M., & Filion, D. L. (1990). The electrodermal system. In J. T. Cacioppo & L. G. Tassinary (Eds.), *Principles of psychophysiology physical, social, and inferential elements* (pp. 295–324). Cambridge: Cambridge University Press.

Dawson, M. E., Schell, A. M., Swerdlow, N. R., & Filion, D. L. (1997). Cognitive, clinical, and neurophysiological implications of startle modification. In P. J. Lang, R. F. Simons, & M. T. Balaban (Eds.), *Attention and orientation: Sensory and motivational processes* (pp. 257–279). Hillsdale, NJ: Erlbaum.

de Jong, P. J., Arntz, A., & Merckelbach, H. (1993). The startle probe response as an instrument for evaluating exposure effects in spider phobia. *Advances in Behaviour Research and Therapy, 15,* 301–316.

de Jong, P. J., Merckelbach, H., & Arntz, A. (1991). Eyeblink startle responses in spider phobics before and after treatment: A pilot study. *Journal of Psychopathology and Behavioral Assessment, 13,* 213–223.

de Jong, P. J., Visser, S., & Merckelbach, H. (1996). Startle and spider phobia: Unilateral probes and the prediction of treatment effects. *Journal of Psychophysiology, 10*.

de Jong, R., Coles, M. G. H., Logan, G. L., & Gratton, G. (1990). In search of the point of no return: The control of response processes. *Journal of Experimental Psychology: Human Perception and Performance, 16*, 164–182.

Deacon, T. W., Eichenbaum, H., Rosenberg, P., & Ecknamm, K. W. (1983). Afferent connections of the perirhinal cortex in the rat. *Journal of Comparative Neurology, 229*, 168–190.

Decker, M. W., Curzon, P., & Brioni, J. D. (1995). Influence of separate and combined septal and amygdala lesions on memory, acoustic startle, anxiety, and locomotor activity in rats. *Neurobiology of Learning and Memory, 64*, 156–168.

DelPezzo, E. M., & Hoffman, H. S. (1980). Attentional factors in the inhibition of a reflex by a visual stimulus. *Science, 210*, 673–674.

Depaulis, A., Keay, K. A., & Bandler, R. (1992). Longitudinal neuronal organization of defensive reactions in the midbrain periaqueductal gray region of the rat. *Experimental Brain Research, 90*, 307–318.

Depaulis, A., Keay, K. A., & Bandler, R. (1994). Quiescence and hyporeactivity evoked by activation of cell bodies in the ventrolateral midbrain periaqueductal gray of the rat. *Experimental Brain Research, 99*, 75–83.

Detenber, B. (1995). *The effects of motion and image size on affective responses to and memory for pictures*. Unpublished doctoral dissertation, Stanford University.

Dickinson, A., & Dearing, M. F. (1979). Appetitive-aversive interactions and inhibitory processes. In A. Dickinson & R. A. Boakes (Eds.), *Mechanisms of learning and motivation* (pp. 203–231). Hillsdale, NJ: Erlbaum.

Docherty, N. M., & Hebert, A. (1996). *Prepulse inhibition, habituation and communication disturbances in schizophrenia*. Paper presented at the 149th annual meeting of the American Psychiatric Association, p. 533.

Dodge, R. (1931). *Conditions and consequences of human variability*. New Haven, CT: Yale University Press.

Donchin, E. (1981). Presidential address, 1980. Surprise! . . . . Surprise? *Psychophysiology, 18*, 493–513.

Donchin, E., & Coles, M. (1988). Is the P300 component a manifestation of context updating? (Commentary on Verleger's critique of the context updating model). *Behavioral and Brain Sciences, 11*, 357–374.

Donchin, E., Karis, D., & Bashore, T. R. (1986). Cognitive psychophysiology and human information processing. In M. G. H. Coles, E. Donchin, & S. W. Porges (Eds.), *Psychophysiology: Systems, processes and application* (pp. 244–267). New York: Guilford Press.

Donchin, E., Kramer, A. F., & Wickens, C. (1986). Applications of brain event-related potentials to problems in engineering psychology. In M. G. H. Coles, E. Donchin, & S. W. Porges (Eds.), *Psychophysiology: Systems, processes and application* (pp. 702–718). New York: Guilford Press.

Drobes, D. J., Hillman, C., Bradley, M. M., Cuthbert, B. N., & Lang, P. J. (1995). Effects of food deprivation on affective startle modulation and eating behavior [Abstract]. *Psychophysiology, 32* (Suppl. 1), S28.

Duffy, E. (1957). The psychological significance of the concept of "arousal" or "activation." *Psychological Review, 64*, 265–275.

Dulawa, S. C., Hen, R., Scearce, K., & Geyer, M. A. (1995). Characterization of serotonin 1B receptor contribution to startle amplitude and prepulse inhibition in wild type and serotonin 1B minus mice. *Society for Neuroscience Abstracts, 21,* 1693.

Dulawa, S. C., Hen, R., Scearce, K., & Geyer, M. A. (1996). Effects of RU24969, 8-OH-DPAT, and GR127935 on prepulse inhibition in wild type and serotonin 1B minus mice. *Proceedings of the Society for Neurosciences, 22,* 2066.

Dunn, A. J., & Berridge, C. W. (1990). Physiological and behavioral responses to corticotropin-releasing factor administration: Is CRF a mediator of anxiety or stress responses? *Brain Research Reviews, 15,* 71–100.

Dykman, B. M., & Ison, J. R. (1979). Temporal integration of acoustic stimulation obtained in reflex inhibition in rats and humans. *Journal of Comparative and Physiological Psychology, 93,* 939–945.

Early, T. S., Relman, E. M., Raichle, M. E., & Spitzmagel, E. L. (1987). Left globus pallidus abnormality in newly medicated patients with schizophrenia. *Proceedings of the National Academy of Sciences, USA, 84,* 561.

Eccles, J. C., & Granit, R. (1929). Crossed extensor reflexes and their interactions. *Journal of Physiology, 67,* 97–118.

Eccles, J. C., & Sherrington, C. S. (1930). Reflex summation in the ipsilateral spinal flexion reflex. *Journal of Physiology, 69,* 1–28.

Eckblad, M., & Chapman, L. J. (1983). Magical ideation as an indicator of schizotypy. *Journal of Consulting and Clinical Psychology, 51,* 215–225.

Ellenbroek, B. A., Budde, S., & Cools, A. R. (1995). The role of dopamine D1 and D2 receptors in the medial prefrontal cortex in prepulse inhibition. *Society for Neuroscience Abstracts, 21,* 747.

Elmasian, R., Galambos, R., & Bernheim, A. (1980). Loudness enhancement and decrement in four paradigms. *Journal of the Acoustical Society of America, 67,* 601–607.

Enright, S. J., & Beech, A. (1993a). Reduced cognitive inhibition in obsessive–compulsive disorder. *British Journal of Clinical Psychology, 32,* 67–74.

Enright, S. J., & Beech, A. (1993b). Further evidence of reduced cognitive inhibition in obsessive-compulsive disorder. *Personality and Individual Differences, 14,* 387–395.

Erickson, L. M., Levenston, G. K., Curtin, J., Goff, A., & Patrick, C. J. (1995). Affect and attention in startle modulation: Picture perception and anticipation [Abstract]. *Psychophysiology, 32* (Suppl. 1), S30.

Erlichman, H., Brown, S., Zhu, J., & Warrenburg, S. (1995). Startle reflex modulation during exposure to pleasant and unpleasant odors. *Psychophysiology, 32,* 150–154.

Evinger, C., Shaw, M. D., Peck, C. K., Manning, K. A., & Baker, R. (1984). Blinking and associated eye movements in humans, guinea pigs, and rabbits. *Journal of Neurophysiology, 52,* 323–339.

Exner, J. E. (1986). *The Rorschach: A comprehensive system: Volume 1. Basic foundations* (2nd ed.). New York: Wiley.

Fallon, J. H., & Genevento, L. A. (1977). Auditory–visual interaction in cat orbito-insular cortex. *Neuroscience Letters, 6,* 143–149.

Falls, W. A., & Davis, M. (1994a). Fear-potentiated startle using three conditioned stimulus modalities. *Animal Learning and Behavior, 22,* 379–383.

Falls, W. A., & Davis, M. (1994b). Visual cortex ablations do not prevent extinction of fear-potentiated startle using a visual conditioned stimulus. *Behavioral and Neural Biology, 60,* 259–270.

Fanselow, M. S. (1994). Neural organization of the defensive behavior system responsible for fear. *Psychonomic Bulletin and Review, 1,* 429–438.

Farber, I. B., & Churchland, P. S. (1995). Consciousness and the neurosciences: Philosophical and theoretical issues. In M. S. Gazzaniga (Ed.), *The cognitive neurosciences* (pp. 1295–1306). Cambridge, MA: MIT Press.

Fearing, F. (1930). *Reflex action.* Baltimore, MD: Williams & Wilkins.

Fechter, L. D., & Young, J. S. (1983). Discrimination of auditory from nonauditory toxicity by reflex modification audiometry: Effects of triethyltin. *Toxicology and Applied Pharmacology, 70,* 216–227.

Feifel, D., & Minor, K. L. (1997). Cysteamine reverses amphetamine-induced deficts in sensorimotor gating. *Pharmacology, Biochemistry and Behavior, 58,* 689–693.

Feifel, D., Dulawa, S., Taaid, N., & Swerdlow, N. R. (1995). Effects of nucleus accumbens injections of neurotensin on sensorimotor gating. *Society for Neuroscience Abstracts, 27,* 756.

Felsten, G., & Wasserman, G. S. (1980). Visual masking: Mechanisms and theories. *Psychological Bulletin, 88,* 329–353.

Fendt, M., Koch, M., & Schnitzler, H.-U. (1994a). Lesions of the central grey block sensitization and fear potentiation of the acoustic startle response in rats. *Society for Neuroscience Abstracts, 20,* 1954.

Fendt, M., Koch, M., & Schnitzler, H.-U. (1994b). Sensorimotor gating deficits after lesions of the superior colliculus. *NeuroReport, 5,* 1725–1728.

Fey, E. T. (1951). The performance of young schizophrenics and young normals on the Wisconsin Card Sorting Test. *Journal of Consulting Psychology, 15,* 311–319.

Filion, D. L., & Ciranni, M. (1994). The functional significance of prepulse inhibition: A test of the protection of processing theory [Abstract]. *Psychophysiology, 31* (Suppl. 1), S46.

Filion, D. L., Dawson, M. E., & Schell, A. M. (1993). Modification of the acoustic startle-reflex eyeblink: A tool for investigating early and late attentional processes. *Biological Psychology, 35,* 185–200.

Filion, D. L., Dawson, M. E., & Schell, A. M. (1994). Probing the orienting response with startle modification and secondary reaction time. *Psychophysiology, 31,* 68–78.

Filion, D. L., Dawson, M. E., & Schell, A. M. (1998). The psychological significance of human startle eyeblink modification: A review. *Biological Psychology, 47,* 1–43.

Filion, D. L., & McDowd, J. M. (1991, October). *Startle modification and selective attention deficits in aging.* Paper presented at the annual meeting of the Society for Psychophysiological Research, Chicago, IL.

Filion, D. L., & McDowd, J. M. (1992). Startle modification and negative priming: Converging measures of inhibitory function in young and older adults [Abstract]. *Psychophysiology, 29* (Suppl. 1), S32.

Flaten, M. A. (1993). Startle reflex facilitation as a function of classical eyeblink conditioning in humans. *Psychophysiology, 30,* 581–588.

Flaten, M. A., & Hugdahl, K. (1991). Does classical eyeblink conditioning generate sensitization of the neural pathway of the conditioned stimulus (CS+)? *Psychobiology, 19,* 51–57.

Fleshler, M. (1965). Adequate acoustic stimulus for startle reaction in the rat. *Journal of Comparative and Physiological Psychology, 15,* 492–495.

Florentine, M., Fastl, H., & Buus, S. (1988). Temporal integration in normal hearing, cochlear impairment, and impairment simulated by masking. *Journal of the Acoustical Society of America, 84,* 195–203.

Ford, J. M., & Pfefferbaum, A. (1991). Event-related potentials and eyeblink responses in automatic and controlled processing: Effects of age. *Electroencephalography & Clinical Neurophysiology, 78,* 361–377.

Ford, J. M., Roth, W. T., Bell, C. M., Li, Y., & Jain, S. (1996). Prepulse inhibition of ERP components elicited by startling noises [Abstract]. *Psychophysiology, 33* (Suppl. 1), S37.

Ford, J. M., Roth, W. T., Isaacks, B. G., Tinklenberg, J., Yesavage, J., & Pfefferbaum, A. (1997). Automatic and effortful processing in aging and dementia: Event-related brain potentials. *Neurobiology of Aging, 18,* 169–180.

Ford, J. M., Roth, W. T., & Kopell, B. S. (1976). Attention effects on auditory evoked potentials to infrequent events. *Biological Psychology, 4,* 65–77.

Ford, J. M., Sullivan, E. V., Marsh, L., White, P. K., Lim, K. O., & Pfefferbaum, A. (1994). The relationship between P300 amplitude and regional gray matter volumes depends upon the attentional system engaged. *Electroencephalography & Clinical Neurophysiology, 90,* 214–228.

Fowles, D. C. (1980). The three arousal model: Implications of Gray's two-factor learning theory for heart rate, electrodermal activity, and psychopathy. *Psychophysiology, 17,* 87–104.

Franks, R. D., Adler, L. E., Waldo, M. C., Alpert, J., & Freedman, R. (1983). Neurophysiological studies of sensory gating in mania: Comparison with schizophrenia. *Biological Psychiatry, 18,* 989–1005.

Freedman, R., Adler, L. E., Waldo, M. C., Pachtman, E., & Franks, R. D. (1983). Neurophysiological evidence for a defect in inhibitory pathways in schizophrenia: Comparison of medicated and drug-free patients. *Biological Psychiatry, 18,* 537–552.

Freedman, R., Adler, L., & Waldo, M. (1987). Gating of the auditory evoked potential in children and adults. *Psychophysiology, 24,* 223–227.

Freedman, R., Coon, H., Myles-Worsley, M., Orr-Urtreger, A., Olincy, A., Davis A., Polymeropoulos, M., Holik, J., Hopkins, J., Hoff, M., Rosenthal, J., Waldo M. C., Reimherr, F., Wender, P., Yaw, J., Young, D. A., Breese, C. R., Adams, C., Patterson, D., Adler, L. E., Kruglyak, L., Leonard, S., & Byerley W. (1997). Linkage of a neurophysiological deficit in schizophrenia to a chromosone 15 locus. *Proceedings of the National Academy of Sciences, 94,* 587–592.

Frick, P. J. (in press). Callous–unemotional traits and conduct problems: Applying the two-factor model of psychopathy to children. In D. J. Cooke, A. Forth, & R. D. Hare (Eds.), *Psychopathy: Theory, research, and implications for society.* Dordrecht, The Netherlands: Kluwer Press.

Fridlund, A. J., & Cacioppo, J. T. (1986). Guidelines for human electromyographic research. *Psychophysiology, 23,* 567–589.

Frith, C. D. (1979). Consciousness, information processing and schizophrenia. *British Journal of Psychiatry, 134,* 225–235.

Fuster, J. M. (1989). *The prefrontal cortex: Anatomy, physiology, and neuropsychology of the frontal lobe* (2nd ed.). New York: Raven Press.

Gainotti, G. (1989). Disorders of emotions and affect after unilateral damage. In F.

Boller & J. Grafman (Eds.), *Handbook of clinical neuropsychology. Vol. 3: Emotional behavior and Its disorders.* New York: Elsevier.

Gautier, C. H., & Cook, E. W., III (1997). Relationships between cardiovascular reactivity and startle reflex modulation. *Psychophysiology, 34,* 87–96.

Gelfland, S. A. (1990). *Hearing: An introduction to psychological and physiological acoustics* (2nd ed.). New York: Dekker.

Gersuni, G. V. (1971). Temporal organization of the auditory function. In G. V. Gersuni (Ed.), *Sensory processes at the neuronal and behavioral levels* (pp. 85–114). New York: Academic Press.

Gescheider, G. A., Hoffman, K. E., Harrison, M. A., Travis, M. L., & Bolanowski, S. J. (1994). The effects of masking on vibrotactile temporal summation in the detection of sinusoidal and noise signals. *Journal of the Acoustical Society of America, 95,* 1001–1016.

Gewirtz, J. C., & Davis, M. (1995). Habituation of prepulse inhibition of the startle reflex using an auditory prepulse close to background noise. *Behavioral Neuroscience, 109,* 388–395.

Geyer, M. A., & Braff, D. L. (1982). Habituation of the blink reflex in normals and schizophrenic patients. *Psychophysiology, 19,* 1–6.

Geyer, M. A., & Braff, D. L. (1987). Startle habituation and sensorimotor gating in schizophrenia and related animal models. *Schizophrenia Bulletin, 13,* 643–668.

Geyer, M. A., Swerdlow, N. R., Mansbach, R. S., & Braff, D. L. (1990). Startle response models of sensorimotor gating and habituation deficits in schizophrenia. *Brain Research Bulletin, 25,* 485–498.

Geyer, M. A., Wilkinson, L. S., Humby, T., & Robbins, T. W. (1993). Isolation rearing of rats produces a deficit in prepulse inhibition of acoustic startle similar to that in schizophrenia. *Biological Psychiatry, 34,* 361–372.

Globisch, J., Hamm, A. O., Esteves, F., & Öhman, A. (1994). Timecourse of the startle reflex modulation during short versus sustained visual stimulation in simple phobics and normals [Abstract]. *Psychophysiology, 31* (Suppl. 1), S90.

Gottschalk, L. A., Haer, J. L., & Bates, D. E. (1972). Effect of sensory overload on psychological state. *Archives of General Psychiatry, 27,* 451–457.

Gouras, P. (1985). Oculomotor system. In E. R. Kandel & J. H. Schwartz (Eds.), *Principles of neural science* (pp. 571–583). Amsterdam: Elsevier.

Graham, F. K. (1975). The more or less startling effects of weak prestimulation. *Psychophysiology, 12,* 238–248.

Graham, F. K. (1979). Distinguishing among orienting, defense, and startle reflexes. In H. D. Kimmel, E. H. van Olst, & J. F. Orlebeke (Eds.), *The orienting reflex in humans* (pp. 137–167). Hillsdale, NJ: Erlbaum.

Graham, F. K. (1980). Control of blink reflex excitability. In R. F. Thompson, L. H. Hicks, & V. B. Shvyrkov (Eds.), *Neural mechanisms of goal-directed behavior and learning* (pp. 511–519). New York: Academic Press.

Graham, F. K. (1992). Attention: The heartbeat, the blink, and the brain. In B. A. Campbell, H. Hayne, & R. Richardson (Eds.), *Attention and information processing in infants and adults: Perspectives from human and animal research* (pp. 3–29). Hillsdale, NJ: Lawrence Erlbaum Associates.

Graham, F. K. (1997). Afterword: Pre-attentive processing and passive and active attention. In P. J. Lang, R. F. Simons, & M. T. Balaban (Eds.), *Attention and orienting: Sensory and motivational processes* (pp. 417–452). Hillsdale, NJ: Lawrence Erlbaum Associates.

Graham, F. K., & Clifton, R. K. (1966). Heart rate change as a component of the orienting response. *Psychological Bulletin, 65,* 305–320.

Graham, F. K., & Hackley, S. A. (1991). Passive and active attention to input. In J. R. Jennings & M. G. H. Coles (Eds.), *Handbook of cognitive psychophysiology* (pp. 251–356). New York: John Wiley.

Graham, F. K., & Murray, G. M. (1977). Discordant effects of weak prestimulation on magnitude and latency of the reflex blink. *Physiological Psychology, 5,* 108–114.

Graham, F. K., Putnam, L. E., & Leavitt, L. A. (1975). Lead stimulation effects on human cardiac orienting and blink reflexes. *Journal of Experimental Psychology: Human Perception and Performance, 104,* 161–169.

Graham, F. K., Strock, B. D., & Zeigler, B. L. (1981). Excitatory and inhibitory influences on reflex responsiveness. In W. A. Collins (Ed.), *Aspects of the development of competence, the Minnesota symposium on child psychology* (pp. 1–38). Hillsdale, NJ: Lawrence Erlbaum.

Grandy, D. K., Kelly, M. A., Rubinstein, M., Saez, C., Bunzow, J. R., Zhang, G., Larson, J. L., Unteustch, A., Garfinkle, J. S., Feddern, C., Japon, M., Civelli, O., Dulawa, S. C., Geyer, M. A., & Low, M. J. (1995). Generation and characterization of dopamine D2 and D4 receptor-deficient transgenic mice. *Proceedings of the American College of Neuropsychopharmacology, 179.*

Grant, D. A., & Berg, E. A. (1948). A behavioral analysis of degree of reinforcement and ease of shifting to new responses in a Weigl type card sorting problem. *Journal of Experimental Psychology, 38,* 404–411.

Gratton, G. (1997). Attention and probability effects in the human occipital cortex: An optical imaging study. *NeuroReport, 8,* 1749–1753.

Gratton, G., Coles, M. G. H., & Donchin, E. (1983). A new method for offline removal of ocular artifact. *Electroencephalography & Clinical Neurophysiology, 55,* 468–484.

Green, D. M. (1973). Minimum integration time. In A. R. Moller (Ed.), *Basic mechanisms in hearing.* New York: Academic Press.

Green, M. F., Nuechterlein, K. H., & Mintz, J. (1994). Backward masking in schizophrenia and mania: II. Specifying the visual channels. *Archives of General Psychiatry, 51,* 945–951.

Greenwald, M., Bradley, M., Cuthbert, B. N., & Lang, P. (1990). The acoustic startle response indexes aversive learning [Abstract]. *Psychophysiology, 27,* S36.

Greenwald, M. K., Cook, E. W., & Lang, P. J. (1989). Affective judgment and psychophysiological response: Dimensional covariation in the evaluation of pictorial stimuli. *Journal of Psychophysiology, 3,* 51–64.

Grillon, C., Ameli, R., Charney, D. S., Krystal, J., & Braff, D. L. (1992). Startle gating deficits occur across prepulse intensities in schizophrenic patients. *Biological Psychiatry, 32,* 939–943.

Grillon, C., Ameli, R., Foot, M., & Davis, M. (1993). Fear-potentiated startle: Relationships to the level of state/trait anxiety in healthy subjects. *Biological Psychiatry, 33,* 566–574.

Grillon, C., Ameli, R., Goddard, A., Woods, S., & Davis, M. (1994). Baseline and fear-potentiated startle in panic disorder patients. *Biological Psychiatry, 35,* 431–439.

Grillon, C., Ameli, R., Merikangas, K., Woods, S. W., & Davis, M. (1993). Measuring the time course of anticipatory anxiety using the fear-potentiated startle reflex. *Psychophysiology, 30,* 340–346.

Grillon, C., Ameli, R., Woods, S. W., Merikangas, K., & Davis, M. (1991). Fear-potentiated startle in humans: Effects of anticipatory anxiety on the acoustic blink reflex. *Psychophysiology, 28,* 588–595.

Grillon, C., & Davis, M. (1995). Acoustic startle and anticipatory anxiety in humans: Effects of monaural right and left ear stimulation. *Psychophysiology, 32,* 155–161.

Grillon, C., Falls, W. A., Ameli, R., & Davis, M. (1994). Safety signals and human anxiety: A fear-potentiated startle study. *Anxiety, 1,* 13–21.

Grillon, C., & Morgan, C. A., III (1997). Fear-potentiated startle conditioning to explicit and contextual cues in Gulf War veterans with posttraumatic stress disorder. Manuscript submitted for publication.

Grillon, C., Morgan, C. A., Southwick, S. M., Davis, M., & Charney, D. (1996). Baseline startle response and prepulse inhibition in Vietnam veterans with PTSD. *Psychiatry Research, 64,* 169–178.

Grillon, C., Morgan, C. A., Davis, M., & Southwick, S. M. (in press). Effects of experimental context and explicit threat cues on acoustic startle in Vietnam veterans with posttraumatic stress disorder. *Biological Psychiatry.*

Groves, P. M. (1983). A theory of the functional organization of the neostriatum and the neostriatal control of voluntary movement. *Brain Research Reviews, 5,* 109–132.

Groves, P. M., & Thompson, R. F. (1970). Habituation: A dual-process theory. *Psychological Review, 77,* 419–450.

Guldin, W. O., & Markowitsch, H. J. (1983). Cortical and thalamic afferent connections of the insular and adjacent cortex of the rat. *Journal of Comparative Neurology, 215,* 135–153.

Guterman, Y., Josiassen, R. C., & Bashore, T. R. (1992). Attentional influence on the P50 component of the auditory event-related brain potential. *International Journal of Psychophysiology, 12,* 197–209.

Hackley, S. A. (1993). An evaluation of the automaticity of sensory processing using event-related potentials and brain-stem reflexes. *Psychophysiology, 30,* 415–428.

Hackley, S. A., & Boelhouwer, A. J. W. (1997). The more or less startling effects of weak prestimulation – Revisited: Prepulse modulation of multicomponent blink reflexes. In P. J. Lang, R. F. Simons, & M. T. Balaban (Eds.), *Attention and orienting: Sensory and motivational processes* (pp. 205–227). Hillsdale, NJ: Erlbaum.

Hackley, S. A., & Burke, J. (1992). Visuospatial attention effects on voluntary and reflexive reactions [Abstract]. *Psychophysiology, 29,* S36.

Hackley, S. A., & Graham, F. K. (1983). Early selective attention effects on cutaneous and acoustic blink reflexes. *Physiological Psychology, 11,* 235–242.

Hackley, S. A., & Graham, F. K. (1987). Effects of attending selectively to the spatial position of reflex-eliciting and reflex-modulating stimuli. *Journal of Experimental Psychology: Human Perception and Performance, 13,* 411–424.

Hackley, S. A., & Graham, F. K. (1991). Passive and active attention to input: Active (voluntary) attention and localized, selective orienting. In J. R. Jennings & M. G. H. Coles (Eds.), *Handbook of cognitive psychophysiology* (pp. 299–356). Chichester: Wiley.

Hackley, S. A., & Johnson, L. N. (1996). Distinct early and late subcomponents of the photic blink reflex: Response characteristics in patients with retrogeniculate lesions. *Psychophysiology, 33,* 239–251.

Hackley, S. A., Sollers, J., & Stafford-Segert, I. (1991). Motor preparation and the visual blink reflex [Abstract]. *Psychophysiology, 28,* S27.

Hackley, S. A., Woldorff, M., & Hillyard, S. A. (1987). Combined use of microreflexes and event-related brain potentials as measures of auditory selective attention. *Psychophysiology, 24,* 632–647.

Hackley, S. A., Woldorff, M., & Hillyard, S. A. (1990). Cross-modal selective attention effects on retinal, myogenic, brainstem, and cerebral evoked potentials. *Psychophysiology, 27,* 195–208.

Haerich, P. (1994). Startle reflex modification: Effects of attention vary with emotional valence. *Psychological Science, 5,* 407–410.

Hall, G. (1995). Pavlovian conditioning: Laws of association. In N. J. Mackintosh (Ed.), *Animal learning and cognition* (pp. 15–44). New York, NY: Academic Press.

Hamm, A. O., Cuthbert, B. N., Globisch, J., & Vaitl, D. (1997). Fear and the startle reflex: Blink modulation and autonomic response patterns in animal and mutilation fearful subjects. *Psychophysiology, 34,* 97–107.

Hamm, A. O., Greenwald, M. K., Bradley, M. M., & Lang, P. J. (1993). Emotional learning, hedonic change, and the startle reflex. *Journal of Abnormal Psychology, 102,* 453–465.

Hamm, A. O., & Stark, R. (1993). Sensitization and aversive conditioning: Effects on the startle reflex and electrodermal responding. *Integrative Physiological and Behavioral Science, 28,* 171–176.

Hamm, A. O., & Vaitl, D. (1993). Affective associations: The conditioning model and the organization of emotions. In N. Birbaumer & A. Öhman (Eds.), *The organization of emotions* (pp. 203–217). Toronto: Hogrefe.

Hamm, A. O., & Vaitl, D (1996). Affective learning: Awareness and aversion. *Psychophysiology, 33,* 698–711.

Harbin, T. J., & Berg, W. K. (1983). The effects of age and prestimulus duration upon reflex inhibition. *Psychophysiology, 20,* 603–610.

Hare, R. D. (1978). Electrodermal and cardiovascular correlates of psychopathy. In R. D. Hare & D. Schalling (Eds.), *Psychopathic behavior: Approaches to research* (pp. 107–143). Chichester: Wiley.

Hare, R. D. (1980). A research scale for the assessment of psychopathy in criminal populations. *Personality and Individual Differences, 1,* 111–119.

Hare, R. D. (1986). Twenty years of experience with the Cleckley psychopath. In W. H. Reid, D. Dorr, J. I. Walker, & J. W. Bonner (Eds.), *Unmasking the psychopath* (pp. 3–27). New York: W. W. Norton & Co.

Hare, R. D. (1991). *The Hare Psychopathy Checklist – Revised.* Toronto: Multi-Health Systems.

Hare, R. D., Hart, S. D., & Harpur, T. J. (1991). Psychopathy and the proposed DSM-IV criteria for antisocial personality disorder. *Journal of Abnormal Psychology, 100,* 391–398.

Harpur, T. J., Hakstian, A. R., & Hare, R. D. (1988). Factor structure of the psychopathy checklist. *Journal of Consulting and Clinical Psychology, 56,* 741–747.

Harpur, T. J., Hare, R. D., & Hakstian, A. R. (1989). Two-factor conceptualization of psychopathy: Construct validity and assessment implications. *Psychological Assessment: A Journal of Consulting and Clinical Psychology, 1,* 6–17.

Harrison, J. M., & Warr, W. B. (1962). A study of the cochlear nucleus and ascending auditory pathways of the medulla. *Journal of Comparative Neurology, 119,* 341–379.

Hart, S., Zreik, M., Carper, R., & Swerdlow, N. R. (1996). Localizing drug effects on sensorimotor gating in a predictive model of antipsychotic potency. *Society for Neuroscience Abstracts, 22,* 481.

Hatanaka, T., Yasuhara, A., & Kobayashi, Y. (1990). Electrically and mechanically elicited blink reflexes in infants and children – Maturation and recovery curves of blink reflex. *Electroencephalography & Clinical Neurophysiology, 76,* 39–46.

Hawk, L. W., & Cook, E. W., III (1993, October). *Affective modulation of unilateral tactile startle.* Paper presented at the Thirty-Third Annual Meeting of the Society for Psychophysiological Research, Rottach-Egern, Germany.

Hawk, L. W., & Cook, E. W., III (1997). Affective modulation of tactile startle. *Psychophysiology, 34,* 23–31.

Hawk, L. W., Cook, E. W., III, & Goates, D. W. (1995). Relationships between valence modulation and prepulse inhibition of startle [Abstract]. *Psychophysiology, 32* (Suppl. 1), S39.

Hawk, L. W., Stevenson, V. E., & Cook, E. W., III (1992). The effects of eyelid closure on affective imagery and eyeblink startle. *Journal of Psychophysiology, 6,* 299–310.

Hebb, D. O. (1949). *The organization of behavior: A neuropsychological theory.* New York: Wiley.

Hebb, D. O. (1955). Drives and the C.N.S. (conceptual nervous system). *Psychological Review, 62,* 243–254.

Heilman, K., & Bowers, D. (1990). Neuropsychological studies of emotional changes induced by right and left hemisphere lesions. In N. Stein, B. Leventhal, & T. Trabasso (Eds.), *Psychological and biological approaches to emotion* (pp. 97–113). Hillsdale, N.J: Erlbaum.

Hetrick, W. P., Sandman, C. A., Bunney, W. E., Gin, Y., Potkin, S. G., & White, M. (1996). Gender differences in the gating of the auditory evoked potential in normal subjects. *Biological Psychiatry, 39,* 51–58.

Hierholzer, R., Munsoon, J., Peabody, C., & Rosenberg, J. (1992). Clinical presentation of PTSD in World War II combat veterans. *Hospital & Community Psychiatry, 43,* 816–820.

Hilgard, E. R. (1933). Reinforcement and inhibition of eyelid reflexes. *Journal of General Psychology, 8,* 85–113.

Hilgard, E. R., & Wendt, G. R. (1933). The problem of reflex sensitivity to light studied in a case of hemianopsia. *Yale Journal of Biology and Medicine, 5,* 373–385.

Hinrichsen, C. F. L., & Watson, C. D. (1983). Brain stem projections to the facial nucleus of the rat. *Brain Behavior and Evolution, 22,* 153–163.

Hirano, C., Russell, A. T., Ornitz, E. M., & Liu M. (1996). Habituation of P300 and reflex motor (startle blink) responses to repetitive startling stimuli in children. *International Journal of Psychophysiology, 33,* 507–513.

Hitchcock, J. M., & Davis, M. (1986). Lesions of the amygdala, but not of the cerebellum or red nucleus, block conditioned fear as measured with the potentiated startle paradigm. *Behavioral Neuroscience, 100,* 11–22.

Hitchcock, J. M., & Davis, M. (1987). Fear-potentiated startle using an auditory conditioned stimulus: Effect of lesions of the amygdala. *Physiology and Behavior, 39,* 403–408.

Hitchcock, J. M., & Davis, M. (1991). Efferent pathway of the amygdala involved in conditioned fear as measured with the fear-potentiated startle paradigm. *Behavioral Neuroscience, 105,* 826–842.

Hitchcock, J. M., Sananes, C. B., & Davis, M. (1989). Sensitization of the startle reflex by footshock: Blockade by lesions of the central nucleus of the amygdala or its efferent pathway to the brainstem. *Behavioral Neuroscience, 103,* 509–518.

Hodes, R. L., Cook, E. W., III, & Lang, P. J. (1985). Individual differences in autonomic response: Conditioned association or conditioned fear? *Psychophysiology, 22,* 545–560.

Hoffman, D. C., & Donovan, H. (1994). D1 and D2 dopamine receptor antagonists reverse prepulse inhibition deficits in an animal model of schizophrenia. *Psychopharmacology, 115,* 447–453.

Hoffman, H. S. (1984). Methodological factors in the behavioral analysis of startle. In R. Eaton (Ed.), *Neural mechanisms of startle behavior* (pp. 267–285). New York: Plenum Press.

Hoffman, H. S., Cohen, M. E., & Anday, E. (1987). Inhibition of the eyeblink reflex in the human infant. *Developmental Psychobiology, 20,* 277–283.

Hoffman, H. S., Cohen, M. E., & Corso, C. (1984). Reflex modification during habituation of a startle response. *Bulletin of the Psychonomic Society, 22,* 574–576.

Hoffman, H. S., Cohen, M. E., & English, L. M. (1985). Reflex modification by acoustic signals in newborn infants and in adults. *Journal of Experimental Child Psychology, 39,* 562–579.

Hoffman, H. S., Cohen, M. E., & Stitt, C. L. (1981). Acoustic augmentation and inhibition of the human eyeblink. *Journal of Experimental Psychology: Human Perception and Performance, 7,* 1357–1362.

Hoffman, H. S., & Fleshler, M. (1963). Startle reaction: Modification by background acoustic stimulation. *Science, 141,* 928–930.

Hoffman, H. S., & Ison, J. R. (1980). Reflex modification in the domain of startle: I. Some empirical findings and their implications for how the nervous system processes sensory input. *Psychological Review, 87,* 175–189.

Hoffman, H. S., & Ison, J. R. (1992). Reflex modification and the analysis of sensory processing in developmental and comparative research. In B. A. Campbell, H. Hayne, & R. Richardson (Eds.), *Attention and information processing in infants and adults* (pp. 83–111). Hillsdale, NJ: Erlbaum.

Hoffman, H. S., Marsh, R. R., & Stein, N. (1969). Persistence of background acoustic stimulation in controlling startle. *Journal of Comparative and Physiological Psychology, 68,* 280–283.

Hoffman, H. S., & Searle, J. R. (1965). Acoustic variables in the modification of startle reaction in the rat. *Journal of Comparative and Experimental Psychology, 60,* 53–58.

Hoffman, H. S., & Searle, J. L. (1968). Acoustic and temporal factors in the evocation of startle. *Journal of the Acoustical Society of America, 43,* 269–282.

Hoffman, H. S., & Wible, B. L. (1969). Temporal parameters in startle facilitation by steady background signals. *Journal of the Acoustical Society of America, 45,* 7–12.

Hoffman, H. S., & Wible, B. L. (1970). Role of weak signals in acoustic startle. *Journal of the Acoustical Society of America, 47,* 489–497.

Holloway, F. A. (1994). *Low-dose alcohol effects on human performance: A review of post-1984 research.* (Office of Aviation Medicine Report No. DOT/FAA/AM-94/24). Washington, DC: Federal Aviation Administration.

Holstege, G., Tan, J., Van Ham, J., & Bos, A. (1984). Mesencephalic projections to the facial nucleus in the cat. An autoradiographic tracing study. *Brain Research, 311,* 7–22.

Holstege, G., Van Ham, J. J., & Tan, J. (1986). Afferent projections to the orbicularis oculi motoneuronal cell group. An autoradiographical tracing study in the cat. *Brain Research, 374,* 306–320.

Hopf, H. D., Bier, J., Breurer, B., & Scheerer, W. (1973). The blink reflex induced by photic stimuli: Parameters, thresholds, and reflex times. In J. E. Desmedt (Ed.), *New developments in electromyography and clinical neurophysiology: Vol. 3. Human reflexes, pathophysiology of motor systems, methodology of human reflexes* (pp. 666–672). Basel: Karger.

Hori, A., Yasuhara, A., Naito, H., & Yasuhara, M. (1986). Blink reflex elicited by auditory stimulation in the rabbit. *Journal of the Neurological Sciences, 76,* 49–59.

Howard, L., & Polich, J. (1985). P300 latency and memory span development. *Developmental Psychology, 21,* 283–289.

Hull, C. L. (1943). *Principles of behavior.* New York: Appleton-Century.

Hull, J. G. (1981). A self-awareness model of the causes and effects of alcohol consumption. *Journal of Abnormal Psychology, 90,* 586–600.

Humby, T., Wilkinson, L. S., Robbins, T. W., & Geyer, M. A. (1996). Prepulses inhibit startle-induced reductions of extracellular dopamine in the nucleus accumbens of rat. *Journal of Neuroscience, 16,* 2149–2156.

Humphreys, L. G. (1943). Measures of strength of conditioned eyelid responses. *Journal of General Psychiatry, 40,* 557–565.

Inagaki, M., Takeshita, K., Nakao, S., Shiraishi, Y., & Oikawa, T. (1989). An electrophysiologically defined trigemino-reticulo-facial pathway related to the blink reflex in the cat. *Neuroscience Letters, 96,* 64–69.

Inhelder, B., & Piaget, J. (1958) *The growth of logical thinking from childhood to adolescence* (A. Parsons & S. Milgram, Trans.). New York: Basic Books, Inc. (Original work published 1951.)

Ison, J. R. (1978). Reflex inhibition and reflex elicitation by acoustic stimuli differing in abruptness of onset and peak intensity. *Animal Learning and Behavior, 6,* 106–110.

Ison, J. R., Bowen, G. P., O'Connor, K. (1991). Reflex modification produced by visual stimuli in the rat following functional decortication. *Psychobiology, 19,* 122–126.

Ison, J. R., & Hammond, G. R. (1971). Modification of the startle reflex in the rat by changes in the auditory and visual environments. *Journal of Comparative and Physiological Psychology, 75,* 435–452.

Ison, J. R., Hammond, G. R., & Krauter, E. E. (1973). Effects of experience on stimulus-produced reflex inhibition in the rat. *Journal of Comparative and Physiological Psychology, 83,* 324–336.

Ison, J. R., & Hoffman, H. S. (1983). Reflex modification in the domain of startle: II. The anomalous history of a robust and ubiquitous phenomenon. *Psychological Review, 94,* 3–17.

Ison, J. R., & Leonard, D. W. (1971). Effects of auditory stimuli on the amplitude of the nictitating membrane reflex of the rabbit (oryctoleagus cuniculus). *Journal of Comparative and Physiological Psychology, 75,* 157–164.

Ison, J. R., McAdam, D. W., & Hammond, G. R. (1973). Latency and amplitude changes in the acoustic startle reflex of the rat produced by variation in auditory prestimulation. *Physiology and Behavior, 10,* 1035–1039.

Ison, J. R., O'Connor, K., Bowen, G., & Bocirnea, A. (1991). Temporal resolution of gaps in noise by the rat is lost with functional decortication. *Behavioral Neuroscience, 105,* 33–40.

Ison, J. R., Reiter, L. A., & Warren, M. (1979). Modulation of the acoustic startle reflex in humans in the absence of anticipatory changes in the middle ear reflex. *Journal of Experimental Psychology: Human Perception and Performance, 5,* 639–642.

Ison, J. R., & Pinckney, L. A. (1990). Inhibition of the cutaneous eyeblink reflex by unilateral and bilateral acoustic input: The persistence of contralateral antagonism in auditory processing. *Perception and Psychophysics, 47,* 337–341.

Ison, J. R., Sanes, J. N., Foss, J. A., & Pinckney, L. A. (1990). Facilitation and inhibition of the human startle blink reflexes by stimulus anticipation. *Behavioral Neuroscience, 104, 3,* 418–429.

Itoh, K., Takada, M., Yasui, Y., & Mizuno, N. (1983). A pretectofacial projection in the cat: Possible link in the visually triggered blink reflex pathways. *Brain Research, 274,* 332–335.

Jacobson, R. (1986). Disorders of facial recognition, social behaviour and affect after combined bilateral amygdalotomy and subcaudate tractotomy – A clinical and experimental study. *Psychological Medicine, 16,* 439–450.

Jancke, L., Bauer, A., & von Giesen, H. (1994). Modulation of the electrically evoked blink reflex by different levels of tonic preinnervation of the orbicularis oculi muscle. *International Journal of Neuroscience, 78,* 215–222.

Jansen, D. M., & Frijda, N. H. (1994). Modulation of the acoustic startle response by film-induced fear and sexual arousal. *Psychophysiology, 31,* 565–571.

Jaspers, R. M., Muijser, H., Lammers, J. H., & Kulig, B. M. (1993). Mid-frequency hearing loss and reduction of acoustic startle responding in rats following trichloroethylene exposure. *Neurotoxicology and Teratology, 15,* 407–412.

Javitt, D. C., & Zukin, S. R. (1991). Recent advances in the phencyclidine model of schizophrenia. *American Journal of Psychiatry, 148,* 1301–1308.

Jennings, P. D., Schell, A. M., Filion, D. L., & Dawson, M. E. (1996). Tracking early and late stages of information processing: Contributions of startle eyeblink reflex modification. *Psychophysiology, 33,* 148–155.

Jepsen, O. (1963). Middle-ear muscle reflexes in man. In J. Jerger (Ed.), *Modern developments in audiology* (pp. 193–239). New York: Academic Press.

Jerger, K., Biggins, C., & Fein, G. (1992). P50 suppression is not affected by attentional manipulations. *Biological Psychiatry, 31,* 365–377.

Judd, L. L., McAdams, L. A., Budnick, G., & Braff, D. L. (1992). Sensory gating deficits in schizophrenia: New results. *American Journal of Psychiatry, 149,* 488–493.

Kadlac, J. A., & Grant, D. A. (1977). Eyelid response topography in differential interstimulus interval conditioning. *Journal of Experimental Psychology: Human Learning & Memory, 3,* 345–355.

Kahneman, D. (1968). Method, findings, and theory in studies of visual masking. *Psychological Bulletin, 70,* 404–414.

Kalman, G. (1977). On combat neurosis: Psychiatric experience during the recent Middle East War. *International Journal of Social Psychiatry, 23,* 195–203.

Kandel, E. R. (1978). *A cell biological approach to learning.* Bethesda: Grass Lecture Monograph.

Kandel, E. R., & Schwartz, M. H. (1985). *Principles of neural science* (pp. 816–834). Amsterdam: Elsevier.

Karper, L. P., Grillon, C., Charney, D. S., & Krystal, J. H. (1994). The effect of ketamine on pre-pulse inhibition and attention. *Proceedings of the American College of Neuropsychopharmacology,* 124.

Karson, C. N., Garcia-Rill, E., Biedermann, J., Mrak, R. E., Husain, M. M., & Skinner, R. D. (1991). The brainstem reticular formation in schizophrenia. *Psychiatry Research, 40,* 31–48.

Kaskey, G. B., Salzman, L. F., Klorman, R., & Pass, H. L. (1980). Relationships between stimulus intensity and amplitude of visual and auditory event related potentials. *Biological Psychology, 10,* 115–125.

Keane, J. R. (1979). Blinking to sudden illumination: A brain stem reflex present in neocortical death. *Archives of Neurology, 36,* 52–53.

Kehne, J. H., & Davis, M. (1984). Strychnine increases acoustic startle amplitude but does not alter short-term or long-term habituation. *Behavioral Neuroscience, 6,* 955–968.

Kehne, J. H., McCloskey, T. C., Taylor, V. L., Black, C. K., Fadayel, G. M., & Schmidt, C. T. (1992). Effects of serotonin releasers 3,4 methylenedioxymethamphetamine (MDMA), 4-chloroamphetamine (PCA) and fenfluramine on acoustic and tactile startle reflexes in rat. *Journal of Pharmacology and Experimental Therapeutics, 260,* 78–89.

Keith, V. A., Mansbach, R. S., & Geyer, M. A. (1991). Failure of haloperidol to block the effects of phencyclidine and dizocilpine on prepulse inhibition of startle. *Biological Psychiatry, 30,* 557–566.

Kendler, K. S., Gruenberg, A. M., & Kinney, D. K. (1994). Independent diagnoses of adoptees and relatives as defined by DSM-III in the provincial and nation samples of the Danish adoption study of schizophrenia. *Archives of General Psychiatry, 51,* 456–468.

Kim, J. J., Rison, R. A., & Fanselow, M. S. (1993). Effects of amygdala, hippocampus, and peri-aqueductal gray lesions on short- and long-term contextual fear. *Behavioral Neuroscience, 107,* 1093–1098.

Kim, M., Campeau, S., Falls, W. A., & Davis, M. (1993). Infusion of the non-NMDA receptor antagonist CNQX into the amygdala blocks the expression of fear-potentiated startle. *Behavioral and Neural Biology, 59,* 5–8.

Kimura, J. (1992). The blink reflex as a clinical test. In M. J. Aminoff (Ed.), *Electrodiagnosis in clinical neurology* (pp. 369–402). London: Churchill Livingstone.

Kimura, J., & Harada, O. (1976). Recovery curves of the blink reflex during wakefulness and sleep. *Journal of Neurology, 213,* 189–198.

Kinsbourne, M., & Bemporad, B. (1984). Lateralization of emotion: a model and the evidence. In N. Fox & R. Davidson (Eds.), *The psychobiology of affective development.* Hillsdale, NJ: Erlbaum.

Kinzie, J. D., Fredrickson, R. H., Ben, R., Fleck, J., & Karls, W. (1984). Posttraumatic stress disorder among survivors of Cambodian concentration camps. *American Journal of Psychiatry, 14,* 645–650.

Klorman, R., Weerts, T. C., Hastings, J. E., Melamed, B. G., & Lang, P. J. (1974). Psychometric description of some specific-fear questionnaires. *Behavior Therapy, 5,* 401–409.

Klorman, R., Wiesenfeld, A., & Austin, M. L. (1975). Autonomic responses to affective visual stimuli. *Psychophysiology, 12,* 553–560.

Knight, R. A., & Roff, R. D. (1985). Affectivity in schizophrenia. In M. Alpert (Ed.), *Controversies in schizophrenia: Changes and constancies* (pp. 337–364). New York: Guilford.

Knight, R. T., Scabini, D., Woods, D. L., & Clayworth, C. (1988). The effects of lesions of superior temporal gyrus and inferior parietal lobe on temporal and vertex components of the human AEP. *Electroencephalography & Clinical Neurophysiology, 70,* 499–509.

Koch, M. (1996). The septohippocampal system is involved in prepulse inhibition of the acoustic startle response in rats. *Behavioral Neuroscience, 110,* 468–477.

Koch, M., & Bubser, M. (1994). Deficient sensorimotor gating after 6-hydroxy-dopamine lesion of the rat medial prefrontal cortex is reversed by haloperidol. *European Journal of Neuroscience, 6,* 1837–1845.

Koch, M., & Friauf, E. (1995). Glycine receptors in the caudal pontine reticular formation: Are they important for the inhibition of the acoustic startle response? *Brain Research, 671,* 63–72.

Koch, M., Kungel, M., & Herbert, H. (1993). Cholinergic neurons in the pedunculopontine tegmental nucleus are involved in the mediation of prepulse inhibition of the acoustic startle response in the rat. *Experimental Brain Research, 97,* 71–82.

Koch, M., Lingenhöhl, K., & Pilz, P. K. D. (1992). Loss of the acoustic startle response following neurotoxic lesions of the caudal pontine reticular formation: Possible role of giant neurons. *Neuroscience, 49,* 617–625.

Kodera, K., Hink, R. F., Yamada, O., & Suzuki, J. I. (1979). Effects of rise time on simultaneously recorded auditory-evoked potentials from the early, middle and late ranges. *Audiology, 18,* 395–402.

Kodsi, M. H., & Swerdlow, N. R. (1994). Quinolinic acid lesions of the ventral striatum reduce sensorimotor gating of acoustic startle in rats. *Brain Research, 643,* 59–65.

Kodsi, M., & Swerdlow, N. R. (1995). Prepulse inhibition in the rat is regulated by ventral and caudodorsal striato-pallidal circuitry. *Behavioral Neuroscience, 109,* 912–928.

Kodsi, M. H., Taaid, N., Hartston, H. J., Zisook, D., Wan, F. J., & Swerdlow, N. R. (1995). Regulation of prepulse inhibition in the rat by ventral pallidal projections. *Society for Neuroscience Abstracts, 21,* 1659.

Konorski, J. (1967). *Integrative activity of the brain: An interdisciplinary approach.* Chicago: University of Chicago Press.

Kraepelin, E. (1921). *Clinical psychiatry: A textbook for students and physicians* (A. R. Defendorf, Trans.). New York: Macmillan.

Krase, W., Koch, M., & Schnitzler, H.-U. (1994). Substance P is involved in the sensitization of the acoustic startle response by footshock in rats. *Behavioral Brain Research, 63,* 81–88.

Krauter, E. E. (1987). Reflex modification of the human auditory startle blink by antecedent interruption of a visual stimulus. *Perceptual and Motor Skills, 64,* 727–738.

Krauter, E. E., Leonard, D. W., & Ison, J. R. (1973). Inhibition of human eyeblink by brief acoustic stimulus. *Journal of Comparative and Physiological Psychology, 84,* 216–251.

Kring, A. M., & Neale, J. M. (1996). Do schizophrenic patients show a disjunctive relationship among expressive, experiential, and psychophysiological components of emotion? *Journal of Abnormal Psychology, 105,* 249–257.

Kugelberg, E. (1952). Facial reflexes. *Brain, 75,* 385–396.

Kumari, V., Checkley, S. A., & Gray, J. A. (1996). Effect of cigarette smoking on prepulse inhibition of the acoustic startle reflex in healthy male smokers. *Psychopharmacology, 128,* 54–60.

Kutas, M., McCarthy, G., & Donchin, E. (1977). Augmenting mental chronometry: The P300 as a measure of stimulus evaluation time. *Science, 197,* 792–795.

Lacey, J. I., Kagan, J., Lacey, B. C., & Moss, H. A. (1963). The visceral level: Situational determinants and behavioral correlates of autonomic response patterns. In P. Knapp (Ed.), *Expression of the emotions in man* (pp. 161–196). New York: International Universities Press.

Lacey, J. I., & Lacey, B. C. (1970). Some autonomic–central nervous system interrelationships. In P. Black (Ed.), *Physiological correlates of emotion* (pp. 205–227). New York: Academic.

Lamb, M. R., & Robertson, L. C. (1987). Effect of alcohol on attention and processing of hierarchical patterns. *Alcoholism: Clinical and Experimental Research, 11,* 243–248.

Landis, C., & Hunt, W. A. (1939). *The startle pattern.* New York: Farrar & Rinehart.

Lane, S. J., Ornitz, E. M., & Guthrie, D. (1991). Modulatory influence of continuous tone, tone offset, and tone onset on the human acoustic startle response. *Psychophysiology, 28,* 579–587.

Lang, A. R. (1985). The social psychology of drinking and human sexuality. *Journal of Drug Issues, 15,* 273–289.

Lang, A. R. (1993). Alcohol-related violence: Psychological perspectives. In S. Martin (Ed.), *Alcohol and interpersonal violence: Fostering interdisciplinary perspectives* (NIAAA Research Monograph No. 24, pp. 121–148). Washington, DC: DHHS Publications.

Lang, P. J. (1980). Behavioral treatment and bio-behavioral assessment: Computer applications. In J. B. Sidowski, J. H. Johnson, & T. A. Williams (Eds.), *Technology in mental health care delivery systems* (pp. 119–137). Norwood, NJ: Ablex.

Lang, P. J. (1989). What are the data of emotion? In V. Hamilton, G. H. Bower, & N. Frijda (Eds.), *Cognitive perspectives on emotion and motivation* (pp. 173–191). Boston: Martinus Nijhoff.

Lang, P. J. (1994). The motivational organization of emotion: Affect-reflex connections. In S. Van Goozen, N. E. Van de Poll, & J. A. Sergeant (Eds.), *The emotions: Essays on emotion theory* (pp. 61–93). Hillsdale, NJ: Erlbaum.

Lang, P. J. (1995). The emotion probe: Studies of motivation and attention. *American Psychologist, 50,* 372–385.

Lang, P. J., Bradley, M. M., & Cuthbert, B. N. (1990). Emotion, attention, and the startle reflex. *Psychological Review, 97,* 377–395.

Lang, P. J., Bradley, M. M., & Cuthbert, B. N. (1992). A motivational analysis of emotion: Reflex-cortex connections. _Psychological Science, 3,_ 44–49.

Lang, P. J., Bradley, M. M., & Cuthbert, B. N. (1995). _International affective picture system (IAPS): Technical manual and affective ratings._ Gainesville, FL: The Center for Research in Psychophysiology, University of Florida.

Lang, P. J., Bradley, M. M., & Cuthbert, B. N. (1997). Motivated attention: Affect, activation, and action. In P. J. Lang, R. F. Simons, & M. T. Balaban (Eds.), _Attention and orienting: Sensory and motivational processes_ (97–136). Hillsdale, NJ: Erlbaum.

Lang, P. J., Bradley, M. M., Drobes, D. J., & Cuthbert, B. N. (1995). Emotional perception: Fearful beasts, scary people, sex, sports, disgust, and disasters [Abstract]. _Psychophysiology, 32_ (Suppl. 1), S48.

Lang, P. J., Greenwald, M. K., Bradley, M. M., & Hamm, A. O. (1993). Looking at pictures: Affective, facial, visceral, and behavioral reactions. _Psychophysiology, 30,_ 261–273.

Lang, P. J., Öhman, A., & Vaitl, D. (1988). _The international affective picture system_ [photographic slides]. Gainesville, FL: Center for Research in Psychophysiology, University of Florida.

Langley, M. K. (1982). Post traumatic stress disorders among Vietnam combat veterans. _Social Casework, 63,_ 593–598.

Larsen, R. J., & Diener, E. (1992). Promises and problems with the circumplex model of emotion. In M. S. Clark (Ed.), _Review of personality and social psychology_ (Vol. 13, pp. 25–59). Newbury Park, CA: Sage Publications.

Leaton, R. N., & Borszcz, G. S. (1985). Potentiated startle: Its relation to freezing and shock intensity in rats. _Journal of Experimental Psychology: Animal Behavior Processes, 11,_ 421–428.

Leaton, R. N., Cassella, J. V., & Borszcz, G. S. (1985). Short-term and long-term habituation of the acoustic startle response in chronic decerebrate rats. _Behavioral Neuroscience, 99,_ 901–912.

LeBar, K. S., LeDoux, J. E., Spencer, D. D., & Phelps, E. A. (1995). Impaired fear conditioning following unilateral temporal lobectomy in humans. _Journal of Neuroscience, 15,_ 6846–6855.

LeDoux, J. E. (1990). Information flow from sensation to emotion: Plasticity in the neural computation of stimulus value. In M. Gabriel & J. Moore (Eds.), _Learning and computational neuroscience: Foundations of adaptive networks_ (pp. 3–52). Cambridge, MA: MIT Press.

LeDoux, J. E. (1995). Emotion: Clues from the brain. _Annual Review of Psychology, 46,_ 209–235.

LeDoux, J. E., Cicchetti, P., Xagoraris, A., & Romanski, L. M. (1990). The lateral amygdaloid nucleus, sensory interface of the amygdala in fear conditioning. _Journal of Neuroscience, 10,_ 1062–1069.

LeDoux, J. E., Iwata, J., Cicchetti, P., & Reis, D. J. (1988). Different projections of the central amygdaloid nucleus mediate autonomic and behavioral correlates of conditioned fear. _Journal of Neuroscience, 8,_ 2517–2529.

Lee, Y., & Davis, M. (1996). The role of bed nucleus of the stria terminalis in CRH-enhanced startle: An animal model of anxiety. _Society for Neuroscience Abstracts, 22,_ 465.

Lee, Y., Lopez, D. E., Meloni, E. G., & Davis, M. (1996). A primary acoustic startle circuit: Obligatory role of cochlear root neurons and the nucleus reticularis pontis caudalis. *Journal of Neuroscience, 16,* 3775–3789.

Leitner, D. S., & Cohen, M. E. (1985). Role of the inferior colliculus in the inhibition of acoustic startle in the rat. *Physiology and Behavior, 34,* 65–70.

Leitner, D. S., Powers, A. S., Stitt, C. L., & Hoffman, H. S. (1981). Midbrain reticular formation involvement in the inhibition of acoustic startle. *Physiology and Behavior, 26,* 259–268.

Lenzenweger, M. F. (1991). Confirming schizotypic personality configurations in hypothetically psychosis-prone university students. *Psychiatry Research, 37,* 81–96.

Liang, K. C., Melia, K. R., Campeau, S., Falls, W. A., Miserendino, M. J. D., & Davis, M. (1992). Lesions of the central nucleus of the amygdala, but not of the paraventricular nucleus of the hypothalamus, block the excitatory effects of corticotropin releasing factor on the acoustic startle reflex. *Journal of Neuroscience, 12,* 2313–2320.

Liang, K. C., Melia, K. R., Miserendino, M. J. D., Falls, W. A., Campeau, S., & Davis, M. (1992). Corticotropin-releasing factor: Long-lasting facilitation of the acoustic startle reflex. *Journal of Neuroscience, 12,* 2303–2312.

Liegois-Chauvel, C., Morin, C., Musolino, A., Bancaud, J., & Chauvel, P. (1989). Evidence for the contribution of the auditory cortex to audiospinal facilitation in man. *Brain, 112,* 375–391.

Lindsley, D. B. (1957). Psychophysiology and motivation. In M. R. Jones (Ed.), *Nebraska symposium on motivation* (pp. 44–105). Lincoln: University of Nebraska Press.

Lingenhohl, K., & Friauf, E. (1994). Giant neurons in the rat reticular formation: A sensorimotor interface in the elementary acoustic startle circuit? *Journal of Neuroscience, 14,* 1176–1194.

Lipp, O. V., Arnold, S. L., Siddle, D. A. T., & Dawson, M. E. (1994). The effect of repeated prepulse-blink reflex trials on blink reflex modulation at short lead intervals. *Biological Psychology, 38,* 19–36.

Lipp, O. V., Krinitzky, S. P., & Siddle, D. A. T. (1996). The effect of repeated prepulse and reflex stimulus presentations on startle prepulse inhibition [Abstract]. *Psychophysiology, 33* (Suppl. 1), S56.

Lipp, O. V., Sheridan, J., & Siddle, D. A. T. (1994). Human blink startle during aversive and nonaversive Pavlovian conditioning. *Journal of Experimental Psychology: Animal Behavior Processes, 20,* 380–389.

Lipp, O. V., Siddle, D. A. T., & Dall, P. J. (1997). The effect of emotional and attentional processes on blink startle modulation and on electrodermal responses. *Psychophysiology, 34,* 340–347.

Lipp, O. V., Siddle, D. A. T., & Dall, P. J. (1998). Effects of stimulus modality and task condition on blink startle modification and on electrodermal responses. *Psychophysiology, 35,* 452–461.

Lipp, O. V., & Vaitl, D. (1990). Reaction time task as unconditional stimulus: Comparing aversive and non-aversive unconditional stimuli. *Pavlovian Journal of Biological Science, 25,* 77–83.

Lipska, B. K., Swerdlow, N. R., Geyer, M. A., Jaskiw, G. E., Braff, D. L., & Weinberger, D. R. (1995). Neonatal excitotoxic hippocampal damage in rats causes post-pubertal changes in prepulse inhibition of startle and its disruption by apomorphine. *Psychopharmacology, 122,* 35–43.

Lister, R. G., Eckardt, M. J., & Weingartner, H. (1987). Ethanol intoxication and memory: Recent developments and new directions. In M. Galanter (Ed.), *Recent developments in alcoholism* (Vol. 5, pp. 111–126). New York: Plenum.

Loe, P. R., & Benevento, L. A. (1969). Auditory-visual interaction in single units in the orbito-insular cortex of the cat. *Electroencephalography & Clinical Neurophysiology, 26,* 395–398.

Loeb, M., & Holding, D. H. (1975). Backward interference by tones or noise in pitch perception as a function of practice. *Perception and Psychophysics, 18,* 205–208.

Lopez, D. E., Merchan, M. A., Bajo, V. M., & Saldana, E. (1993). The cochlear root neurons in the rat, mouse and gerbil. In M. A. Merchan (Ed.), *The mammalian cochlear nuclei: Organization and function* (pp. 291–301). New York: Plenum Press.

Loveless, N. E., & Brunia, C. H. M. (1990). Effects of rise-time on late components of the auditory evoked potential. *Journal of Psychophysiology, 4,* 369–380.

Low, K. A., Larson, S. L., Burke, J., & Hackley, S. A. (1996). Alerting effects on choice reaction time and the photic eyeblink reflex. *Electroencephalography & Clinical Neurophysiology, 98,* 385–393.

Lykken, D. T. (1957). A study of anxiety in the sociopathic personality. *Journal of Abnormal and Clinical Psychology, 55,* 6–10.

Lykken, D. T. (1995). *The antisocial personalities.* Hillsdale, NJ: Erlbaum.

Mackintosh, N. J. (1974). *The psychology of animal learning.* London: Academic Press.

Mackintosh, N. J. (1983). *Conditioning and associative learning.* London: Oxford University Press.

Maher, B. A., McKean, K. O., & McLaughlin, B. (1966). Studies in psychotic language. In P. J. Stone (Ed.), *The general inquirer: A computer approach to content analysis.* Boston, MA: MIT Press.

Malmo, H. P. (1974). On frontal lobe functions: Psychiatric patient controls. *Cortex, 10,* 231–237.

Malmo, R. B. (1958). Measurement of drive: An unsolved problem in psychology. In M. R. Jones (Ed.), *Nebraska symposium on motivation* (pp. 229–265). Lincoln: University of Nebraska Press.

Mangun, G. R. (1995). Neural mechanisms of visual selective attention. *Psychophysiology, 32,* 4–18.

Mangun, G. R., Hansen, J. C., & Hillyard, S. A. (1987). The spatial orienting of attention: Sensory facilitation or response bias? In R. Johnson, J. W. Rohrbaugh, & R. Parasuraman (Eds.), *Event-related brain potentials: Basic issues and applications* (pp. 178–209). New York: Oxford University Press.

Manning, K. A., & Evinger, C. (1986). Different forms of blinks and their two-stage control. *Experimental Brain Research, 64,* 579–588.

Mansbach, R. S., Braff, D. L., & Geyer, M. A. (1989). Prepulse inhibition of the acoustic startle response is disrupted by N-ethyl-3,4-methylenedioxy-amphetamine (MDEA) in the rat. *European Journal of Pharmacology, 167,* 49–55.

Mansbach, R. S., & Geyer, M. A. (1989). Effects of phencyclidine and phencyclidine biologs on sensorimotor gating in the rat. *Neuropsychopharmacology, 2,* 299–308.

Mansbach, R. S., & Geyer, M. A. (1991). Parametric determinants of pre-stimulus modification of acoustic startle: Interactions with ketamine. *Psychopharmacology, 105,* 162–168.

Mansbach, R. S., Geyer, M. A., & Braff, D. L. (1988). Dopaminergic stimulation disrupts sensorimotor gating in the rat. *Psychopharmacology, 94,* 507–514.

Marsh, R. R., & Hoffman, H. S. (1981). Eye blink elicitation and measurement in the human infant: A circuit modification. *Behavioral Research Methods and Instrumentation, 13,* 707.

Marsh, R. R., Hoffman, H. S., & Stitt, C. L. (1973). Temporal integration in the acoustic startle reflex of the rat. *Journal of Comparative and Physiological Psychology, 82,* 507–511.

Marsh, R. R., Hoffman, H. S., & Stitt, C. L. (1978). Reflex inhibition audiometry: A new objective technique. *Acta Otolaryngolia, 85,* 336–341.

Marsh, R. R., Hoffman, H. S., & Stitt, C. L. (1979). Eyeblink elicitation and measurement in the human infant. *Behavior Research Methods and Instrumentation, 11,* 498–502.

Massaro, D. W., & Kahn, B. J. (1973). Effects of central processing on auditory recognition. *Journal of Experimental Psychology, 97,* 51–58.

Masterson, F. A., & Crawford, M. (1982). The defense motivation system: A theory of avoidance behavior. *Behavioral and Brain Sciences, 5,* 661–696.

Matthews, D. B., Best, P. J., White, A. M., Vandergriff, J. L., & Simson, P. E. (1996). Ethanol impairs spatial cognitive processing: New behavioral and electrophysiological findings. *Current Directions in Psychological Science, 5,* 111–115.

Matthews, D. B., Simson, P. E., & Best, P. J. (1995). Acute ethanol impairs spatial memory but not stimulus/response memory in the rat. *Alcoholism: Clinical and Experimental Research, 19,* 902–909.

Mayford, M., Bach, M. E., Huang, Y., Wang, L., Hawkins, R. D., & Kandel, E. R. (1996). Control of memory formation through regulated expression of a CaMKII transgene. *Science, 274,* 1678–1683.

McAndrew, C., & Edgerton, R. (1969). *Drunken comportment: A social explanation.* Chicago: Aldine Press.

McCaughey, B. G. (1986). The psychological symptomatology of a U.S. Naval disaster. *Military Medicine, 151,* 162–165.

McDonald, A. J., & Jackson, T. R. (1987). Amygdaloid connections with posterior insular and temporal cortical areas in the rat. *Journal of Comparative Neurology, 262,* 59–77.

McDowd, J. M., Filion, D. L., Harris, M. J., & Braff, D. L. (1993). Sensory gating and inhibitory function in late-life schizophrenia. *Schizophrenia Bulletin, 19,* 733–46.

McGhie, A., & Chapman, J. (1961). Disorders of attention and perception in early schizophrenia. *British Journal of Medical Psychology, 34,* 103–116.

McKellar, P. (1957). *Imagination and thinking.* London: Cohen and West.

McManis, M. H., Bradley, M. M., Cuthbert, B. N., & Lang, P. J. (1995). Kids have feelings too: Children's physiological responses to affective pictures [Abstract]. *Psychophysiology, 33* (Suppl. 1), S53.

McManis, M. H., Bradley, M. M., Cuthbert, B. N., & Lang, P. J. (1997). *Kids' reactions to affective pictures: A 3-systems study.* Manuscript submitted for publication.

Melia, K., Corodimas, K., Ryabinin, A., Wilson, M., & LeDoux, J. (1994). Ethanol (ETOH) pre-treatment selectively impairs classical conditioning of contextual cues: Possible involvement of the hippocampus. *Society for Neuroscience Abstracts, 24,* 1007.

Meloni, E. G., & Davis, M. (1992). Anatomical connections mediating the pinna component of the acoustic startle reflex in the rat. *Society for Neuroscience Abstracts, 18,* 1547.

Mennemeier, M. S., Chatterjee, A., Watson, R. T., Wertman, E., Carter, L. P., & Heilman, K. M. (1994). Contributions of the parietal and frontal lobes to sustained attention and habituation. *Neuropsychologia, 12,* 703–716.

Merchan, M. A., Collia, F., Lopez, D. E., & Saldana, E. (1988). Morphology of cochlear root neurons in the rat. *Journal of Neurocytology, 17,* 711–725.

Miller, G. A., Gratton, G., & Yee, C. M. (1988). Generalized implementation of an eye movement correction procedure. *Psychophysiology, 25,* 241–243.

Miller, M. W., Levenston, G. K., Geddings, V. J., & Patrick, C. J. (1994). Affect and startle modulation during imagery of personal experiences [Abstract]. *Psychophysiology, 31* (Suppl. 1), S68.

Miller, M. W., Curtin, J. J., & Patrick, C. J. (in press). A startle-probe methodology for investigating the effects of active avoidance on stress reactivity. *Biological Psychology.*

Miltner, W. (1994). Emotional qualities of odors and their influence on the startle reflex in humans. *Psychophysiology, 31,* 107–110.

Miltner, W., Matjak, M., Braun, C., Diekmann, H., & Brody, S. (1994). Emotional qualities of odours and their influence on the startle reflex in humans. *Psychophysiology, 31,* 107–110.

Mineka, M. (1992). *Evolutionary memories, emotional processing, and the emotional disorders. The psychology of learning and motivation* (Vol. 28, pp. 161–206). Orlando, FL: Academic.

Miserendino, M. J. D., & Davis, M. (1988). Blockade of the acoustic startle reflex by local infusion of excitatory amino acid antagonists into the ventral cochlear nucleus. *Society for Neuroscience Abstracts, 14,* 1263.

Miserendino, M. J. D., & Davis, M. (1993). NMDA and non-NMDA antagonists infused into the nucleus reticularis pontis caudalis depress the acoustic startle reflex. *Brain Research, 623,* 215–222.

Miserendino, M. J. D., Sananes, C. B., Melia, K. R., & Davis, M. (1990). Blocking of acquisition but not expression of conditioned fear-potentiated startle by NMDA antagonists in the amygdala. *Nature, 345,* 716–718.

Mizuno, N. (1979). Mesencephalic and pontine afferent fiber system to the facial nucleus in the cat: A study using horseradich peroxidase and silver impregnation techniques. *Experimental Neurology, 66,* 330–342.

Mogenson, G. J., & Nielsen, M. (1984). A study of the contribution of hippocampal–accumbens–subpallidal projections to locomotor activity. *Behavioral and Neural Biology, 42,* 38–51.

Moran, J., & Desimone, R. (1985). Selective attention gates visual processing in the extrastriate cortex. *Science, 229,* 782–784.

Morgan, C. A., III, Grillon, C., Southwick, S. M., Davis, M., & Charney, D. S. (1995). Fear-potentiated startle in posttraumatic stress disorder. *Biological Psychiatry, 38,* 378–385.

Morgan, C. A., III, Grillon, C., Southwick, S. M., Davis, M., & Charney, D. S. (1996). Exaggerated acoustic startle reflex in Gulf War veterans with posttraumatic stress disorder. *American Journal of Psychiatry, 153,* 64–68.

Morgan, C. A., III, Grillon, C., Southwick, S. M., Nagy, L. M., Davis, M., Krystal, J. H., & Charney, D. S. (1995). Yohimbine facilitated acoustic startle in combat veterans with post-traumatic stress disorder. *Psychopharmacology, 117,* 466–471.

Morris, M., Bradley, M., Bowers, D., Lang, P., & Heilman, K. (1991). *Valence-specific hypoarousal following right temporal lobectomy.* Paper presented at the Nineteenth Annual Meeting of the International Neuropsychological Society, San Antonio, Texas.

Morton, J. (1979). Word recognition. In J. Morton & J. C. Marshall (Eds.), *Psycholinguistics: Vol. 2. Structures and processes.* London: Elek & Cambridge.

Morton, N., Chaudhuri, K. R., Ellis, C., Gray, N. S., & Toone, B. K. (1995). The effects of apomorphine and L-dopa challenge on prepulse inhibition in patients with Parkinson's disease. *Schizophrenia Research, 15,* 181.

Morton, N., Gray, N. S., Mellers, J., Toone, B., Lishman, W. A., & Gray, J. A. (1994). Prepulse inhibition in temporal lobe epilepsy. *Proceedings of the European Behavioral Pharmacology Society,* 191.

Moulder, B., Bradley, M. M., & Lang, P. J. (1996). It's shocking: Conditioning affective categories. *Psychophysiology, 33* (Suppl. 1), S64.

Murray, N. M. F. (1992). Motor evoked potentials. In M. J. Aminoff (Ed.), *Electrodiagnosis in clinical neurology* (pp. 605–626). London: Churchill-Livingstone.

Muse, K. B., Weike, A. I., & Hamm, A. O. (1996). Individual differences and startle response modulation [Abstract]. *Psychophysiology, 33* (Suppl. 1), S64.

Mussat-Whitlow, B. J., & Blumenthal, T. D. (1997). Impact of acoustic and vibrotactile prepulses on acoustic and electrical blink reflexes: Startle inhibition and task accuracy results [Abstract]. *Psychophysiology, 34* (Suppl. 1), S66.

Näätänen, R., & Picton, T. (1987). The N1 wave of the human electric and magnetic response to sound: A review and an analysis of the component structure. *Psychophysiology, 24,* 375–425.

Nadel, L., & Willner, J. (1980). Context and conditioning: A place for space. *Physiological Psychology, 8,* 218–228.

Nagamoto, H. T., Adler, L. E., Waldo, M. C., & Freedman, R. (1989). Sensory gating in schizophrenics and normal controls: Effects of changing stimulation interval. *Biological Psychiatry, 25,* 549–561.

Nagamoto, H. T., Adler, L. E., Waldo, M. C., Griffith, J., & Freedman, R. (1991). Gating of auditory response in schizophrenics and normal controls – Effects of recording site and stimulation interval on the P50 wave. *Schizophrenia Research, 4,* 31–40.

Nakashima, K., Shimoyama, Y., Yokoyama, Y., & Takahashi, K. (1993). Auditory effects on the electrically elicited blink reflex in patients with Parkinson's disease. *Electroencephalography & Clinical Neurophysiology, 89,* 108–112.

Newman, J. P., & Kosson, D. S. (1986). Passive avoidance learning in psychopathic and nonpsychopathic offenders. *Journal of Abnormal Psychology, 95,* 252–256.

Newman, J. P., Widom, C. S., & Nathan, S. (1985). Passive avoidance in syndromes of disinhibition: Psychopathy and extraversion. *Journal of Personality and Social Psychology, 48,* 1316–1327.

Norris, C. M., & Blumenthal, T. D. (1996). A relationship between inhibition of the acoustic startle response and the protection of prepulse processing. *Psychobiology, 24,* 160–168.

Nuechterlein, K. H., & Dawson, M. E. (1984). Information processing and attentional functioning in the developmental course of schizophrenic disorders. *Schizophrenia Bulletin, 10,* 160–203.

Öhman, A. (1983). The orienting response during Pavlovian conditioning. In D. A. T. Siddle (Ed.), *Orienting and habituation: Perspectives in human research* (pp. 315–370). Chichester: John Wiley.

Öhman, A. (1992). Orienting and attention: Preferred preattentive processing of potentially phobic stimuli. In B. A. Campbell, H. Hayne, & R. Richardson (Eds.), *Attention and information processing in infants and adults: Perspectives from human and animal research* (pp. 263–296). Hillsdale, NJ: Erlbaum.

Öhman, A. (1997). As fast as the blink of an eye: Evolutionary preparedness for preattentive processing of threat. In P. J. Lang, R. F. Simons, & M. T. Balaban (Eds.), *Attention and orienting: Sensory and motivational processes* (pp. 165–184). Hillsdale, NJ: Erlbaum.

Oltmanns, T. F., & Neale, J. M. (1975). Schizophrenic performance when distractors are present: Attentional deficits or differential task difficulty? *Journal of Abnormal Psychology, 84,* 205–209.

Ongerboer de Visser, B. W. (1983a). Anatomical and functional organization of reflexes involving the trigeminal system in man: Jaw reflex, blink reflex, corneal reflex, and exteroceptive suppression. In J. E. Desmedt (Ed.), *Motor control mechanisms in health and disease* (pp. 727–738). New York: Raven Press.

Ongerboer de Visser, B. W. (1983b). Comparative study of corneal and blink reflex latencies in patients with segmental or with cerebral lesions. In J. E. Desmedt (Ed.), *Motor control mechanisms in health and disease* (pp. 757–772). New York: Raven Press.

Ongerboer de Visser, B. W., & Kuypers, H. G. J. M. (1978). Late blink reflex changes in lateral medullary lesions. *Brain, 101,* 285–294.

Ornitz, E. M. (1996a). Interaction of emotion with magnitude, habituation, and relationships of P300 and startle response in children [Abstract]. *Psychophysiology, 33* (Suppl. 1), S66.

Ornitz, E. M. (1996b). Developmental aspects of neurophysiology. In M. Lewis (Ed.), *Child and adolescent psychiatry: A comprehensive textbook* (pp. 39–51), Baltimore, MD: Williams & Wilkins.

Ornitz, E. M., & Guthrie, D. (1989). Long-term habituation and sensitization of the acoustic startle response in the normal adult human. *Psychophysiology, 26,* 166–173.

Ornitz, E. M., Guthrie, D., Kaplan, A. R., Lane, S. J., & Norman, R. J. (1986). Maturation of startle modulation. *Psychophysiology, 23,* 624–634.

Ornitz, E. M., Guthrie, D., Lane, S. J., & Sugiyama, T. (1990). Maturation of startle facilitation by sustained prestimulation. *Psychophysiology, 27,* 298–308.

Ornitz, E. M., Guthrie, D., Sadeghpour, M., & Sugiyama, T. (1991). Maturation of prestimulation-induced startle modulation in girls. *Psychophysiology, 28,* 11–20.

Ornitz, E. M., Hanna, G. L., & de Traversay, J. (1992). Prestimulation-induced startle modulation in attention-deficit hyperactivity disorder and nocturnal enuresis. *Psychophysiology, 29,* 437–451.

Ornitz, E. M., & Pynoos, R. S. (1989). Startle modulation in children with posttraumatic stress disorder. *American Journal of Psychiatry, 146,* 866–870.

Ornitz, E. M., Russell, A. T., & Hirano, C. (1997). [Startle habituation in preschool and school-aged boys]. Unpublished raw data.

Ornitz, E. M., Russell, A. T., Yuan, H., & Liu M. (1996). Autonomic, electroencephalographic, and myogenic activity accompanying startle and its habituation during mid-childhood. *Psychophysiology, 33,* 507–513.

Orr, S. P., Lasko, N. B., Shalev, A. Y., & Pitman, R. K. (1995). Physiologic responses to loud tones in Vietnam veterans with posttraumatic stress disorder. *Journal of Abnormal Psychology, 104,* 75–82.

Ortony, A., Clore, G. L., & Collins, A. (1988). *The cognitive structure of emotions.* Cambridge: Cambridge University Press.

Osgood, C. E., Suci, G. J., & Tannenbaum, P. H. (1957). *The measurement of meaning.* Urbana: University of Illinois Press.

Palmatier, A. D., Goates, D. W., & Cook, E. W., III (1995). Spontaneous eyeblink: Electromyographic measurement and affective modulation [Abstract]. *Psychophysiology, 32* (Suppl. 1), S58.

Palomba, D., Angrilli, A., & Mini, A. (1997). Visual evoked potentials, heart rate responses and memory to emotional pictorial stimuli. *International Journal of Psychophysiology, 27,* 55–67.

Panneton, W. M., & Martin, G. F. (1983). Brainstem projections to the facial nucleus of the opposum. A study using axonal transport techniques. *Brain Research, 267,* 19–33.

Pardo, J. V., Pardo, K., Janer, K., & Raichle, M. E. (1990). The anterior cingulate cortex mediates processing selection in the Stroop attention conflict paradigm. *Proceedings of the National Academy of Sciences, 87,* 256–259.

Parisi, T., & Ison, J. R. (1979). Development of the acoustic startle response in the rat: Ontogenetic changes in the magnitude of inhibition by prepulse stimulation. *Developmental Psychobiology, 12,* 219–230.

Pashler, H. (1984). Processing stages in overlapping tasks: Evidence for a central bottleneck. *Journal of Experimental Psychology: Human Perception and Performance, 10,* 358–377.

Passler, M. A., Isaac, W., & Hynd, G. W. (1985). Neuropsychological development of behavior attributed to frontal lobe functioning in children. *Developmental Neuropsychology, 1,* 349–370.

Patrick, C. J. (1994). Emotion and psychopathy: Startling new insights. *Psychophysiology, 31,* 319–330.

Patrick, C. J. (1995). Emotion and temperament in psychopathy. *Clinical Science,* 5–8.

Patrick, C. J., & Berthot, B. D. (1995). Startle potentiation during anticipation of a noxious stimulus: Active versus passive response sets. *Psychophysiology, 32,* 72–80.

Patrick, C. J., Berthot, B., & Moore, J. D. (1996). Diazepam blocks fear-potentiated startle in humans. *Journal of Abnormal Psychology, 105,* 89–96.

Patrick, C. J., Bradley, M. M., & Lang, P. J. (1993). Emotion in the criminal psychopath: Startle reflex modulation. *Journal of Abnormal Psychology, 102,* 82–92.

Patrick, C. J., Cuthbert, B. N., & Lang, P. J. (1994) Emotion in the criminal psychopath: Fear image processing. *Journal of Abnormal Psychology, 103,* 523–534.

Patrick, C. J., Zempolich, K. A., & Levenston, G. K. (1997). Emotionality and violent behavior in psychopaths: A biosocial analysis. In A. Raine, P. Brennan, D. Farrington, & S. A. Mednick (Eds.), *Unlocking crime: The biosocial key* (pp. 145–161). New York: Plenum.

Patterson, C. M., & Newman, J. P. (1993). Reflectivity and learning from aversive events: Toward a psychological mechanism for the syndromes of disinhibition. *Psychological Review, 100,* 716–736.

Payne, R. W., Mattussek, P., & George, E. I. (1959). An experimental study of schizophrenic thought disorder. *Journal of Mental Science, 105,* 440.

Pearce, J. M., & Hall, G. (1980). A model for Pavlovian learning: Variation in the effectiveness of conditioned but not of unconditioned stimuli. *Psychological Review, 87,* 532–552.

Penders, C. A., & Delwaide, P. J. (1973). Physiological approach to the human blink reflex. In J. E. Desmedt (Ed.), *New developments in electromyography and clinical neurophysiology: Vol. 3. Human reflexes, pathophysiology of motor systems, methodology of human reflexes* (pp. 649–657). Basel: Karger.

Peng, R. Y., Mansbach, R. S., Braff, D. L., & Geyer, M. A. (1990). A D2 dopamine receptor agonist disrupts sensorimotor gating in rats: Implications for dopaminergic abnormalities in schizophrenia. *Neuropsychopharmacology, 3,* 211–218.

Perlstein, W. M., Fiorito, E., Simons, R. F., & Graham, F. K. (1993). Lead stimulation effects on reflex blink, exogenous brain potentials, and loudness judgments. *Psychophysiology, 30,* 347–358.

Pernanen, K. (1976). Alcohol and crimes of violence. In B. Kissin & H. Begleiter (Eds.), *The biology of alcoholism* (Vol. 4, pp. 344–351). New York: Plenum.

Perry, W., & Braff, D. L. (1994). Information-processing deficits and thought disorder in schizophrenia. *American Journal of Psychiatry, 151,* 363–367.

Perry, W., & Braff, D. (1996). Disturbed thought and information processing deficits in schizophrenia. *Biological Psychiatry, 39,* 549.

Perry, W., & Viglione, D. J. (1991). The Ego Impairment Index as a predictor of outcome in melancholic depressed patients treated with tricyclic antidepressants. *Journal of Personality Assessment, 56,* 487–501.

Perry, W., Viglione, D., & Braff, D. (1992). The Ego Impairment Index and schizophrenia: A validation study. *Journal of Personality Assessment, 59,* 165–175.

Peterson, J. B., Rothfleisch, J., Zelazo, P. D., & Pihl, R. O. (1990). Acute alcohol intoxication and cognitive functioning. *Journal of Studies on Alcohol, 51,* 114–122.

Phillips, R. G., & LeDoux, J. E. (1992). Differential contribution of amygdala and hippocampus to cued and contextual fear conditioning. *Behavioral Neuroscience, 106,* 274–285.

Pihl, R. O., & Peterson, J. B. (1993). Alcohol and aggression: Three potential mechanisms of the drug effect. In S. Martin (Ed.), *Alcohol and interpersonal violence: Fostering interdisciplinary perspectives.* (NIAAA Research Monograph No. 24, pp. 149–159). Washington, DC: DHHS Publications.

Pihl, R. O., Peterson, J. B., & Lau, M. (1993). A biosocial model of the alcohol-aggression relationship. *Journal of Studies on Alcohol* (Suppl. 11), 128–139.

Plant, Y., & Hammond, G. (1989). Temporal integration of acoustic and cutaneous stimuli shown in the blink reflex. *Perception and Psychophysics, 45,* 258–264.

Plourde, G., Joffe, D., Villemure, C., & Trahan, M. (1993). The P3a wave of the auditory event-related potential reveals registration of pitch change during sufentanil anesthesia for cardiac surgery. *Anaesthesiology, 78,* 498–509.

Pohorecky, L. A. (1991). Stress and alcohol interaction: An update of human research. *Alcoholism: Clinical and Experimental Research, 15,* 438–459.

Pohorecky, L. A., Cagan, M., Brick, J., & Jaffe, L. S. (1976). The startle response in rats: Effects of ethanol. *Pharmacology: Biochemistry and Behavior, 4,* 311–316.

Polich, J. (1989). P300 from a passive auditory paradigm. *Electroencephalography & Clinical Neurophysiology, 74,* 312–320.

Polich, J., Aung, M., & Dalessio, D. J. (1988). Long latency auditory evoked potentials: Intensity, inter-stimulus interval, and habitation. *Pavlovian Journal of Biological Science, 23,* 35–40.

Polich, J., & Kok, A. (1995). Cognitive and biological determinants of P300: An integrative review. *Biological Psychology, 41,* 103–146.

Posner, M. I. (1978). *Chronometric explorations of mind.* Hillsdale, NJ: Erlbaum.

Posner, M. I. (1980). Orienting of attention. *Quarterly Journal of Experimental Psychology, 32,* 3–25.

Posner, M. I. (1995). Attention in cognitive neuroscience: An overview. In M. S. Gazzaniga (Ed.), *The cognitive neurosciences* (pp. 615–624). Cambridge, MA: MIT Press.

Posner, M. I., & Cohen, Y. (1984). Components of attention. In H. Bousma & D. Bowhuis (Eds.), *Attention and performance X* (pp. 531–556). Hillsdale, NJ: Erlbaum.

Posner, M. I., & Petersen, S. E. (1990). The attention system of the human brain. *Annual Review of Neuroscience, 13,* 25–42.

Posner, M. I., Rafal, R. D., Choate, L., & Vaughan, J. (1985). Inhibition of return: Neural basis and function. *Cognitive Neuropsychology, 2,* 211–228.

Prins, A., Kaloupek, D. G., & Keane, T. M. (1995). Psychophysiological evidence for autonomic arousal and startle in traumatized adult populations. In M. J. Friedman, D. S. Charnet, & A. Y. Deutch (Eds.), *Neurobiological and clinical consequences of stress* (pp. 291–314). Philadelphia: Lippincott-Raven.

Pritchard, W. S. (1981). Psychophysiology of P300. *Psychological Bulletin, 89,* 506–540.

Prokasy, W. F., & Kumpfer, K. L. (1973). Classical conditioning. In W. F. Prokasy & D. C. Raskin (Eds.), *Electrodermal activity in psychological research* (pp. 157–202). New York: Academic Press.

Putnam, L. E. (1975). *The human startle reaction: Mechanisms of modification by background acoustic stimulation.* Unpublished doctoral dissertation, University of Wisconsin, Madison.

Putnam, L. E. (1990). Great expectations: Anticipatory responses of the heart and brain. In R. Johnson, J. W. Rohrbaugh, R. Parasuraman, & R. Johnson, Jr. (Eds.), *Event-related brain potentials: Basic issues and applications* (pp. 178–209). New York: Oxford University Press.

Putnam, L. E., Butler, G. H., & Anthony, B. J. (1978). Reflex facilitation accompanying anticipatory HR deceleration in a forewarned startle paradigm [Abstract]. *Psychophysiology, 15,* 285.

Putnam, L. E., & Roth, W. T. (1987). Heart rate responses to startling stimuli that evoke P300: Evidence for a defensive response? *Psychophysiology, 24,* 607–608.

Putman, L. E., & Roth, W. T. (1990). Effects of stimulus repetition, duration and rise time on startle blink and automatically elicited P300. *Psychophysiology, 27,* 275–297.

Rabinowicz, T. (1986). The differentiated maturation of the cerebral cortex. In F. Falkner & J. M. Tanner (Eds.), *Human growth: A comprehensive treatise* (pp. 385–410). New York: Plenum.

Raine, A. (1993). *The psychopathology of crime.* San Diego: Academic Press.

Rauch, S. L., Jenike, M. J., Alpert, N. A., Baer, L., Breiter, H. C. R., & Fischman, A. J. (1994). Regional cerebral blood flow measured during symptom provocation in obsessive–compulsive disorder using 15 0-labeled co2 and position emission tomography. *Archives of General Psychiatry, 51,* 62–70.

Raymond, J. E., Shapiro, K. L., & Arnell, K. M. (1992). Temporary suppression of visual processing in an RSVP task: An attentional blink? *Journal of Experimental Psychology: Human Perception and Performance, 18,* 849–860.

Raymond, J. E., Shapiro, K. L., & Arnell, K. M. (1995). Similarity determines the attentional blink. *Journal of Experimental Psychology: Human Perception and Performance, 21,* 653–662.

Reese, N. B., Garcia-Rill, E., & Skinner, R. D. (1995). Auditory input to the pedunculopontine nucleus: II. Unit responses. *Brain Research Bulletin, 37,* 265–273.

Reeves, A., & Sperling, G. (1986). Attention gating in short-term visual memory. *Psychological Review, 93,* 180–206.

Reijmers, L. G., Vanderheyden, P. M., & Peeters, B. W. (1995). Changes in prepulse inhibition after local administration of NMDA receptor ligands in the core region of the rat nucleus accumbens. *European Journal of Pharmacology, 272,* 131–138.

Reite, M., Teale, P., Zimmerman, J., Davis, K., Whalen, J., & Edrich, J. (1988). Source origin of a 50-msec latency auditory evoked field component in young schizophrenic men. *Biological Psychiatry, 24,* 495–506.

Reiter, L. A. (1977). *Development and evaluation of reflex modulation as an objective audiometric procedure.* Unpublished doctoral dissertation, University of Rochester.

Reiter, L. A. (1981). Experiments re: clinical application of reflex modulation audiometry. *Journal of Speech and Hearing Research, 24,* 92–98.

Reiter, L. A., Goetzinger, C. P., & Press, S. E. (1981). Reflex modulation: A hearing test for the difficult-to-test. *Journal of Speech and Hearing Disorders, 24,* 262–266.

Reiter, L. A., & Ison, J. R. (1977). Inhibition of the human eyeblink reflex: An evaluation of the sensitivity of the Wendt–Yerkes method for threshold detection. *Journal of Experimental Psychology: Human Perception and Performance, 3,* 325–336.

Rescorla, R. A., & Wagner, A. R. (1972). A theory of Pavlovian conditioning: Variations in the effectiveness of reinforcement and nonreinforcement. In A. H. Black & W. F. Prokasy (Eds.), *Classical conditioning II: Current research and theory* (pp. 64–99). New York: Appleton-Century-Crofts.

Riede, K. (1993). Prepulse inhibition of the startle reaction in the locust *Locusta migratoria* (Insecta: Orthoptera: Acridoidea). *Journal of Comparative Physiology A, 172,* 351–358.

Rigdon, G. (1990). Differential effects of apomorphine on prepulse inhibition of acoustic startle reflex in two rat strains. *Psychopharmacology, 102,* 419–421.

Rigdon, G. C., & Viik, K. (1991). Prepulse inhibition as a screening test for potential antipsychotics. *Drug Development Research, 23,* 91–99.

Rigdon, G. C., & Weatherspoon, J. (1992). 5HT1A receptor agonists block prepulse inhibition of the acoustic startle reflex. *Journal of Pharmacology and Experimental Therapeutics, 263,* 486–493.

Rimpel, J., Geyer, D., & Hopf, H. C. (1982). Changes in the blink response to combined trigeminal, acoustic and visual repetitive stimulation, studied in the human subject. *Electroencephalography & Clinical Neurophysiology, 54,* 552–560.

Ritter, W., Vaughan, H. G., & Costa, L. D. (1968). Orienting and habituation to auditory stimuli: A study of short term changes in average evoked responses. *Electroencephalography & Clinical Neurophysiology, 25,* 550–556.

Robinson, C. J., & Burton, H. (1980). Somatic submodality distribution within the second somatosensory (SII), 7b, retroinsular, postauditory, and granular insular cortical areas of M. fascicularis. *Journal of Comparative Neurology, 192,* 93–108.

Roedema, T., & Simons, R. F. (1994). Imagery and emotion in anhedonia: Blink-reflex modulation [Abstract]. *Psychophysiology, 31* (Suppl. 1), S82.

Rosen, J. B., Hitchcock, J. M., Miserendino, M. J. D., Falls, W. A., Campeau, S., & Davis, M. (1992). Lesions of the perirhinal cortex but not of the frontal, medial prefrontal, visual, or insular cortex block fear-potentiated startle using a visual conditioned stimulus. *Journal of Neuroscience, 12,* 4624–4633.

Rosen, J. B., Hitchcock, J. M., Sananes, C. B., Miserendino, M. J. D., & Davis, M. (1991). A direct projection from the central nucleus of the amygdala to the acoustic startle pathway: Anterograde and retrograde tracing studies. *Behavioral Neuroscience, 105,* 817–825.

Ross, L. E. (1961). Conditioned fear as a function of CS-UCS and probe stimulus intervals. *Journal of Experimental Psychology, 61,* 265–273.

Ross, L. E., & Nelson, M. N. (1973). The role of awareness in differential conditioning. *Psychophysiology, 10,* 91–94.

Rossi, B., Risaliti, R., & Rossi, A. (1989). The R3 component of the blink reflex in man: A reflex response induced by activation of high threshold cutaneous afferents. *Electroencephalography & Clinical Neurophysiology, 73,* 334–340.

Rossi, B., Vista, M., Farnetani, W., Gabrielli, L., Vignocchi, G., Bianchi, F., Berton, F., & Francesconi, W. (1995). Modulation of electrically elicited blink reflex components by visual and acoustic prestimuli in man. *International Journal of Psychophysiology, 20,* 177–187.

Roth, W. T., Dorato, K. H., & Kopell, B. S. (1984). Intensity and task effects on evoked physiological responses to noise bursts. *Psychophysiology, 21,* 466–481.

Rudy, J. W., & Sutherland, R. J. (1992). Configural and elemental associations and the memory coherence problem. *Journal of Cognitive Neuroscience, 4,* 208–216.

Russell, J. A. (1980). A circumplex model of affect. *Journal of Personality and Social Psychology, 39,* 1161–1178.

Russell, J. A., & Mehrabian, A. (1977). Evidence for a three-factor theory of emotions. *Journal of Research in Personality, 11,* 273–294.

Russell, J. F. (1984). The captivity experience and its psychological consequences. *Psychiatric Annals, 14,* 250–254.

Sabatinelli, D., Bradley, M. M., Cuthbert, B. N., & Lang, P. J. (1996). Wait and see: Aversion and activation in anticipation and perception [Abstract]. *Psychophysiology, 33* (Suppl. 1), S72.

Saitoh, K., Tilson, H. A., Shaw, S., & Dyer, R. S. (1987). Possible role of the brainstem in the mediation of prepulse inhibition in the rat. *Neuroscience Letters, 75,* 216–222.

Sananes, C. B., & Davis, M. (1992). N-Methyl-D-aspartate lesions of the lateral and basolateral nuclei of the amygdala block fear-potentiated startle and shock sensitization of startle. *Behavioral Neuroscience, 106,* 72–80.

Sanders, A. F. (1980). Stage analysis of reaction processes. In G. E. Stelmach & J. Requin (Eds.), *Tutorials in motor behavior* (pp. 331–354). Amsterdam: North-Holland.

Sanders, A. F. (1983). Towards a model of stress and human performance. *Acta Psychologica, 53,* 61–97.

Sanes, J. N. (1984). Voluntary movements and excitability of cutaneous eyeblink reflexes. *Psychophysiology, 21,* 653–664.

Sanes, J. N., & Ison, J. R. (1979). Conditioning auditory stimuli and the cutaneous eyeblink reflex in humans: Differential effects according to oligosynaptic or polysynaptic central pathways. *Electroencephalography & Clinical Neurophysiology, 47,* 546–555.

Sanford, L. D., Ball, W. A., Morrison, A. R., & Ross, R. J. (1992). Peripheral and central components of alerting: Habituation of acoustic startle, orienting responses, and elicited waveforms. *Behavioral Neuroscience, 106,* 112–120.

Sarno, A. J., Blumenthal, T. D., & Boelhouwer, A. J. W. (1996, March). *Modification of the electrically-elicited startle response by visual stimuli.* Paper presented at the Southeastern Psychological Association Meeting, Norfolk, VA.

Sayette, M. A. (1993). An appraisal-disruption model of alcohol's effects on stress response in social drinkers. *Psychological Bulletin, 114,* 459–476.

Schall, U., & Ward, P. B. (1996). "Prepulse inhibition" facilitates a liberal response bias in an auditory discrimination task. *NeuroReport, 7,* 652–656.

Schall, U., Schön, A., Zerbin, D., Effers, C., & Oades, R. D. (1996). Event-related potentials during an auditory discrimination with prepulse inhibition in patients with schizophrenia, obsessive–compulsive disorder and healthy subjects. *International Journal of Neuroscience, 84,* 15–33.

Schell, A. M., Dawson, M. E., Hazlett, E. A., & Filion, D. L. (1995). Attentional modulation of startle in psychosis-prone college students. *Psychophysiology, 32,* 266–273.

Schlenker, R., Cohen, R., & Hopmann, G. (1993). Affective modulation of the startle reflex in schizophrenic patients. *European Archives of Psychiatry and Clinical Neuroscience, 245,* 309–318.

Schlosberg, H. (1952). The description of facial expression in terms of two dimensions. *Journal of Experimental Psychology, 44,* 229–237.

Schmidtke, K., & Büttner-Ennever, J. A. (1992). Nervous control of eyelid function: A review of clinical, experimental and pathological data. *Brain, 115,* 227–247.

Schmolesky, M. T., Boelhouwer, A. J. W., & Blumenthal, T. D. (1996). The effect of acoustic pulse intensity upon the electrically elicited blink reflex at positive and negative stimulus onset asynchronies. *Biological Psychology, 44,* 69–84.

Schneider, W., Dumais, S. T., & Shiffrin, R. M. (1984). Automatic and controlled processing and attention. In R. Parasuraman & J. Davies (Eds.), *Varieties of attention* (pp. 1–27). Orlando, FL: Academic Press.

Schneirla, T. (1959). An evolutionary and developmental theory of biphasic processes underlying approach and withdrawal. In M. Jones (Ed.), *Nebraska symposium on motivation* (pp. 1–42). Lincoln: University of Nebraska Press.

Schupp, H. T., Cuthbert, B. N., Bradley, M. M., Birbaumer, N., & Lang, P. J. (1997). Probe P3 and blinks: Two measures of affective startle modulation. *Psychophysiology, 34,* 1–6.

Schupp, H. T., Cuthbert, B. N., Hillman, C., Raymann, R., Bradley, M. M., & Lang, P. J. (1996). ERP's and blinks: Sex differences in response to erotic and violent picture content [Abstract]. *Psychophysiology, 33* (Suppl. 1), S75.

Schwartz, J. M., Stoessel, P. W., Baxter, L. R. J., Martin, K. M., & Phelps, M. E. (1996). Systematic changes in cerebral glucose metabolic rate after successful behavior modification treatment of obsessive–compulsive disorder. *Archives of General Psychiatry, 53,* 109–113.

Schwartz, S. H., & Loop, M. S. (1984). Effect of duration on detection by the chromatic and achromatic systems. *Perception & Psychophysics, 36,* 65–67.

Schwarzkopf, S. B., Bruno, J. P., & Mitra, T. (1993). Effects of haloperidol and SCH 23390 on acoustic startle and prepulse inhibition under basal and stimulated conditions. *Progress in Neuro-Psychopharmacology and Biological Psychiatry, 17,* 1023–1036.

Schwarzkopf, S. B., Ison, J. R., Taylor, M. K., & Barlow, J. (1994). Apomorphine disrupts prepulse facilitation and inhibition of startle. *Biological Psychiatry, 35,* 630.

Schwarzkopf, S. B., Lamberti, J. S., & Smith, D. A. (1993). Concurrent assessment of acoustic startle and auditory P50 evoked potential measures of sensory inhibition. *Biological Psychiatry, 33,* 815–828.

Schwarzkopf, S. B., McCoy, L., Smith, D. A., & Boutros, N. N. (1993). Test–retest reliability of prepulse inhibition of the acoustic startle response. *Biological Psychiatry, 34,* 896–900.

Schwarzkopf, S. B., Mitra, T., & Bruno, J. P. (1992). Sensory gating in rats depleted of dopamine as neonates: Potential relevance to findings in schizophrenic patients. *Biological Psychiatry, 31,* 759–773.

Schwent, V. L., Snyder, E., & Hillyard, S. A. (1976). Auditory evoked potentials during multichannel selective listening: Role of pitch and localization cues. *Journal of Experimental Psychology: Human Perception and Performance, 2,* 313–325.

Semba, K., & Egger, M. D. (1986). The facial "motor" nerve of the rat: Control of vibrissa and examination of motor and sensory components. *Journal of Comparative Neurology, 247,* 144–158.

Shagass, C. (1977). Early evoked potentials. *Schizophrenia Bulletin, 3,* 80–92.

Shahani, B. T., & Young, R. R. (1972). Human orbicularis oculi reflexes. *Neurology, 22,* 149–154.

Shahani, B. T., & Young, R. R. (1973). Blink reflexes in orbicularis oculi. In J. E. Desmedt (Ed.), *New developments in electromyography and clinical neurophysiology: Vol. 3. Human reflexes, pathophysiology of motor systems, methodology of human reflexes* (pp. 641–648). Basel: Karger.

Shalev, A. Y., & Rogel-Fuchs, Y. (1993). Psychophysiology of the posttraumatic stress disorder: From sulfur fumes to behavioral genetics. *Psychosomatic Medicine, 55,* 413–423.

Shanks, D. R., & Dickinson, A. (1990). Contingency awareness in evaluative conditioning: A comment on Baeyens, Eelen, and Van den Bergh. *Cognition and Emotion, 4,* 19–30.

Shapiro, K. L., Raymond, J. E., & Arnell, K. M. (1994). Attention to visual pattern information produces the atttentional blink in rapid serial visual presentation. *Journal of Experimental Psychology: Human Perception and Performance, 20,* 357–371.

Sharf, B. (1970). Critical bands. In J. V. Tobias (Ed.), *Foundations of modern auditory theory* (Vol. 1). New York: Academic Press.

Shenton, M. E., Kirkinis, R., & Jolesz, F. A. E. A. (1992). Abnormalities of the left temporal lobe and thought disorder in schizophrenia. *New England Journal of Medicine, 327,* 604–612.

Sher, K. (1987). Stress-response dampening. In H. Blane & K. Leonard (Eds.), *Psychological theories of alcoholism* (pp. 227–271). New York: Guilford.

Sherrington, C. (1906). *The integrative action of the nervous system.* New York: Scribner's.

Shi, C., & Davis, M. (1996). Anatomical tracing and lesion studies of visual pathways involved in fear conditioning measured with fear potentiated startle. *Society for Neuroscience Abstracts, 22,* 1115.

Shortley, B. M., & Berg, W. K. (1996). Avoiding noise artifacts in airpuff startle stimuli [Abstract]. *Psychophysiology, 33* (Suppl. 1), S77.

Siddle, D. A. T. (1991). Orienting, habituation, and resource allocation: An associative analysis. *Psychophysiology, 28,* 245–259.

Siddle, D. A. T., Lipp, O. V., & Dall, P. J. (1997). The effect of unconditional stimulus modality and intensity on blink startle and electrodermal responses. *Psychophysiology, 34,* 406–413.

Siddle, D. A. T., & Trasler, G. B. (1981). The psychophysiology of psychopathic behavior. In M. J. Christie & P. G. Mellett (Eds.), *Foundations of psychosomatics* (pp. 283–303). New York: Wiley.

Siegel, C., Waldo, M., Mizner, G., Adler, L. E., & Freedman, R. (1984). Deficits in sensory gating in schizophrenic patients and their relatives: Evidence obtained with auditory evoked responses. *Archives of General Psychiatry, 41,* 607–612.

Siever, L. J. (1991). The biology of the boundaries of schizophrenia. In C. A. Tamminga & S. C. Schulz (Eds.), *Advances in neuropsychiatry and psychopharmacology: Vol. 1. Schizophrenia research* (pp. 181–192). New York: Raven Press Ltd.

Silverstein, L. D., & Graham, F. K. (1978). Eyeblink EMG: A miniature eyelid electrode for recording from orbicularis oculi. *Psychophysiology, 15,* 377–379.

Silverstein, L. D., Graham, F. K., & Bohlin, G. (1981). Selective attention effects on the reflex blink. *Psychophysiology, 18,* 240–247.

Silverstein, L. D., Graham, F. K., & Calloway, J. M. (1980). Preconditioning and excitability of the human orbicularis oculi reflex as a function of state. *Electroencephalography & Clinical Neurophysiology, 48,* 406–417.

Simmons, F. B. (1959). Middle ear muscle activity at moderate sound levels. *Annals of Otology, Rhinology, and Laryngology, 68,* 1126–1144.

Simons, R. F., & Giardina, B. D. (1992). Reflex modification in psychosis-prone young adults. *Psychophysiology, 29,* 8–16.

Simons, R. F., & Perlstein, W. M. (1997). A tale of two reflexes: An ERP analysis of prepulse inhibition and orienting. In P. J. Lang, R. F. Simons, & M. T. Balaban (Eds.), *Attention and orienting: Sensory and motivational processes* (pp. 229–255). Hillsdale, NJ: Erlbaum.

Simons, R. F., & Zelson, M. F. (1985). Engaging visual stimuli and reflex blink modification. *Psychophysiology, 22,* 44–49.

Sipes, T. A., & Geyer, M. A. (1994). Multiple serotonin receptor subtypes modulate prepulse inhibition of the startle response in rats. *Neuropsychopharmacology, 33,* 441–448.

Smith, S. S., & Newman, J. P. (1990). Alcohol and drug abuse – Dependence disorders in psychopathic and nonpsychopathic criminal offenders. *Journal of Abnormal Psychology, 99,* 430–439.

Smulders, F. T. Y., Kenemans, J. L., & Kok, A. (1995). The locus of effect of stage manipulations as indexed by the latencies of lateralized readiness potential and P300. *Acta Psychologica, 90*, 119–127.

Snow, B. J., & Frith, R. W. (1989). The relationship of eyelid movement to the blink reflex. *Journal of the Neurological Sciences, 91*, 179–189.

Sokolov, Y. N. (1963). *Perception and the conditioned reflex* (S. W. Waydenfeld, Trans.). New York: Macmillan. (Original work published 1958.)

Sollers, J. J., & Hackley, S. A. (1997). Effects of foreperiod duration on reflexive and voluntary responses to intense noise bursts. *Psychophysiology, 34*, 518–526.

Sonnenberg, D. C., Low, K. A., & Hackley, S. A. (1996). Visuospatial attention effects on brainstem reflexes and cortical event-related potentials [Abstract]. *Psychophysiology, 33* (Suppl. 1), S80.

Spence, E., & Lang, P. J. (1990). Reading affective text: The startle probe response [Abstract]. *Psychophysiology, 27*, S65.

Spence, E. L., Vrana, S. R., & Lang, P. J. (1987). Effects of attention and emotion on the acoustic startle response. *Psychophysiology, 24*, 613.

Spence, K. W., & Runquist, W. N. (1958). Temporal effects of conditioned fear on the eyelid reflex. *Journal of Experimental Psychology, 55*, 613–616.

Spetch, M. L., Wilkie, D. M., & Pinel, J. P. J. (1981). Backward conditioning: A reevaluation of the empirical evidence. *Psychological Bulletin, 89*, 163–175.

Spitzer, R. L., Endicott, J., & Gibbon, M. (1979). Crossing the border into borderline personality and borderline schizophrenia: The development of criteria. *Archives of General Psychiatry, 36*, 17–24.

Squire, L. R. (1992). Memory and the hippocampus: A synthesis from findings with rats, monkeys, and humans. *Psychological Review, 99*, 195–231.

Squires, N. K., Squires, K. C., & Hillyard, S. A. (1975). Two varieties of long-latency positive waves evoked by unpredictable auditory stimuli in man. *Electroencephalography & Clinical Neurophysiology, 38*, 387–401.

Stafford, I. L., & Jacobs, B. L. (1990). Noradrenergic modulation of the masseteric reflex in behaving cats. II. Physiologic studies. *Journal of Neuroscience, 10*, 99–107.

Steele, C. M., & Josephs, R. A. (1988). Drinking your troubles away. II: An attention-allocation model of alcohol's effect on psychological stress. *Journal of Abnormal Psychology, 97*, 196–205.

Steele, C. M., & Josephs, R. A. (1990). Alcohol myopia: Its prized and dangerous effects. *American Psychologist, 45*, 921–933.

Stein, P. S. G. (1989). Spinal cord circuits for motor pattern selection in the turtle. *Annals of the New York Academy of Sciences, 563*, 1–10.

Stephens, S. D. G. (1976). Auditory temporal summation in patients with central nervous system lesions. In S. D. G. Stephens (Ed.), *Disorders of auditory function* (Vol. 2, pp. 231–241). New York: Academic Press.

Sternberg, S. (1969). The discovery of processing stages: Extensions of Donder's method. In W. G. Koster (Ed.), *Attention and performance II* (pp. 276–315). Amsterdam: North-Holland.

Stevenson, V. E., & Cook, E. W., III (1997). *Affective modulation of startle in fearful and schizotypal college students.* Manuscript submitted for publication.

Stevenson, V. E., Cook, E. W., III, & Hawk, L. W. (1991). Specificity of affective modulation of acoustic startle [Abstract]. *Psychophysiology, 28* (Suppl. 1), S53.

Stitt, C. L., Hoffman, H. S., Marsh, R., & Boskoff, K. J. (1974). Modification of the rat's startle reaction by an antecedent change in the acoustic environment. _Journal of Comparative and Physiological Psychology, 86_, 826–836.

Stoerig, P. (1996). Varieties of vision: From blind responses to conscious recognition. _Trends in Neuroscience, 19_, 401–406.

Stoerig, P., & Cowey, A. (1989). Wavelength sensitivity in blindsight. _Nature, 342_, 916–918.

Stritzke, W. G. K., Lang, A. R., & Patrick, C. J. (1996). Beyond stress and arousal: A reconceptualization of alcohol-emotion relations with special reference to psychophysiological methods. _Psychological Bulletin, 120_, 376–395.

Stritzke, W. G. K., Patrick, C. J., & Lang, A. R. (1995). Alcohol and human emotion: A multidimensional analysis incorporating startle-probe methodology. _Journal of Abnormal Psychology, 104_, 114–122.

Sugawara, M., Sadeghpour, M., de Traversay, J., & Ornitz, E. M. (1984). Prestimulation-induced modulation of the P300 component of event related potentials accompanying startle in children. _Electroencephalography & Clinical Neurophysiology, 90_, 201–213.

Swerdlow, N. R., Auerbach, P., Monroe S. M., Hartston, H., Geyer, M. A., & Braff, D. L. (1993). Men are more inhibited than women by weak prepulses. _Biological Psychiatry, 34_, 253–260.

Swerdlow, N. R., Bakshi, V., & Geyer, M. A. (1996). Seroquel restores sensorimotor gating in phencyclidine (PCP)-treated rats. _Journal of Pharmacology and Experimental Therapeutics, 279_, 1290–1299.

Swerdlow, N. R., Benbow, C. H., Zisook, S., Geyer, M. A., & Braff, D. L. (1993). A preliminary assessment of sensorimotor gating in patients with obsessive compulsive disorder (OCD). _Biological Psychiatry, 33_, 298–301.

Swerdlow, N. R., Braff, D. L., & Geyer, M. A. (1990). GABAergic projection from nucleus accumbens to ventral pallidum mediates dopamine-induced sensorimotor gating deficits of acoustic startle in rats. _Brain Research, 532_, 146–150.

Swerdlow, N. R., Braff, D. L., Geyer, M. A., & Koob, G. F. (1986). Central dopamine hyperactivity in rats mimics abnormal acoustic startle response in schizophrenics. _Biological Psychiatry, 21_, 23–33.

Swerdlow, N. R., Braff, D. L., Masten, V. L., & Geyer, M. A. (1990). Schizophrenic-like sensorimotor gating abnormalities in rats following dopamine infusion into the nucleus accumbens. _Psychopharmacology, 101_, 414–420.

Swerdlow, N. R., Braff, D. L., Taaid, N., & Geyer, M. A. (1994). Assessing the validity of an animal model of deficient sensorimotor gating in schizophrenic patients. _Archives of General Psychiatry, 51_, 139–154.

Swerdlow, N. R., Caine, S. B., Braff, D. L., & Geyer, M. A. (1992). The neural substrates of sensorimotor gating of the startle reflex: A review of recent findings and their implications. _Journal of Psychopharmacology, 6_, 176–190.

Swerdlow, N. R., Caine, S. B., & Geyer, M. A. (1992). Regionally selective effects of intracerebral dopamine infusion on sensorimotor gating of the startle reflex in rats. _Psychopharmacology, 108_, 189–195.

Swerdlow, N. R., Filion, D., Geyer, M. A., & Braff, D. L. (1995). "Normal" personality correlates of sensorimotor, cognitive, and visuospatial gating. _Biological Psychiatry, 37_, 286–299.

Swerdlow, N. R., & Geyer, M. A. (1993). Prepulse inhibition of acoustic startle in rats after lesions of the pedunculopontine nucleus. *Behavioral Neuroscience, 107,* 104–117.

Swerdlow, N. R., Geyer, M., Braff, D., & Koob, G. F. (1986). Central dopamine hyperactivity in rats mimics abnormal acoustic startle in schizophrenics. *Biological Psychiatry, 21,* 23–33.

Swerdlow, N. R., Geyer, M. A., Vale, W. W., & Koob, G. F. (1986). Corticotropin-releasing factor potentiates acoustic startle in rats: Blockade by chlordiazepoxide. *Psychopharmacology, 88,* 147–152.

Swerdlow, N. R., Hartman, P. L., & Auerbach, P. P. (1997). Changes in sensorimotor inhibition across the menstrual cycle: Implications for neuropsychiatric disorders. *Biological Psychiatry, 41,* 452–460.

Swerdlow, N. R., Keith, V. A., Braff, D. L., & Geyer, M. A. (1991). The effects of spiperone, raclopride, SCH 23390 and clozapine on apomorphine-inhibition of sensorimotor gating of the startle response in the rat. *Journal of Pharmacology and Experimental Therapeutics, 256,* 530–536.

Swerdlow, N. R., & Koob, G. F. (1987). Dopamine, schizophrenia, mania and depression: Toward a unified hypothesis of cortico-striato-pallido-thalamic function. *Behavioral and Brain Sciences, 10,* 197–245.

Swerdlow, N. R., Lipska, B. K., Weinberger, D. R., Braff, D. L., Jaskiw, G. E., & Geyer, M. A. (1995). Increased sensitivity to the gating-disruptive effects of apomorphine after lesions of the medial prefrontal cortex or ventral hippocampus in adult rats. *Psychopharmacology, 122,* 27–34.

Swerdlow, N. R., Mansbach, R. S., Geyer, M. A., Pulvirenti, L., Koob, G. F., & Braff, D. L. (1990). Amphetamine disruption of prepulse inhibition of acoustic startle is reversed by depletion of mesolimbic dopamine. *Psychopharmacology, 100,* 413–416.

Swerdlow, N. R., Paulsen, J., Braff, D. L., Butters, N., Geyer, M. A., & Swenson, M. R. (1995). Impaired prepulse inhibition of acoustic and tactile startle in patients with Huntington's disease. *Journal of Neurology, Neurosurgery and Psychiatry, 58,* 192–200.

Swerdlow, N. R., Wan, F., Kodsi, M., Hartston, H., & Caine, S. B. (1993). Limbic cortico-striato-pallido-pontine substrates of startle gating. *Biological Psychiatry, 33,* 62A.

Swerdlow, N. R., Zisook, D., & Taaid, N. (1994). Seroquel (ICI 204, 636) restores prepulse inhibition of acoustic startle in apomorphine-treated rats: Similarities to clozapine. *Psychopharmacology, 114,* 675–678.

Takeuchi, Y., Nakano, K., Uemura, M., Kojyuro, M., Matsushima, R., & Mizuno, N. (1979). Mesencephalic and pontine afferent fiber system to the facial nucleus in the cat: A study using horseradish peroxidase and silver impregnation techniques. *Experimental Neurology, 66,* 330–342.

Takmann, W., Ettlin, T., & Barth, R. (1982). Blink reflexes elicited by electrical, acoustic and visual stimuli. *European Neurology, 21,* 210–216.

Tavy, D. L. J., van Woerkom, C. A. M., Bots, G. T. A. M., & Endtz, L. J. (1984). Persistence of the blink reflex to sudden illumination in a comatose patient. *Archives of Neurology, 41,* 323–324.

Tellegen, A. (1982). *Brief manual for the Multidimensional Personality Questionnaire.* Unpublished manuscript.

Tellegen, A. (1985). Structures of mood and personality and their relevance to assessing anxiety, with an emphasis on self-report. In A. H. Tuma & J. D. Maser (Eds.), *Anxiety and the anxiety disorders* (pp. 681–706). Hillsdale, NJ: Lawrence Erlbaum.

Thompson, R. F. (1986). Neurobiology of learning and memory. *Science, 233,* 941–947.

Thompson, R. F., Berry, S. D., Rinaldi, P. C., & Berger, T. W. (1979). Habituation and the orienting reflex: The dual process theory revisted. In H. D. Kimmel, E. H. Van Olst, & J. F. Orlebeke (Eds.), *The orienting reflex in humans* (pp. 21–60). Hillsdale, NJ: Erlbaum.

Thompson, R. F., Groves, P. M., Teyler, T. J., & Roemer, R. A. (1973). A dual-process theory of habituation: Theory and behavior. In H. V. S. Peeke & M. J. Herz (Eds.), *Habituation* (pp. 239–271). New York: Academic Press.

Tipper, S. A. (1985). The negative priming effect: Inhibitory effects of ignored primes. *Quarterly Journal of Experimental Psychology, 37A,* 571–590.

Tranel, D., & Damasio, H. (1994). Neuroanatomical correlates of electrodermal skin conductance responses. *Psychophysiology, 31,* 427–438.

Tranel, D., & Hyman, B. T. (1990). Neuropsychological correlates of bilateral amygdala damage. *Archives of Neurology, 47,* 349–355.

Tucker, D. M. (1981). Lateral brain function, emotion, and conceptualization. *Psychological Bulletin, 89,* 19–46.

Valle-Inclan, F., & Hackley, S. A. (1996). Accessory stimulus (prepulse) effects on the lateralized motor readiness potential [Abstract]. *Psychophysiology, 33* (Suppl. 1), S85.

van Boxtel, A., Boelhouwer, A. J. W., & Bos, A. R. (1996). Optimal recording of electric, acoustic, and visual blink reflexes: Effects of EMG signal bandwidth and inter-electrode distance [Abstract]. *Psychophysiology, 32* (Suppl. 1), S12–13.

van Boxtel, A., Goudswaard, P., & Schomaker, L. R. B. (1984). Amplitude and bandwidth of the frontalis surface EMG: Effects of electrode parameters. *Psychophysiology, 21,* 699–707.

Vandergriff, J. L., Matthews, D. B., Best, P. J., & Simson, P. E. (1995). Effect of ethanol and diazepam on spatial and non-spatial tasks in rats on an 8-arm radial arm maze. *Alcoholism: Clinical and Experimental Research, 19,* 64.

Vanman, E. J., Boehmelt, A. H., Dawson, M. E., & Schell, A. M. (1996). The varying time courses of attentional and affective modulation of the startle eyeblink reflex. *Psychophysiology, 33,* 691–698.

Varty, G. B., Hayes, A. G., & Higgins, G. A. (1995). Pharmacological characterisation of various dopamine (DA) agonists in two putative models of D3 receptor function: Comparison with effect on prepulse inhibition (PPI). *Society for Neuroscience Abstracts, 21,* 1133.

Varty, G. B., & Higgins, G. A. (1995). Examination of drug-induced and isolation-induced disruptions of prepulse inhibition as models to screen antipsychotic drugs. *Psychopharmacology, 122,* 15–26.

Venables, P. H., & Christie, M. J. (1973). Mechanisms, instrumentation, scoring techniques, and quantification of responses. In W. F. Prokasy & D. C. Raskin (Eds.), *Electrodermal activity in psychological research* (pp. 1–124). New York: Wiley.

Verleger, R. (1988). Event-related potentials and cognition: A critique of the context updating hypothesis and an alternative interpretation of P3. *Behavioral and Brain Sciences, 11,* 343–427.

Vollema, M. G., & van den Bosch, R. J. (1995). The multidimensionality of schizotypy. *Schizophrenia Bulletin, 21,* 19–31.

Vrana, S. R. (1995). Emotional modulation of skin conductance and eyeblink responses to a startle probe. *Psychophysiology, 32,* 351–357.

Vrana, S. R., Constantine, J. A., & Westman, J. S. (1992). Startle reflex modification as an outcome measure in the treatment of phobia: Two case studies. *Behavioral Assessment, 14,* 279–291.

Vrana, S. R., & Lang, P. J. (1990). Fear imagery and the startle-probe reflex. *Journal of Abnormal Psychology, 99,* 189–197.

Vrana, S. R., Spence, E. L., & Lang, P. J. (1988). The startle probe response: A new measure of emotion? *Journal of Abnormal Psychology, 97,* 487–491.

Wagner, A. R. (1963). Conditioned frustration as a learned drive. *Journal of Experimental Psychology, 66,* 142–148.

Wagner, A. R. (1978). Expectancies and the priming of STM. In S. H. Hulse, H. Fowler, & W. K. Honig (Eds.), *Cognitive processes in animal behavior* (pp. 177–209). Hillsdale, NJ: Erlbaum.

Walker, D. L., Cassella, J. V., Lee, Y., de Lima, T. C. M., & Davis, M. (1997). Opposing roles of the amygdala and dorsolateral periaqueductal gray in fear-potentiated startle. *Brain Research Bulletin, 21,* 743–753.

Walker, D. L., & Davis, M. (1995). Involvement of the periaqueductal gray in fear-potentiated startle. *Society for Neuroscience Abstracts, 21,* 1936.

Walker, D. L., & Davis, M. (1996). Inactivation of the bed nucleus of the stria terminalis (BNST), but not the central nucleus of the amygdala (CNA) disrupts light-enhanced startle: A novel paradigm for the assessment of anxiety in rats. *Society for Neuroscience Abstracts, 22,* 1117.

Walker, D. L., & Davis, M. (1997). Anxiogenic effects of high illumination levels assessed with the acoustic startle paradigm. *Biological Psychiatry, 42,* 461–471.

Wan, F. J., Caine, S. B., & Swerdlow, N. R. (1996). The ventral subiculum modulation of prepulse inhibition is not mediated via dopamine D2 or nucleus accumbens non-NMDA glutamate receptor activity. *European Journal of Pharmacology, 314,* 9–18.

Wan, F. J., Geyer, M. A., & Swerdlow, N. R. (1994). Accumbens D2 substrates of sensorimotor gating: Assessing anatomical localization. *Pharmacology, Biochemistry and Behavior, 49,* 155–263.

Wan, F. J., Geyer, M. A., & Swerdlow, N. R. (1995). Presynaptic dopamine–glutamate interactions in the nucleus accumbens regulate sensorimotor gating. *Psychopharmacology, 120,* 433–441.

Wan, F. J., & Swerdlow, N. R. (1994). Intra-accumbens infusion of quinpirole impairs sensorimotor gating of acoustic startle in rats. *Psychopharmacology, 113,* 103–109.

Wan, F. J., & Swerdlow, N. R. (1996). Sensorimotor gating in rats is regulated by different dopamine–glutamate interactions in the nucleus accumbens core and shell subregions. *Brain Research, 722,* 168–176.

Wan, F. J., & Swerdlow, N. R. (1996). The basolateral amygdala regulates sensorimotor gating of acoustic startle in the rat. *Neuroscience, 76,* 715–724.

Wan, F. J., Taaid, N., & Swerdlow, N. R. (1995). Do D1/D2 interactions regulate prepulse inhibition in rats? *Neuropsychopharmacology, 14,* 265–274.

Watson, D., Clark, L. A., & Carey, A. (1988). Positive and negative affectivity and their relation to anxiety and depressive disorders. *Journal of Abnormal Psychology, 97,* 346–353.

Watson, D., Clark, L. A., & Tellegen, A. (1988). Development and validation of brief measures of positive and negative affect: The PANAS scales. *Journal of Personality and Social Psychology, 54,* 1063–1070.

Watson, D., & Tellegen, A. (1985). Toward a consensual structure of mood. *Psychological Bulletin, 98,* 219–235.

Webb, R. A., & Obrist, P. A. (1970). The physiological concomitants of reaction time performance as a function of preparatory interval and preparatory interval series. *Psychophysiology, 6,* 398–403.

Wecker, J. R., Ison, J. R., & Foss, J. A. (1985). Reflex modification as a test for sensory function. *Neurobehavioral Toxicology and Teratology, 7,* 733–738.

Weichselgartner, E., & Sperling, G. (1987). Dynamics of automatic and controlled visual attention. *Science, 238,* 778–780.

Weinberger, D. R. (1987). Implications of normal brain development for the pathogenesis of schizophrenia. *Archives of General Psychiatry, 44,* 660–669.

Weinberger, D. R., Berman, K. F., & Illowsky, B. P. (1988). Physiological dysfunction of dorsolateral prefrontal cortex in schizophrenia: III. A new cohort and evidence for a monoaminergic mechanism. *Archives of General Psychiatry, 45,* 609–615.

Weiskrantz, L. (1986). *Blindsight: A case study and implications.* Oxford: Oxford University Press.

Wilson, G. T. (1988). Alcohol and anxiety. *Behavior Research and Therapy, 26,* 369–381.

Winton, W. M., Putnam, L. E., & Krauss, R. M. (1984). Facial and autonomic manifestations of the dimensional structure of emotion. *Journal of Experimental Social Psychology, 20,* 195–216.

Witvliet, C., & Vrana, S. R. (1995). Psychophysiological responses as indicators of affective dimensions. *Psychophysiology, 32,* 436–443.

Woldorff, M. G. (1993). Distortion of ERP averages due to overlap from temporally adjacent ERPs – Analysis and correction. *Psychophysiology, 30,* 98–119.

Woldorff, M., Hansen, J. C., & Hillyard, S. A. (1987). Evidence for effects of selective attention in the mid-latency range of the human auditory event-related potential. In R. Johnson, Jr., J. W. Rohrbaugh, & R. Parasuraman (Eds.), *Current trends in event-related potential research* (EEG Suppl. 40). North Holland: Elsevier Science Publishers.

Wolpe, J., & Lang, P. J. (1964). A fear survey schedule for use in behaviour therapy. *Behaviour Research and Therapy, 2,* 27–30.

Woods, D. L., & Courchesne, E. (1986). The recovery functions of auditory event-related potentials during split-second discriminations. *Electroencephalography & Clinical Neurophysiology, 65,* 304–315.

Woods, D. L., Clayworth, C. C., Knight, R. T., Simpson, G. V., & Naeser, M. A. (1987). Generators of middle- and long-latency auditory evoked potentials: Implications from studies of patients with bitemporal lesions. *Electroencephalography & Clinical Neurophysiology, 68,* 132–148.

Wootton, J. M., Frick, P. J., Shelton, K. K., & Silverthorn, P. (1997). Ineffective parenting and childhood conduct problems: The moderating role of callous-unemotional traits. *Journal of Consulting and Clinical Psychology, 65.*

Wu, M.-F., Kreuger, J., Ison, J. R., & Gerrard, R. L. (1984). Startle reflex inhibition in the rat: Its persistence after extended repetition of the inhibitory stimulus. *Journal of Experimental Psychology: Animal Behavior Processes, 10,* 221–228.

Wu, M.-F., Suzuki, S. S., & Siegel, J. M. (1988). Anatomical distribution and response patterns of reticular neurons active in relation to acoustic startle. *Brain Research, 457,* 399–406.

Wynn, J. K., Schell, A. M., & Dawson, M. E. (1996). Effects of prehabituation of the prepulse on startle eyeblink modification [Abstract]. *Psychophysiology, 33* (Suppl. 1), S92.

Yantis, S., & Hillstrom, A. P. (1994). Stimulus-driven attentional capture: Evidence from equiluminant visual objects. *Journal of Experimental Psychology: Human Perception and Performance, 20,* 95–107.

Yantis, S., & Jonides, J. (1990). Abrupt visual onsets and selective attention: Voluntary versus automatic allocation. *Journal of Experimental Psychology: Human Perception and Performance, 16,* 121–134.

Yasgan, M. Y., Peterson, B., Wexler, B. E., & Leckman, J. F. (1995). Behavioral laterality in individuals with Gilles de la Tourette's syndrome and basal ganglia alterations: A preliminary report. *Biological Psychiatry, 38,* 386–390.

Yates, S. K., & Brown, W. F. (1981). Light-stimulus-evoked blink reflex: Methods, normal values, relation to other blink reflexes, and observations in multiple sclerosis. *Neurology, 31,* 272–281.

Yeomans, J. S., & Franklin, P. W. (1994). Synapses in the rostrolateral midbrain mediate "fear" potentiation of acoustic startle and electrically evoked startle. *Society for Neuroscience Abstracts, 20,* 1753.

Yerkes, R. M. (1905). The sense of hearing in frogs. *Journal of Comparative Neurology and Psychology, 15,* 279–304.

Yerkes, R. M., & Dodson, J. D. (1908). The relation of strength of stimulus to rapidity of habit-formation. *Journal of Comparative and Neurological Psychology, 18,* 459–482.

Yingling, C. D., Hosobuchi, Y., & Harrington, M. (1990). P300 as a predictor of recovery from coma. *Lancet, 336,* 873.

Young, A. W., Aggleton, J. P., Hellawell, D. J., Johnson, M., Broks, P., & Hanley, J. R. (1995). Face processing impairments after amygdalotomy. *Brain, 118,* 15–24.

Young, J. S., & Fechter, L. D. (1983). Reflex inhibition procedures for animal audiometry: A technique for assessing ototoxicity. *Journal of the Acoustical Society of America, 73,* 1686–1693.

Young, R. A., Cegavske, C. F., & Thompson, R. F. (1976). Tone-induced changes in excitability of abducens motoneurons and of the reflex path of nictitating membrane response in rabbit. *Journal of Comparative and Physiological Psychology, 90,* 424–434.

Zeichner, A., Allen, J. D., Petrie, C. D., Rasmussen, P. R., & Giancola, P. R. (1993). Attention allocation: Effects of alcohol and information salience on attentional processes in male social drinkers. *Alcoholism: Clinical and Experimental Research, 17,* 727–732.

Zeichner, A., & Pihl, R. O. (1979). Effects of alcohol and behavior contingencies on human aggression. *Journal of Abnormal Psychology, 88,* 153–160.

Zeichner, A., & Pihl, R. O. (1980). Effects of alcohol and instigator intent on human aggression. *Journal of Studies on Alcohol, 41,* 265–276.

Zhang, J., Engel, J. A., Hjorth, S., & Svensson, L. (1995). Changes in the acoustic startle response and prepulse inhibition of acoustic startle in rats after local injection of
pertussis toxin into the ventral tegmental area. *Psychopharmacology, 119,* 71–78.

Zigun, J., & Weinberger, D. R. (1992). In vivo studies of brain morphology in patients
with schizophrenia. In J.-P. Lindenmayer & S. R. Kay (Eds.), *New biological vistas
on schizophrenia* (pp. 57–81). New York: Brunner Mazel.

Zwislocki, J. J. (1969). Temporal summation of loudness: An analysis. *Journal of the
Acoustical Society of America, 46,* 320–328.

Zwislocki, J. J. (1983). Group and individual relations between sensation magnitudes
and their numerical estimates. *Perception & Psychophysics, 33,* 460–468.

Zwislocki, J. J., & Sokolich, W. G. (1974). On loudness enhancement of a tone burst by
a preceding tone burst. *Perception & Psychophysics, 16,* 87–90.

Author Index

365

Subject Index